Kernel Methods in Bioengineering, Signal and Image Processing

Gustavo Camps-Valls, Universitat de València, Spain

José Luis Rojo-Álvarez, Universidad Rey Juan Carlos, Spain

Manel Martínez-Ramón, Universidad Carlos III de Madrid, Spain

T0321982

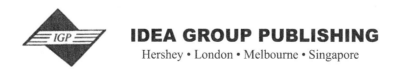

IDEA GROUP PUBLISHING

Hershey • London • Melbourne • Singapore

Acquisition Editor:	Kristin Klinger
Senior Managing Editor:	Jennifer Neidig
Managing Editor:	Sara Reed
Assistant Managing Editor:	Sharon Berger
Development Editor:	Kristin Roth
Copy Editor:	Shanelle Ramelb
Typesetter:	Jamie Snavely
Cover Design:	Lisa Tosheff
Printed at:	Integrated Book Technology

Published in the United States of America by
Idea Group Publishing (an imprint of Idea Group Inc.)
701 E. Chocolate Avenue
Hershey PA 17033
Tel: 717-533-8845
Fax: 717-533-8661
E-mail: cust@idea-group.com
Web site: http://www.idea-group.com

and in the United Kingdom by
Idea Group Publishing (an imprint of Idea Group Inc.)
3 Henrietta Street
Covent Garden
London WC2E 8LU
Tel: 44 20 7240 0856
Fax: 44 20 7379 3313
Web site: http://www.eurospan.co.uk

Library of Congress Cataloging-in-Publication Data

Kernel methods in bioengineering, signal and image processing / Gustavo Camps-Valls, José Luis Rojo-Álvarez and Manel Martínez-Ramón, editors.
    p. cm.
  Summary: "This book presents an extensive introduction to the field of kernel methods and real world applications. The book is organized in four parts: the first is an introductory chapter providing a framework of kernel methods; the others address Bioegineering, Signal Processing and Communications and Image Processing"-- Provided by publisher.
  Includes bibliographical references and index.
  ISBN 1-59904-042-5 (hardcover) -- ISBN 1-59904-043-3 (softcover) -- ISBN 1-59904-044-1 (ebook)
  1. Engineering mathematics. 2. Biomedical engineering--Mathematics. 3. Signal processing--Mathematics. 4. Cellular telephone systems--Mathematics. 5. Image processing--Mathematics. 6. Kernel functions. I. Camps-Valls, Gustavo, 1972- II. Rojo-Alvarez, Jose Luis, 1972- III. Martínez-Ramón, Manel, 1968-
  TA335.K47 2006
  610.28--dc22
                           2006027728

British Cataloguing in Publication Data
A Cataloguing in Publication record for this book is available from the British Library.

Kernel Methods in Bioengineering, Signal and Image Processing

Table of Contents

Section II: Signal Processing

Foreword

The editors have kindly invited me to contribute a foreword to the book you are holding in your hands. This being my first such invitation, two questions entered my mind. First, how does one write a foreword? A Web site with the promising name *Fashioning Fabulous Forewords* recommends to "write a short anecdote about something that happened in your life that has some bearing, no matter how far-fetched, on the book"—and off we go. Last year, I was invited to give a talk at a conference in Spain. During the opening night, I was having a drink with a few attendees. At some point, most had already left and I announced that I better leave now, too, since I would have to give the first talk the next morning. An attendee replied that I must be mistaken for the first speaker was Schölkopf. When I told him that I was Schölkopf, he laughed, shook his head, and said, "No, you are not—Schölkopf is a monster."

The second question entering my mind was, why me? Categorically rejecting the thought that this may be due to my questionable reputation in the editors' home country, I decided it must have been the beer I bought two of the editors when they visited Tübingen.

Judging from the present volume, the editors probably have not had much time for drinking during the past year (and they deserve to be generously compensated on their next visit). They have done an admirable job in soliciting and collecting a variety of chapters from many intriguing application domains. As a late chapter coauthor, reviewer, and foreword writer, I can moreover testify that they have done their job with the utmost patience and diplomatic nous.

I was privileged to follow the development of the field of kernel machines from its early days. Initially confined to machine learning, the area has since broadened. On the theoretical side, significant interest from mathematics promises to deepen and expand the foundations of the field. At the same time, kernel methods are entering the standard engineering toolbox—a development that is particularly prominent in Spain, as witnessed by the present collection including a number of studies in signal and image processing. A different but equally popular and promising direction is computational biology and medical research. These areas, too, are represented in this book by some excellent contributions. I very much look forward to seeing this book in print, and to reading up in detail on the various exciting applications that are being discussed.

Let me close with a quote from Vladimir Vapnik, the field's real "monster" in the Spanish sense of the word. It is taken from the second edition of *Estimating Dependences Based on Empirical Data:*

"Looking back, one can see how rapidly life and technology have changed, and how slow and difficult it is to change the theoretical foundation of the technology and its philosophy."

Bernhard Schölkopf

Max-Planck-Institute for Biological Cybernetics, Tübingen

August 2006

Preface

Machine learning experienced a great advance in the '80s and '90s due to the active research in *artificial neural networks, adaptive schemes, and fuzzy systems*. These tools have demonstrated good results in many real applications, especially for classification and regression tasks, since neither a *priori* knowledge about the distribution of the available data nor the relationships among the independent variables should be necessarily assumed. Neural networks, however, have found some difficulties in their way. For example, their use in scenarios with high input-space dimensionality is not easy. Other common problems of neural networks are the possibility of overfitting, the lack of interpretation of the neural-network structure and functionality and, in many cases, the local minima phenomenon, which lead to suboptimal solutions. Despite their good performance in many fields and applications, these theoretical problems must be solved through the regularization of the minimization functional, feature selection and extraction techniques used prior to the design of the network, or the development of techniques to identify feature relevance in the problem at hand. These additional techniques increase the number of free parameters to be tuned, typically through heuristic rules. Some of these issues can be alleviated by the introduction of the so-called *kernel methods*.

Kernel methods are emerging and innovative techniques that can be simply viewed as a first step that consists of mapping the data from the original input space to a *kernel* feature space of higher dimensionality through a nonlinear function, and then a second step of solving a *linear* problem in that space. These methods allow us to design and interpret learning algorithms geometrically in the kernel space (which is nonlinearly related to the input space), thus combining statistics and geometry in an effective way, and all of this while still obtaining solutions with that desirable property that is uniqueness. A few sets of free parameters are commonly needed to make the algorithms work properly. In addition, the inclusion of regularization in the function to be optimized becomes a natural and theoretically well-founded task. This theoretical elegance is also matched by the methods' practical performance. Interestingly, this framework allows us to create nonlinear methods from linear well-established ones.

In the last decade, a number of powerful kernel-based learning methods have been proposed in the machine-learning community, for example, support vector machines (SVMs), kernel Fisher discriminant (KFD) analysis, kernel PCA/ICA, kernel mutual information, kernel k-means, or kernel ARMA. Successful applications of these algorithms have been reported in many, many fields, such as medicine, bioengineering, communications, audio and image processing, and computational biology and bioinformatics. In many cases, kernel methods have demonstrated superior results compared to their competitors and also revealed some additional advantages, both theoretical and practical. For instance, kernel methods handle large input spaces efficiently, they deal with noisy samples in a robust way, they commonly yield sparse solutions, and they allow the user to easily introduce knowledge about the problem into the method formulation. The interest of these methods is twofold. On the one hand, the machine-learning community has found in the kernel concept an elegant framework to develop efficient nonlinear learning methods, thus solving complex problems efficiently (e.g., pattern recognition, function approximation, clustering, source independence, and density estimation). On the other hand, these methods can be easily used and tuned in many research areas (e.g., biology, signal and image processing, and communications), which has also captured the attention of many researchers and practitioners in safety-related areas.

In this context, this book is intended to encompass the vast field of kernel methods from a multidisciplinary approach by presenting dedicated chapters to the adaptation and use of kernel methods in the selected areas of bioengineering, signal processing and communications, and image processing. These general areas of application cover a selection of a representative set of real-world applications, such as computational biology, text categorization, time-series prediction, interpolation, system identification, speech recognition, image de-noising, image coding, classification, and segmentation. Methods are presented in a way such that they can be extrapolated to other research areas in which machine-learning methods are needed.

The book is organized in three sections, each dedicated to the selected areas of bioengineering, signal processing, and image processing. These specific application domains are preceded by an introductory chapter presenting the elements of kernel methods, which is intended to help readers from different backgrounds to follow the motivations and technicalities of the chapters. Written by Cristianini, Shawe-Taylor, and Saunders, Chapter I provides the reader with an exhaustive introduction to the framework of kernel methods. The authors address the revision of the main concepts and theoretical derivations, give pointers to useful Web pages, and discuss theoretical and practical issues. Therefore, this introduction can be useful both for the nonexpert reader in kernel methods and for practitioners interested in the theoretical and practical issues of kernel machines. Then, three blocks are devoted to the areas of *bioengineering, signal processing,* and *image processing,* respectively. The 15 chapters of these blocks include a literature review of the specific area, a critical discussion of the needs and demands of each field, novel research contributions, and experimental results to demonstrate method capabilities. Chapters are written by leading experts in their respective fields. A brief description and achievements of each of the chapters follows.

The first block of chapters is devoted to the field of *bioengineering*. This is an active research area for kernel methods due to the special characteristics of the problems. In particular, the fields of computational biology and genomics have given rise to a great number of kernel applications, mainly due to the high dimensionality of the data, the representation as discrete and structured data, and the need for combining heterogeneous information. In Chapter II, Vert surveys some of the most prominent applications published so far in the context of computational biology and genomics while highlighting the particular developments in kernel methods triggered by problems in biology and mentioning a few promising research directions likely to expand in the future. In Chapter III, a specific problem in this context is addressed by Pochet, Ojeda, De Smet, De Bie, Suykens, and De Moor, who introduce the techniques of kernel k-means and spectral clustering for knowledge discovery in clinical microarray data analysis. For this purpose, the authors reformulate some classical clustering assessment techniques (commonly used in the original input space) as a kernel-induced feature space. Further biomedical applications are included in this part. In Chapter IV, Osowski and Markiewicz present an automatic system for white blood cell recognition in the context of leukaemia. The authors exploit the good classification performance of support vector machines and a refined feature selection. In particular, some features of cell texture, geometry, morphology, and statistical description of the image are fed to the linear and nonlinear SVM classifiers. The system finally yields accurate results and may find practical application in hospitals in the diagnosis of patients suffering from leukaemia. The first part of the book is concluded with Chapter V by Martínez-Ramón, Koltchinskii, Heileman, and Posse, in which an Adaboost methodology is presented to improve the classification of multiple interleaved human-brain tasks in functional magnetic resonance imaging (fMRI). The method combines weak region-based classifiers efficiently through segmentation of the brain in functional areas.

The second section of the book is devoted to the field of signal processing and communications, and it covers signal processing theory, multiuser detection, array processing, speech recognition, and text categorization. Chapter VI, by Rojo-Álvarez, Martínez-Ramón, Camps-Valls, Martínez-Cruz, and Figuera, presents a full framework based on support vector machines for signal processing in general terms, which is particularized for (linear and nonlinear) system identification, time-series prediction, filtering, sync-based time interpolation, and convolution. The statement of linear signal models in the primal problem yields a set of robust estimators of the model coefficients in classical digital signal processing problems. Chapter VII, by Fernández-Getino García, Rojo-Álvarez, Gil-Jiménez, Alonso-Atienza, and García-Armada, deals with the state-of-the-art communications problem of coherent demodulation in orthogonal frequency division multiplexing (OFDM) systems. The authors present a new complex-valued SVM formulation that is adapted to a pilot-based OFDM signal, which produces a simple scheme that has better performance in real-life broadband, fixed wireless channel models than the standard least-squares algorithms. A different communications' task is addressed in Chapter VIII by Christodoulou and Martínez-Ramón, in which the authors introduce three novel approaches for antenna array beamforming based on support vector machines: a robust linear SVM-based beamformer, a nonlinear parameter estimator for linear beamformers, and a nonlinear generalization of the linear regressor. They make further use of the background previously given in Chapter VI and of the complex formulation presented in Chapter VII. Chapters IX and X present the applications of Kernel methods to speech recognition from two different, complementary points of view. In Chapter IX, Picone, Ganapathiraju, and Hamaker present a unified framework of kernel methods in the context of speech recognition. In this approach, both generative and discriminative models are motivated from an information-theoretic perspective. The authors introduce the modern statistical approach to speech recognition and discuss how kernel-based methods are used to model knowledge at each level of the problem. Chapter X, by Wan, discusses in a systematic and thorough way the adaptation and application of kernel methods for speech processing in general, and the architecture of some of the most important sequence kernels in particular. This part is concluded with Chapter XI, by Fortuna, Cristianini, and Shawe-Taylor, in which the authors address the challenging signal processing problem of translating text from one natural language to another. For this purpose, the authors make an exhaustive revision of the vast literature, and they present a novel kernel canonical correlation analysis method. Theoretical analysis of this method is surveyed, and application to crosslinguistic retrieval and text categorization is demonstrated through extensive comparison.

The third section of the book is devoted to the field of image processing and includes the four main application branches of this field: image de-noising, image coding, image segmentation, and image classification of both gray-level and multidimensional scenes. Chapter XII, by Bakır, Schölkopf, and Weston, covers the problem of the inversion of nonlinear mappings, known in the kernel community as the pre-image problem. After extensive revision of existing algorithms, a new learning-based approach is presented. All the algorithms are discussed regarding their usability and complexity, and are evaluated on an image de-noising application. After this chapter, Gutiérrez, Gómez-Pérez, Malo, and Camps-Valls, analyze in Chapter XIII the general procedure of image compression based on support vector machines. For this purpose, and to significantly improve the results of a direct exploitation of the sparsity property, the authors take human-vision models into account in image coding based on support vector regression. Chapter XIV, by Odone and Verri, discusses the general problem of image classification and segmentation. Starting from the problem of constructing appropriate image representations, the authors describe and comment on the main properties of various kernel-engineering approaches that have been recently proposed in the computer-vision and machine-learning literature. Current work and some open issues in the literature are discussed and pointed out. Subsequently, Chapter XV, by Cremers and Kohlberger, presents a method of density estimation that is based on an extension of kernel PCA to a probabilistic framework. Applications to the segmentation and tracking of 2-D and 3-D objects demonstrate that the resulting segmentation process can incorporate highly accurate knowledge on a large variety of complex real-world shapes. The presented method makes the segmentation process robust against misleading information due to noise, clutter, and occlusion. Finally, this part is concluded with Chapter XVI, by Bruzzone, Gómez-Chova, Marconcini, and Camps-Valls, in which the authors focus on the classification of high-dimensional hyperspectral satellite images by means of kernel methods. After introducing the reader to the general framework of remote sensing and the imposed problems and constraints, an extensive comparison of kernel methods is performed. Finally, two novel kernel approaches, aiming to exploit the special characteristics of hyperspectral images, are presented: a transductive approach to deal with the high number of unlabeled samples, and a composite kernel family to exploit the spatial coverage in images.

Finally, we would like to note the fact that some of the chapters in different domains are related in the conception and application of kernel methods. For instance, one can see tight relationships between bioinformatics, text retrieval, and speech recognition tasks when dealing with string objects. Also, clear relationships appear when dealing with images; almost all chapters in the third section deal with the search for a proper image representation and the exploitation of its properties in a transformed domain. Certainly, the main goal of the book you are holding in your hands is to identify common techniques used in different domains, which could help tackling problems under different perspective and sets of tools. Rephrasing Patrick Haffner, "You'll get a good book if cross-referencing comes natural."

We hope this has been achieved.

Gustavo Camps-Valls, José Luis Rojo-Álvarez, and Manel Martínez-Ramón
Editors

Acknowledgments

The editors would like to acknowledge the help of all involved in the collation and review process of the book, without whose support the project could not have been satisfactorily completed. A further special note of thanks goes also to all the staff at Idea Group Inc., whose contributions throughout the whole process, from inception of the initial idea to final publication, have been invaluable. Special thanks also go to the publishing team at Idea Group Inc., and in particular to Kristin Roth, who continuously prodded via e-mail, keeping the project on schedule.

We wish to thank all of the authors for their insights and excellent contributions to this book. In particular, we wish to especially thank Professors Cristianini, Shawe-Taylor, and Saunders, who enthusiastically took on the important task of writing a comprehensive introductory chapter to kernel methods. Also, we would also like to thank Professor Jesús Cid-Sueiro, who read a semifinal draft of the manuscript and provided helpful suggestions for enhancing its content, structure, and readability.

Most of the authors of chapters included in this book also served as referees for articles written by other authors. Thanks go to all those who provided constructive and comprehensive reviews. In addition, a qualified set of external reviewers participated actively in the revision process. We would like to express our deepest gratitude to them. *For a full list of reviewers, please see the following page.*

And last but not least, we would like to thank Ana, Estrella, and Inma for their unfailing support and encouragement during the months it took to give birth to this book.

Gustavo Camps-Valls, José Luis Rojo-Álvarez, and Manel Martínez-Ramón
Editors

Reviewer	Affiliation
Anthony Gualtieri	NASA/GSFC
Alain Rakotomamonjy	INSA de Rouen, Information Technology Department, France
Anthony Kuh	Department of Electrical Engineering, University of Hawaii at Manoa, USA
Davide Mattera	Dept. Di Ingeneria Elettronica e delle Telecomunicazioni, Università degli Studi di Napoli Federico II, Napoli, Italy
Emilio Parrado	Universidad Carlos III de Madrid, Spain
Francis Bach	Centre de Morphologie Mathématique, Ecole des Mines de Paris, France
Jon A. Benediktson	University of Iceland
Johnny Mariéthoz	IDIAP, Swiss Federal Institute of Technology at Lausanne (EPFL), and the University of Geneva, Switzerland
Jose Principe	Computational NeuroEngineering Laboratory, University of Florida, Gainesville, USA
Luigi Occhipinti	Strategic Alliances & Programs Manager, Corporate R&D (Research and Development), SST Group, STMicroelectronics, Italy
Mário Figueiredo	Technical University of Lisbon, Portugal
Michael Georgio-poulos	Electrical & Computer Engineering Department at University of Central Florida, USA
Mounir Ghogho	Royal Academy of Engineering Research Fellow, School of Electronic and Electrical Engineering, Leeds University, Woodhouse Lane, United Kingdom
Patrick Haffner	Voice Enabled Services Research Lab at AT&T Labs-Research
Stephen M. LaConte	Emory/Georgia Tech Biomedical Imaging Technology Center, Hospital Education Annex, Atlanta, USA
Vojislav Kecman	The University of Auckland, New Zealand
Vito Di Gesù	Dipartimento di Matematica ed Applicazioni, Palermo, Italy
Wang Min	Department of Pathology, Yale University School of Medicine, USA
Wang Shitong	East China Shipbuilding Institute, Zhenjiang, China
Zhang Changsui	Department of Automation, Tsinghua University, China

Chapter I

Kernel Methods:
A Paradigm for Pattern Analysis

Nello Cristianini, University of Bristol, UK

John Shawe-Taylor, University College London, UK

Craig Saunders, University of Southampton, UK

Introduction

During the past decade, a major revolution has taken place in pattern-recognition technology with the introduction of rigorous and powerful mathematical approaches in problem domains previously treated with heuristic and less efficient techniques. The use of convex optimisation and statistical learning theory has been combined with ideas from functional analysis and classical statistics to produce a class of algorithms called kernel methods (KMs), which have rapidly become commonplace in applications. This book, and others, provides evidence of the practical applications that have made kernel methods a fundamental part of the toolbox for machine learning, statistics, and signal processing practitioners. The field of kernel methods has not only provided new insights and therefore new algorithms, but it has also created much discussion on well-established techniques such as Parzen windows and Gaussian processes, which use essentially the same technique but in different frameworks.

This introductory chapter will describe the main ideas of the kernel approach to pattern analysis, and discuss some of the reasons for their popularity. Throughout the chapter, we will assume that we have been given a set of data (be it made of vectors, sequences, documents, or any other format) and that we are interested in detecting relations existing within this data set. The ideas presented here have been introduced by many different researchers, but we will not point out the history behind these ideas, preferring to add pointers to books that address this field in a more coherent way.

The fundamental step of the kernel approach is to embed the data into a (Euclidean) space where the patterns can be discovered as linear relations. This capitalizes on the fact that over the past 50 years, statisticians and computer scientists have become very good at detecting linear relations within sets of vectors. This step therefore reduces many complex problems to a class of well-understood problems.

The embedding and subsequent analysis are performed in a *modular* fashion, as we will see below. The embedding map is defined implicitly by a so-called *kernel function*. This function depends on the specific data type and domain knowledge concerning the patterns that are to be expected in the particular data source. The second step is aimed at detecting relations within the embedded data set. There are many pattern-analysis algorithms that can operate with kernel functions, and many different types of kernel functions, each with different properties. Indeed, one reason for the popularity of the kernel approach is that these algorithms and kernels can be combined in a modular fashion. This strategy suggests a *software engineering approach* to learning systems' design through the breakdown of the task into subcomponents and the reuse of key modules.

In this introductory chapter, through the example of least squares linear regression, we will introduce all of the main ingredients of kernel methods. Though this example means that we will have restricted ourselves to the particular task of supervised regression, four key aspects of the approach will be highlighted.

1. Data items are embedded into a Euclidean space called the feature space.

2. Linear relations are sought among the images of the data items in the feature space.

3. The algorithms are implemented in such a way that the coordinates of the embedded points are not needed, only their pairwise inner products.

4. The pairwise inner products can be computed efficiently directly from the original data items using a kernel function.

These four observations will imply that, despite restricting ourselves to algorithms that optimise linear functions, our approach will enable the development of a rich toolbox of efficient and well-founded methods for discovering nonlinear relations in data through the use of nonlinear embedding mappings.

KMs offer a very general framework for performing pattern analysis on many types of data. The main idea of kernel methods is to embed the data set $S \subseteq X$ into a (possibly high-dimensional) vector space $\mathbb{R}^N$, and then to use linear pattern-analysis algorithms to detect relations in the embedded data. Linear algorithms are extremely efficient and well understood, both from a statistical and computational perspective. The embedding map is denoted here by ϕ, and it is understood that $\phi : X \rightarrow \mathbb{R}^N$ can be any set.

Although formally accurate, the overview given so far of the way kernel methods work does not reflect the way the patterns are actually computed. An important point is that the embedding does not need to be performed explicitly: We do not actually need the coordinates of all the image vectors of the data in the embedding space $\mathbb{R}^N$; we can perform a number of algorithms just knowing their relative positions. To be more accurate, if we know all the pairwise inner products between image vectors for all pairs of data points $\mathbf{x}, \mathbf{z} \in X$ we can perform most linear pattern-discovery methods known from multivariate statistics and machine learning without ever needing the coordinates of such data points.

This point is important because it turns out that it is often easy to compute the inner product in the embedding space, even when the dimensionality N is high and the coordinate vectors are very large (i.e., they would be very high-dimensional vectors). It is often possible to find a (cheaply computable) function that returns the inner product between the images of any two data points in the feature space, and we call it a kernel.

Formally, if we have data $\mathbf{x}, \mathbf{z} \in X$ and a map $\phi : X \to \mathbb{R}^N$, we call a kernel a function such that:

$$K(\mathbf{x}, \mathbf{z}) = \langle \phi(\mathbf{x}), \phi(\mathbf{z}) \rangle$$

for every $\mathbf{x}, \mathbf{z} \in X$. As mentioned above, X and Z can be elements of any set, and in this case study, they will be text documents. On the other hand, their image $\phi(x)$ is a vector in $\mathbb{R}^N$. The matrix $K_{ij} = (\mathbf{x}_i, \mathbf{x}_j)$ (where $\mathbf{x}_i, \mathbf{x}_j$ are data points) is called the kernel matrix.

Armed with this tool, we can look for linear relations in very high-dimensional spaces at a very low computational cost. If the map ϕ is nonlinear, then this will provide us with an efficient way to discover nonlinear relations in the data by using well-understood linear algorithms in a different space. What is even more powerful is that if X is not a vector space itself, the use of kernels enables us to operate on generic entities with essentially algebraic tools.

The kernel matrix contains sufficient information to run many classic and new linear algorithms in the embedding space, including support vector machines (SVMs), Fisher's linear discriminant (FDA), partial least squares (PLS), ridge regression (RR), principal components analysis (PCA), k-means and spectral clustering (SC), canonical correlation analysis (CCA), novelty detection (ND), and many others (often collectively called kernel methods). For more information about all of these methods and their origins, the authors can refer to the textbooks of Cristianini and Shawe-Taylor (2000), Schoelkopf & Smola (2002), Shawe-Taylor and Cristianini (2004), and Vapnik (1998), and the tutorial De Bie, Cristianini, and Rosipal (2004), which discusses the use of eigenproblems for kernel pattern analysis. Owing to the level of maturity already achieved in these algorithmic domains, recently, the focus of kernel methods research has been shifting toward the design of kernels defined on general data types (such as DNA sequences, text documents, trees, and labeled graphs, among others). The Web site http://www.kernel-methods.net provides free software, data sets, and constantly updated pointers to relevant literature.

The rest of this chapter is divided into three main sections.

1. The next section covers the well-known problem of linear regression. This allows us to introduce the key concepts of primal and dual variables, the latter of which allows the application of kernels. The key idea in this section is that in the dual-variable solution, example vectors only appear as inner products, and it is this fact that allows kernels to be used. This duality concept runs through all kernel methods. We end this section with a definition and a brief discussion of kernels (which is then developed later on).

2. After considering the example of linear regression, we take a step back and discuss three groups of learning tasks: classification, regression, and unsupervised learning. We give a brief example of a kernel technique in each domain, namely, SVMs for classification, SVMs for regression, and kernel PCA.

3. The final section of this chapter is devoted to kernels. We start by showing how elementary operations in the feature space can be calculated using kernels, and then move on to a slightly more in-depth discussion of kernel properties for the interested reader.

As mentioned above, we now turn to linear regression in order to give a fundamental example of a kernel method at work.

Example: Linear Regression in Feature Space

Primal Linear Regression

Consider the problem of finding a homogeneous real-valued linear function:

$$g(\mathbf{x}) = \langle \mathbf{w}, \mathbf{x} \rangle = \mathbf{w}'\mathbf{x} = \sum_{i=1}^{n} w_i x_i$$

that best interpolates a given training set $S = \{(\mathbf{x}_1, y_1), ..., (\mathbf{x}_\ell, y_\ell)\}$ of points x_i from $X \subseteq \mathbb{R}^n$ with corresponding labels y_i in $Y \subseteq \mathbb{R}$.[1] Here, we use the notation $\mathbf{x} = (x_1, x_2, ..., x_n)'$ for the n-dimensional input vectors, while w' denotes the transpose of the vector $\mathbf{w} \in \mathbb{R}^n$. This is naturally one of the simplest relations one might find in the source $X \times Y$, namely, a linear function g of the features x matching the corresponding label y, creating a pattern function that should be approximately equal to zero:

$$f((\mathbf{x}, y)) = |y - g(\mathbf{x})| = |y - \langle \mathbf{w}, \mathbf{x} \rangle| \approx 0.$$

This task is also known as *linear interpolation*. Geometrically, it corresponds to fitting a hyperplane through the given n-dimensional points. In the exact case, when the data has been generated in the form $(\mathbf{x}, g(\mathbf{x}))$, where $g(\mathbf{x}) = <\mathbf{w}, \mathbf{x}>$, and there are exactly $\ell = n$ linearly independent points, it is possible to find the parameters $\mathbf{w}$ by solving the system of linear equations:

$$\mathbf{Xw} = \mathbf{y},$$

where we have used $\mathbf{X}$ to denote the matrix whose rows are the row vectors $\mathbf{x'}_1, ..., \mathbf{x'}_\ell$, and y to denote the vector $(y_1, ..., y_\ell)'$.

If there are less points than dimensions, there are many possible $\mathbf{w}$ that describe the data exactly, and a criterion is needed to choose between them. In this situation, we will favour the vector $\mathbf{w}$ with minimum norm. If there are more points than dimensions and there is noise in the generation process, then we should not expect an exact pattern, therefore an approximation criterion is needed. In this situation, we will select the pattern with smallest error. In general, if we deal with noisy, small data sets, a mix of the two strategies is needed: Find a vector $\mathbf{w}$ that has both small norm and small error.

We call ξ the error of the linear function on the particular training example $\xi = (y - g(\mathbf{x}))$. We would like to find a function for which all of these training errors are small. The sum of the squares of these errors is the most commonly chosen measure of the collective discrepancy between the training data and a particular function:

$$L(g, S) = L(\mathbf{w}, S) = \sum_{i=1}^{\ell} (y_i - g(\mathbf{x}_i))^2 = \sum_{i=1}^{\ell} \xi_i^2 = \sum_{i=1}^{\ell} L((\mathbf{x}_i, y_i), g),$$

where we have used the same notation $L((\mathbf{x}_i, y_i), g) = \xi_i^2$ to denote the squared error or loss of g on example $(\mathbf{x}_i, y_i)$, and $L(f, S)$ to denote the collective loss of a function f on the training set S. The learning problem now becomes that of choosing the vector $\mathbf{w} \in W$ that minimises the collective loss. This is a well-studied problem that is applied in virtually every discipline. It was introduced by Gauss and is known as *least squares approximation*.

Using the notation above, the vector of output discrepancies can be written as:

$$\xi = \mathbf{y} - \mathbf{Xw}.$$

Hence, the loss function can be written as:

$$L(\mathbf{w}, S) = \|\xi\|_2^2 = (\mathbf{y} - \mathbf{Xw})'(\mathbf{y} - \mathbf{Xw}). \tag{1}$$

Note that we again use $\mathbf{X'}$ to denote the transpose of $\mathbf{X}$. We can seek the optimal $\mathbf{w}$ by taking the derivatives of the loss with respect to the parameters $\mathbf{w}$ and setting them equal to the zero vector:

$$\frac{\partial L(\mathbf{w}, S)}{\partial \mathbf{w}} = -2\mathbf{X'y} + 2\mathbf{X'Xw} = 0$$

hence obtaining the so-called normal equations:

$$\mathbf{X'Xw} = \mathbf{X'y}. \tag{2}$$

If the inverse of $\mathbf{X'X}$ exists, the solution of the least squares problem can be expressed as:

$$\mathbf{w} = (\mathbf{X'X})^{-1}\mathbf{X'y}.$$

Hence, to minimise the squared loss of a linear interpolation, one needs to maintain as many parameters as dimensions. Solving an $n \times n$ system of linear equations is an operation that has cubic cost n. This cost refers to the number of operations and is generally expressed as a complexity of $O(n^3)$, meaning that the number of operations $t(n)$ required for the computation can be upper bounded by:

$$t(n) \le Cn^3$$

for some constant C.

The predicted output on a new data point can now be computed using the prediction function:

$$g(\mathbf{x}) = \langle \mathbf{w}, \mathbf{x} \rangle.$$

Dual Representation

Notice that if the inverse of $\mathbf{X'X}$ exists, we can express $\mathbf{w}$ in the following way:

$$\mathbf{w} = (\mathbf{X'X})^{-1}\mathbf{X'y} = \mathbf{X'X}(\mathbf{X'X})^{-2}\mathbf{X'y} = \mathbf{X'\alpha},$$

making it a linear combination of the training points $\mathbf{w} = \sum_{i=1}^{\ell} \alpha_i \mathbf{x}_i$.

Pseudo-Inverse

If $\mathbf{X'X}$ is singular, the pseudo-inverse can be used. This finds the $\mathbf{w}$ that satisfies equation (2) with minimal norm. Alternatively, we can trade off the size of the norm against the loss. This is the approach known as ridge regression, which we will describe.

As mentioned earlier, there are, of course, situations where fitting the data exactly may not be possible. Either there is not enough data to ensure that the matrix $\mathbf{X'X}$ is invertible, or there may be noise in the data, making it unwise to try to match the target output exactly. Problems that suffer from this difficulty are known as *ill conditioned* since there is not enough information in the data to precisely specify the solution. In these situations, an approach that is frequently adopted is to restrict the choice of functions in some way. Such a restriction or bias is referred to as *regularisation*. Perhaps the simplest regulariser is to favour functions that have small norms. For the case of least squares regression, this gives the well-known optimisation criterion of ridge regression.

Ridge Regression

Ridge regression corresponds to solving the optimisation:

$$\min_{\mathbf{w}} L_{\lambda}(\mathbf{w}, S) = \min_{\mathbf{w}} \left(\lambda \|\mathbf{w}\|^2 + \sum_{i=1}^{\ell} (y_i - g(\mathbf{x}_i))^2 \right) \tag{3}$$

where λ is a positive number that defines the relative trade-off between norm and loss, and hence controls the degree of regularisation. The learning problem is reduced to solving an optimisation problem over $\mathbb{R}^N$.

Ridge Regression: Primal and Dual

Again taking the derivative of the cost function with respect to the parameters, we obtain the equations:

$$\mathbf{X'Xw} + \lambda \mathbf{w} = (\mathbf{X'X} + \lambda \mathbf{I}_n)\mathbf{w} = \mathbf{X'y}, \tag{4}$$

where $\mathbf{I}_n$ is the $n \times n$ identity matrix. In this case, the matrix $(\mathbf{X'X} + \lambda \mathbf{I}_n)$ is always invertible if $\lambda > 0$, so that the solution is given by:

$$\mathbf{w} = (\mathbf{X'X} + \lambda \mathbf{I}_n)^{-1} \mathbf{X'y}. \tag{5}$$

Solving this equation for $\mathbf{w}$ involves solving a system of linear equations with n unknowns and n equations. The complexity of this task is $O(n^3)$. The resulting prediction function is given by:

$$g(\mathbf{x}) = \langle \mathbf{w}, \mathbf{x} \rangle = \mathbf{y'X}(\mathbf{X'X} + \lambda \mathbf{I}_n)^{-1}\mathbf{x}.$$

Alternatively, we can rewrite equation (4) in terms of $\mathbf{w}$ and use the dual representation to obtain:

$$\mathbf{w} = \lambda^{-1}\mathbf{X}'(\mathbf{y} - \mathbf{Xw}) = \mathbf{X}'\,\alpha,$$

showing that again $\mathbf{w}$ can be written as a linear combination of the training points $\mathbf{w} = \sum_{i=1}^{\ell} \alpha_i \mathbf{x}_i$ with $\alpha = \lambda^{-1}(\mathbf{y} - \mathbf{Xw})$. Hence, we have:

$$\alpha = \lambda^{-1}(\mathbf{y} - \mathbf{Xw})$$
$$\Rightarrow \lambda\,\alpha = (\mathbf{y} - \mathbf{XX}'\alpha)$$
$$\Rightarrow (\mathbf{XX}' + \lambda\mathbf{I}_\ell)\,\alpha = \mathbf{y}$$
$$\Rightarrow \alpha = (\mathbf{G} + \lambda\mathbf{I}_\ell)^{-1}, \tag{6}$$

where $\mathbf{G} = \mathbf{XX}'$ or, component-wise, $\mathbf{G}_{ij} = \langle \mathbf{x}_i, \mathbf{x}_j \rangle$. Solving for α involves solving ℓ linear equations with ℓ unknowns, a task of complexity $O(\ell^3)$. The resulting prediction function is given by:

$$g(\mathbf{x}) = \langle \mathbf{w}, \mathbf{x} \rangle = \left\langle \sum_{i=1}^{\ell} \alpha_i \mathbf{x}_i, \mathbf{x} \right\rangle = \sum_{i=1}^{\ell} \alpha_i \langle \mathbf{x}_i, \mathbf{x} \rangle = \mathbf{y}'(\mathbf{G} + \lambda\mathbf{I}_\ell)^{-1}\mathbf{k}$$

where $k_i = \langle \mathbf{x}_i, \mathbf{x} \rangle$. We have thus found two distinct methods for solving the ridge regression optimisation of equation (3). The first, given in equation (5), computes the weight vector explicitly and is known as the *primal solution*, while equation (6) gives the solution as a linear combination of the training examples and is known as the *dual solution*. The parameters α are known as the *dual variables*.

The crucial observation about the dual solution of equation (6) is that the information from the training examples is given by the inner products between pairs of training points in the matrix $\mathbf{G} = \mathbf{XX}'$. Similarly, the information about a novel example $\mathbf{x}$ required by the predictive function is just the inner products between the training points and the new example $\mathbf{x}$.

The matrix $\mathbf{G}$ is referred to as the *Gram matrix*. The Gram matrix and the matrix $(\mathbf{G} + \lambda\mathbf{I}_\ell)$ have dimensions $\ell \times \ell$. If the dimension n of the feature space is larger than the number ℓ of training examples, it becomes more efficient to solve equation (6) rather than the primal equation (5) involving the matrix $(\mathbf{X}'\mathbf{X} + \lambda\mathbf{I}_n)$ of dimension $n \times n$. Evaluation of the predictive function in this setting is, however, always more costly since the primal involves $O(n)$ operations, while the complexity of the dual is $O(n\ell)$ (assuming that computing the function k is of the order $O(n)$). Despite this, we will later see that the dual solution can offer enormous advantages.

Hence, one of the key findings of this section is that the ridge regression algorithm can be solved in a form that only requires inner products between data points. The primal-dual dynamic described above recurs throughout the theory of kernel methods. It also plays an important role in optimisation, text analysis, and many other problem domains.

Kernel-Defined Non-Linear Feature Mappings

The ridge regression method presented in the previous subsection addresses the problem of identifying linear relations between one selected variable and the remaining features, where the relation is assumed to be functional. The resulting predictive function can be used to estimate the value of the selected variable given the values of the other features. Often, however, the relations that are sought are nonlinear, that is, the selected variable can only be accurately estimated as a nonlinear function of the remaining features. Following our overall strategy, we will map the remaining features of the data into a new feature space in such a way that the sought relations can be represented in a linear form, and hence the ridge regression algorithm described above will be able to detect them. We will consider an embedding map:

$$\phi : \mathbf{x} \in \mathbb{R}^n \mapsto \phi(\mathbf{x}) \in F \subseteq \mathbb{R}^N.$$

The choice of the map ϕ aims to convert the nonlinear relations into linear ones. Hence, the map reflects our expectations about the relation $y = g(\mathbf{x})$ to be learned. The effect of ϕ is to recode our data set S as $\hat{S} = \{(\phi(\mathbf{x}_1), y_1), ..., (\phi(\mathbf{x}_\ell), y_\ell)\}$. We can now proceed as above, looking for a relation of the form:

$$f((\mathbf{x}, y)) = |y - g(\mathbf{x})| = |y - \langle \mathbf{w}, \phi(\mathbf{x}) \rangle| = |\xi|.$$

Although the primal method could be used, problems will arise if N is very large, making the solution of the $N \times N$ system of equation (5) very expensive. If, on the other hand, we consider the dual solution, we have shown that all the information the algorithm needs is the inner products between data points $\langle \phi(\mathbf{x}), \phi(\mathbf{z}) \rangle$ in the feature space F. In particular, the predictive function $g(\mathbf{x}) = \mathbf{y}'(\mathbf{G} + \lambda \mathbf{I}_\ell)^{-1}\mathbf{k}$ involves the Gram matrix $\mathbf{G} = \mathbf{XX}'$ with entries:

$$\mathbf{G}_{ij} = \langle \phi(\mathbf{x}_i), \phi(\mathbf{x}_j) \rangle, \tag{7}$$

where the rows of $\mathbf{X}$ are now the feature vectors $\phi(\mathbf{x}_1)'$, ..., $\phi(\mathbf{x}_\ell)'$, and the vector $\mathbf{k}$ contains the values

$$k_i = \langle \phi(\mathbf{x}_i), \phi(\mathbf{x}) \rangle. \tag{8}$$

When the value of N is very large, it is worth taking advantage of the dual solution to avoid solving the large $N \times N$ system. With the optimistic assumption that the complexity of evaluating ϕ is $O(N)$, the complexity of evaluating the inner products of equations (7) and (8) is still $O(N)$, making the overall complexity of computing the vector α equal to $O(\ell^3 + \ell^2 N)$ while that of evaluating g on a new example is $O(\ell N)$.

We have seen that in the dual solution, we make use of inner products in the feature space. In the above analysis, we assumed that the complexity of evaluating each inner product was proportional to the dimension of the feature space. The inner products can, however, sometimes be computed more efficiently as a direct function of the input features, without explicitly computing the mapping ϕ. In other words, the feature-vector representation step can be bypassed. A function that performs this direct computation is known as a *kernel function*.

Kernel Function

A *kernel* is a function κ that for all $\mathbf{x}, \mathbf{z} \in X$ satisfies:

$$\kappa(\mathbf{x}, \mathbf{z}) = \langle \phi(\mathbf{x}), \phi(\mathbf{z}) \rangle$$

where ϕ is a mapping from X to an (inner product) feature space F

$$\phi : \mathbf{x} \mapsto \phi(\mathbf{x}) \in F.$$

Kernel functions form the basis of the techniques that are presented and applied later on in this book. We shall see many examples of algorithms that can take advantage of them and use them successfully in a wide variety of tasks and application areas. We will see that they make possible the use of feature spaces with an exponential or even infinite number of dimensions, something that would seem impossible if we wish to produce practical algorithms that are computationally efficient. By this we mean algorithms with computation time that scales by polynomials in the number of training examples. Through the use of efficient kernels, however, this can be done. Our aim in this chapter is to give examples to illustrate the key ideas underlying the proposed approach. We therefore now give an example of a kernel function whose complexity is less than the dimension of its corresponding feature space F, hence demonstrating that the complexity of applying ridge regression using the kernel improves on the estimates given earlier that involved the dimension N of F (where F in this case is equal to $\mathbb{R}^N$).

Consider a two-dimensional input space $X \subseteq \mathbb{R}^2$ together with the feature map:

$$\phi : \mathbf{x} = (x_1, x_2) \mapsto \phi(\mathbf{x}) = (x_1^2, x_2^2, \sqrt{2}x_1x_2) \in F = \mathbb{R}^3.$$

The hypothesis space of linear functions in F would then be:

$$g(\mathbf{x}) = w_{11}x_1^2 + w_{22}x_2^2 + w_{12}\sqrt{2}x_1x_2.$$

The feature map takes the data from a two-dimensional to a three-dimensional space in a way that linear relations in the feature space correspond to quadratic relations in the input space. The composition of the feature map with the inner product in the feature space can be evaluated as follows:

$$\langle \phi(\mathbf{x}), \phi(\mathbf{z}) \rangle = \left\langle (x_1^2, x_2^2, \sqrt{2}x_1 x_2), (z_1^2, z_2^2, \sqrt{2}z_1 z_2) \right\rangle$$
$$= x_1^2 z_1^2 + x_2^2 z_2^2 + 2x_1 x_2 z_1 z_2$$
$$= (x_1 z_1 + x_2 z_2)^2 = \langle \mathbf{x}, \mathbf{z} \rangle^2$$

Hence, the function

$$\kappa(\mathbf{x}, \mathbf{z}) = \langle \mathbf{x}, \mathbf{z} \rangle^2$$

is a kernel function with F as its corresponding feature space. This means that we can compute the inner product between the projections of two points into the feature space without explicitly evaluating their coordinates. Note that the same kernel computes the inner product corresponding to the four-dimensional feature map:

$$\phi : \mathbf{x} = (x_1, x_2) \mapsto \phi(\mathbf{x}) = (x_1^2, x_2^2, x_1 x_2, x_2 x_1) \in F = \mathbb{R}^4$$

showing that the feature space is not uniquely determined by the kernel function.

The previous example can readily be generalised to higher dimensional input spaces. Consider an n-dimensional space $X \subseteq \mathbb{R}^n$; then the function:

$$\kappa(\mathbf{x}, \mathbf{z}) = \langle \mathbf{x}, \mathbf{z} \rangle^2$$

is a kernel function corresponding to the feature map

$$\phi : \mathbf{x} \mapsto \phi(\mathbf{x}) = (x_i x_j)_{i,j=1}^n \in F = \mathbb{R}^{n^2}$$

since we have

$$\langle \phi(\mathbf{x}), \phi(\mathbf{z}) \rangle = \left\langle (x_i x_j)_{i,j=1}^n, (z_i z_j)_{i,j=1}^n \right\rangle$$
$$= \sum_{i,j=1}^n x_i x_j z_i z_j = \sum_{i=1}^n x_i z_i \sum_{j=1}^n x_j z_j$$
$$= \langle \mathbf{x}, \mathbf{z} \rangle^2$$

If we now use this kernel in the dual form of the ridge regression algorithm, the complexity of the computation of the vector α is $O(n\ell^2 + \ell^3)$ as opposed to a complexity of $O(n^2\ell^2 + \ell^3)$. If we were analysing 1,000 images, each with 256 pixels, this would roughly correspond to a 50-fold reduction in the computation time. Similarly, the time to evaluate the predictive function would be reduced by a factor of 256.

The example illustrates our second key finding that kernel functions can improve the computational complexity of computing inner products in a feature space, hence rendering algorithms efficient in very high-dimensional feature spaces. The example of dual ridge regression and the polynomial kernel of degree 2 have demonstrated how a linear pattern-analysis algorithm can be efficiently applied in a high-dimensional feature space by using an appropriate kernel function together with the dual form of the algorithm. Note that there was no need to change the underlying algorithm to accommodate the particular choice of kernel function. Clearly, we could use any suitable kernel for the data being considered. Similarly, if we wish to undertake a different type of pattern analysis we could substitute a different algorithm while retaining the chosen kernel. This illustrates the modularity of the approach that makes it possible to consider the algorithmic design and analysis separately from that of the kernel functions.

Learning Tasks

The previous section illustrated how kernel methods can implement nonlinear regression through the use of a kernel-defined feature space. The aim was to show how the key components of the kernel approach fit together in one particular example. In this section, we expand this idea to give a discussion of how kernel methods can be applied to a variety of pattern-analysis tasks. Given that we have already presented an example for regression, in this section, we will focus on classification. We will, however, provide an alternative method for regression, namely, support vector machines, for regression, and also briefly discuss some unsupervised methods.

Classification

Consider now the supervised classification task. Given a set:

$$S = \{(\mathbf{x}_1, y_1), ..., (\mathbf{x}_\ell, y_\ell)\}$$

of points $\mathbf{x}_i$ from $X \subseteq \mathbb{R}^n$ with labels y_i from $Y = \{-1, +1\}$, find a prediction function $g(\mathbf{x}) = sign(\langle \mathbf{w}, \mathbf{x} \rangle - b)$ such that

$$E[0.5|g(\mathbf{x}) - y|]$$

Figure 1. A linear function for classification creates a separating hyperplane

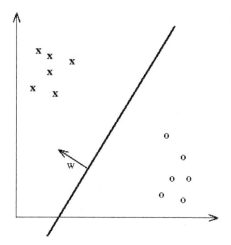

is small, where we will use the convention that $sign(0) = 1$. Note that 0.5 is included to make the loss the discrete loss and the value of the expectation the probability that a randomly drawn example $\mathbf{x}$ is misclassified by g.

Since g is a linear function with a threshold, this can be regarded as learning a hyperplane defined by the equation $\langle \mathbf{w}, \mathbf{x} \rangle = b$ separating the data according to their labels (Figure 1).

Recall that a hyperplane is an affine subspace of dimension n-1 that divides the space into two half spaces corresponding to the inputs of the two distinct classes. For example, in Figure 1, the hyperplane is the dark line, with the positive region above and the negative region below. The vector $\mathbf{w}$ defines a direction perpendicular to the hyperplane, while varying the value of b moves the hyperplane parallel to itself. A representation involving n–1 free parameters therefore can describe all possible hyperplanes in $\mathbb{R}^n$.

Both statisticians and neural network researchers have frequently used this simple kind of classifier, calling them respectively *linear discriminants* and *perceptrons*. The theory of linear discriminants was developed by Fisher in 1936, while neural network researchers studied perceptrons in the early 1960s, mainly due to the work of Rosenblatt. We will refer to the quantity $\mathbf{w}$ as the *weight vector*, a term borrowed from the neural networks literature. There are many different algorithms for selecting the weight vector $\mathbf{w}$, many of which can be implemented in dual form. In order to illustrate this concept, we will now look in more detail at one algorithm that has received a great deal of attention and is probably the most well-known technique in the kernel method toolbox: the support vector machine.

Support Vector Machines for Classification: Maximal Margin Classifier

Let us assume initially that for a given training set for a binary classification problem (i.e., $y_i \in \{1, -1\}$):

$$S = \{(\mathbf{x}_1, y_1), ..., (\mathbf{x}_\ell, y_\ell)\},$$

there exists a linear function of norm 1

$$g(\mathbf{x}) = \langle \mathbf{w}, \phi(\mathbf{x}_i) \rangle + b$$

that is determined by a weight vector $\mathbf{w}$ and threshold b, and in which there exists $\gamma > 0$ such that $\xi_i = (\gamma - y_i g(\mathbf{x}_i))_+ = 0$ for $1 \le i \le \ell$ (where $(\alpha)_+$ is 0 if $\alpha < 0$ and α otherwise). Informally, this implies that the two classes of data can be separated by a hyperplane with a margin of γ as shown in Figure 2.

We will call such a training set *separable* or more precisely *linearly separable* with margin γ. More generally, a classifier is called *consistent* if it correctly classifies all of the training set.

Since the function $\mathbf{w}$ has norm 1, the expression $\langle \mathbf{w}, \phi(\mathbf{x}_i) \rangle$ measures the length of the perpendicular projection of the point $\phi(\mathbf{x}_i)$ onto the ray determined by $\mathbf{w}$, and so:

$$y_i g(\mathbf{x}_i) = y_i(\langle \mathbf{w}, \phi(\mathbf{x}_i) \rangle + b)$$

measures how far the point $\phi(\mathbf{x}_i)$ is from the boundary hyperplane given by

$$\{\mathbf{x} : g(\mathbf{x}) = 0\},$$

Figure 2. Example of large margin hyperplane with support vectors circled

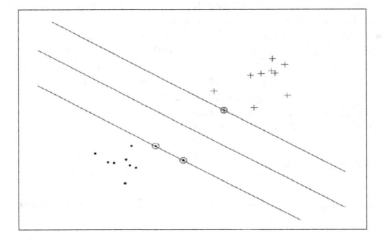

measuring positively in the direction of correct classification. For this reason, we refer to the functional margin of a linear function with norm 1 as the *geometric margin* of the associated classifier. Hence, $m(S, g) \geq \gamma$ implies that S is correctly classified by g with a geometric margin of at least γ.

Based on statistical considerations that we cannot discuss here, our task is to find the linear function that maximises the geometric margin as this has been shown to relate to the generalisation error of the classifier. This function is often referred to as the *maximal margin hyperplane* or the *hard-margin support vector machine*.

Hard-Margin SVM

Hence, the choice of hyperplane should be made to solve the following optimisation problem.

$$\begin{aligned}
\max_{\mathbf{w},b,\gamma} \quad & \gamma \\
\text{subject to} \quad & y_i(\langle\mathbf{w},\phi(\mathbf{x}_i)\rangle+b) \geq \gamma, \, i = 1, ..., \ell \\
\text{and} \quad & \|\mathbf{w}\|^2 = 1.
\end{aligned} \tag{9}$$

This is known as the primal problem as it is formulated in terms of the primal variables **w** and b.

Canonical Hyperplanes

The traditional way of formulating the optimisation problem makes use of the observation that rescaling the weight vector and threshold does not change the classification function. Hence we can fix the functional margin to be 1 and minimise the norm of the weight vector. Here though, we use the more direct method of considering the margin as it gives a clearer presentation.

For the purposes of conversion to the dual, it is better to treat the optimisation as minimising $-\gamma$. In order to arrive at the dual optimisation problem, we derive a Lagrangian. Introducing Lagrange multipliers, we obtain:

$$L(\mathbf{w},b,\gamma,\alpha,\lambda) = -\gamma - \sum_{i=1}^{\ell} \alpha_i[y_i(\langle\mathbf{w},\phi(\mathbf{x}_i)\rangle+b)-\gamma] + \lambda(\|\mathbf{w}\|^2-1).$$

Differentiating with respect to the primal variables gives:

$$\frac{\partial L(\mathbf{w},b,\gamma,\alpha,\lambda)}{\partial\mathbf{w}} = -\sum_{i=1}^{\ell}\alpha_i y_i\phi(\mathbf{x}_i) + 2\lambda\mathbf{w} = 0,$$

$$\frac{\partial L(\mathbf{w},b,\gamma,\alpha,\lambda)}{\partial\gamma} = -1 + \sum_{i=1}^{\ell}\alpha_i = 0, \text{ and}$$

$$\frac{\partial L(\mathbf{w},b,\gamma,\alpha,\lambda)}{\partial b} = -\sum_{i=1}^{\ell} \alpha_i y_i = 0. \tag{10}$$

Substituting, we obtain:

$$
\begin{aligned}
L(\mathbf{w},b,\gamma,\alpha,\lambda) &= -\sum_{i=1}^{\ell} \alpha_i y_i \langle \mathbf{w}, \phi(\mathbf{x}_i) \rangle + \lambda \|\mathbf{w}\|^2 - \lambda \\
&= \left(-\frac{1}{2\lambda} + \frac{1}{4\lambda} \right) \sum_{i,j=1}^{\ell} \alpha_i y_i \alpha_j y_j \langle \phi(\mathbf{x}_i), \phi(\mathbf{x}_j) \rangle - \lambda \\
&= -\frac{1}{4\lambda} \sum_{i,j=1}^{\ell} \alpha_i \alpha_j y_i y_j \kappa(\mathbf{x}_i,\mathbf{x}_j) - \lambda
\end{aligned}
$$

Finally, optimising the choice of λ gives:

$$\lambda = \frac{1}{2}\left(\sum_{i,j=1}^{\ell} \alpha_i \alpha_j y_i y_j \kappa\left(\mathbf{x}_i,\mathbf{x}_j\right) \right)^{1/2},$$

resulting in

$$L(\alpha) = -\left(\sum_{i,j=1}^{\ell} \alpha_i \alpha_j y_i y_j \kappa\left(\mathbf{x}_i,\mathbf{x}_j\right) \right)^{1/2}, \tag{11}$$

where $\alpha_i \geq 0, i = 1,...,\ell$, which we call the dual Lagrangian or *dual problem*. We have therefore derived the algorithm for the hard-margin support vector machine, which is shown in line 3 of the pseudocode.

On Sparseness

The Karush-Kuhn-Tucker (KKT) complementarity conditions provide useful information about the structure of the solution. The conditions state that the optimal solutions $\alpha^*,(\mathbf{w}^*,b^*)$ must satisfy:

$$\alpha_i^*\left[y_i(\langle \mathbf{w}^*,\phi(\mathbf{x}_i) \rangle + b^*) - \gamma^* \right] = 0, i = 1,...,\ell.$$

This implies that only for inputs $\mathbf{x}_i$, for which the geometric margin is γ^* and therefore lie closest to the hyperplane, are the corresponding α_i^* nonzero. All the other parameters α_i^*

Figure 3. Pseudocode for the hard-margin SVM

Input	training set $S = \{(\mathbf{x}_1, y_1), ..., (\mathbf{x}_\ell, y_\ell)\}$, $\delta > 0$
Process maximise	find α^* as solution of the optimisation problem: $W(\alpha) = -\sum_{i,j=1}^{\ell} \alpha_i \alpha_j y_i y_j \kappa(\mathbf{x}_i, \mathbf{x}_j)$
subject to	$\sum_{i=1}^{\ell} y_i \alpha_i = 0$, $\sum_{i=1}^{\ell} \alpha_i = 1$ and $0 \leq \alpha_i$, $i = 1, ..., \ell$.
	$\gamma^* = \sqrt{-W(\alpha^*)}$ choose i such that $0 < \alpha_i^*$ $b = y_i(y^*)^2 - \sum_{j=1}^{\ell} \alpha_j^* y_j \kappa(\mathbf{x}_j, \mathbf{x}_i)$ $f(\cdot) = sgn(\sum_{j=1}^{\ell} \alpha_j^* y_j \kappa(\mathbf{x}_j, \cdot) + b);$ $\mathbf{w} = \sum_{j=1}^{\ell} y_j \alpha_j^* \phi(\mathbf{x}_j)$
Output	weight vector $\mathbf{w}$, dual solution α^*, margin γ^* and function f implementing the decision rule represented by the hyperplane

are zero. The inputs with nonzero α_i^* are called *support vectors* (see Figure 2), and we will denote the set of indices of the support vectors with *sv*.

On Convexity

Note that the requirement that κ is a kernel means that the optimisation problem of the hard-margin SVM is convex since the matrix $\mathbf{G} = (y_i y_j \kappa(\mathbf{x}_i, \mathbf{x}_j))_{i,j=1}^{\ell}$ is also positive semidefinite, as the following computation shows:

$$\beta'\mathbf{G}\beta = \sum_{i,j=1}^{\ell} \beta_i \beta_j y_i y_j \kappa(\mathbf{x}_i, \mathbf{x}_j) = \left\langle \sum_{i=1}^{\ell} \beta_i y_i \phi(\mathbf{x}_i), \sum_{j=1}^{\ell} \beta_j y_j \phi(\mathbf{x}_j) \right\rangle$$

$$= \left\| \sum_{i=1}^{\ell} \beta_i y_i \phi(\mathbf{x}_i) \right\|^2 \geq 0$$

Hence, the property required of a kernel function to define a feature space also ensures that the maximal margin optimisation problem has a unique solution that can be found efficiently. This rules out the problem of local minima often encountered in, for example, training neural networks.

Duality Gap

An important result from optimisation theory states that throughout the feasible regions of the primal and dual problems, the primal objective is always bigger than the dual objective when the primal is a minimisation. This is also indicated by the fact that we are minimising the primal and maximising the dual. Since the problems we are considering satisfy the conditions of strong duality, there is no duality gap at the optimal solution. We can therefore use any difference between the primal and dual objectives as an indicator of convergence. We will call this difference the duality gap. Let $\hat{\alpha}$ be the current value of the dual variables. The possibly still negative margin can be calculated as:

$$\hat{\gamma} = \frac{\min_{y_i=1}\left(\langle \hat{\mathbf{w}}, \phi(\mathbf{x}_i) \rangle\right) - \max_{y_i=-1}\left(\langle \hat{\mathbf{w}}, \phi(\mathbf{x}_i) \rangle\right)}{2},$$

where the current value of the weight vector is $\hat{\mathbf{w}}$. Hence, the duality gap can be computed as

$$-\sqrt{-W(\hat{\alpha})} + \hat{\gamma},$$

where

$$W(\alpha) = -\sum_{i,j=1}^{\ell} \alpha_i \alpha_j y_i y_j \kappa\left(\mathbf{x}_i, \mathbf{x}_j\right).$$

Soft-Margin Classifiers

The maximal margin classifier is an important concept, but it can only be used if the data are separable. For this reason, it is not applicable in many real-world problems where the data are frequently noisy. If we are to ensure linear separation in the feature space in such cases, we will need very complex kernels that may result in overfitting. Since the hard-margin support vector machine always produces a consistent hypothesis, it is extremely sensitive to noise in the training data. The dependence on a quantity like the margin opens the system up to the danger of being very sensitive to a few points. For real data, this will result in a nonrobust estimator.

This problem motivates the development of more robust versions that can tolerate some noise and outliers in the training set without drastically altering the resulting solution. In the above, we assumed that $\xi_i = 0$ for all i. Hence, if we relax this assumption, we will be able to tolerate some misclassification of the training data. We must now optimise a combination of the margin and norm of the vector ξ, where $\xi_i = \xi((y_i, \mathbf{x}_i), \gamma, g) = (\gamma - y_i g(\mathbf{x}_i))_+$. Introducing this vector into the optimisation criterion results in an optimisation problem with what are known as *slack variables* that allow the margin constraints to be violated. For this reason, we often refer to the vector ξ as the *margin slack vector*.

1-Norm Soft-Margin SVM

The 1-norm soft-margin support vector machine is given by the computation:

$$\min_{\mathbf{w}, b, \gamma, \xi} -\gamma + C\sum_{i=1}^{\ell} \xi_i$$
$$\text{subject to } y_i(\langle \mathbf{w}, \phi(\mathbf{x}_i) \rangle + b) \geq \gamma - \xi_i, \; \xi_i \geq 0,$$
$$i = 1, ..., \ell, \text{ and } \|\mathbf{w}\|^2 = 1. \tag{12}$$

The parameter C controls the trade-off between the margin and the size of the slack variables. The optimisation problem in equation (12) controls the norm of the margin slack vector. In order to make use of kernels, we once again introduce a Lagrangian and express this problem in terms of the dual variables.

1-Norm Soft Margin: The Box Constraint

The corresponding Lagrangian for the 1-norm soft-margin optimisation problem is:

$$L(\mathbf{w}, b, \gamma, \xi, \alpha, \beta, \lambda) = -\gamma + C\sum_{i=1}^{\ell} \xi_i - \sum_{i=1}^{\ell} \alpha_i \left[y_i(\langle \phi(\mathbf{x}_i), \mathbf{w} \rangle + b) - \gamma + \xi_i \right]$$
$$- \sum_{i=1}^{\ell} \beta_i \xi_i + \lambda(\|\mathbf{w}\|^2 - 1)$$

with $\alpha_i \geq 0$ and $\beta_i \geq 0$.

One can then differentiate and examine the KKT conditions in a similar fashion to the hard-margin case above in order to create an algorithm for solving the above. The resulting algorithm is shown in Figure 4.

Hence, the most immediate affect of minimising the norm of the slack variables is to place a box constraint on the dual variables α_i, upper bounding them by the value C.

Regression

Regression is another fundamental learning task to which many kernel methods have been applied. The essential difference to that of the classification setting is that the labels y_i are now drawn from the real line, that is, $yi \in \mathbb{R}$. We have already seen one example of a kernel regression technique in this chapter, namely that of ridge regression, so we shall not go into too much detail here. For completeness, however, we shall state the SVM algorithm for regression. This has become another default method in the kernel method toolbox and has proven successful on a wide variety of regression problems.

Figure 4. Pseudocode for the 1-norm soft-margin SVM

Input	training set $S = \{(\mathbf{x}_1, y_1), ..., (\mathbf{x}_\ell, y_\ell)\}$, $\delta > 0$, $C \in [1/\ell, \infty)$
Process	find $\boldsymbol{\alpha}^*$ as solution of the optimisation problem:
maximise	$W(\boldsymbol{\alpha}) = -\sum_{i,j=1}^{\ell} \alpha_i \alpha_j y_i y_j \, \kappa(\mathbf{x}_i, \mathbf{x}_j)$
subject to	$\sum_{i=1}^{\ell} y_i \alpha_i = 0$, $\sum_{i=1}^{\ell} \alpha_i = 1$ and $0 \le \alpha_i \le C, i = 1, ..., \ell$.

$$\lambda^* = \tfrac{1}{2}\left(\sum_{i,j=1}^{\ell} \alpha_i^* \alpha_j^* y_i y_j \, \kappa(\mathbf{x}_i, \mathbf{x}_j)\right)^{\frac{1}{2}}$$

choose i, j such that $-C < \alpha_i^* y_i \, 0 < \alpha_j^* y_j < C$

$$b^* = -\lambda^* \left(\sum_{k=1}^{\ell} \alpha_k^* y_k \, \kappa(\mathbf{x}_k, \mathbf{x}_i) + \sum_{k=1}^{\ell} \alpha_k^* y_k \, \kappa(\mathbf{x}_k, \mathbf{x}_j)\right)$$

$$\gamma^* = 2\lambda^* \sum_{k=1}^{\ell} \alpha_k^* y_k \, \kappa(\mathbf{x}_k, \mathbf{x}_j) + b^*$$

$$f(\cdot) = sgn\left(\sum_{j=1}^{\ell} \alpha_j^* y_j \kappa(\mathbf{x}_j, \cdot) + b^*\right);$$

$$\mathbf{w} = \sum_{j=1}^{\ell} y_j \alpha_j^* \phi(\mathbf{x}_j)$$

Output	weight vector $\mathbf{w}$, dual solution $\boldsymbol{\alpha}^*$, margin γ^* and function f implementing the decision rule represented by the hyperplane

In SVM regression, a different loss function from that used in ridge regression is minimised. We no longer concentrate on the square loss; instead, ε-insensitive loss is used. This is defined as:

$$L^\varepsilon(\mathbf{x}, y, f) = | y - f(\mathbf{x}) |_\varepsilon = \max(0, | y - f(\mathbf{x}) | - \varepsilon) \tag{13}$$

and aids to give a sparse solution. By minimising the quadratic form of this loss and the norm of $\mathbf{w}$, (similar to the classification case) we obtain the following primal optimisation problem:

$$\min_{\mathbf{w}, b, \xi, \hat{\xi}} \ \| \mathbf{w} \|^2 + C \sum_{i=1}^{\ell} (\xi_i + \hat{\xi}_i)$$
$$\text{subject to } \ (\langle \mathbf{w}, \mathbf{x} \rangle + b) - y_i \le \varepsilon + \xi_i, i = 1, ..., \ell$$
$$(\langle \mathbf{w}, \mathbf{x} \rangle + b) - y_i \le \varepsilon + \xi_i, i = 1, ..., \ell$$
$$\xi_i, \hat{\xi}_i \ge 0, i = 1, ..., \ell$$

The dual problem can be derived in a similar fashion to that of the classification case and can be stated as:

$$\max_{\hat{\alpha}, \alpha} \quad \sum_{i=1}^{\ell} y_i (\alpha_i - \hat{\alpha}_i) - \varepsilon \sum_{i=1}^{\ell} y_i (\alpha_i + \hat{\alpha}_i)$$
$$- \frac{1}{2} \sum_{i,j=1}^{\ell} (\alpha_i - \hat{\alpha}_i)(\alpha_j - \hat{\alpha}_j) \kappa(\mathbf{x}_i, \mathbf{x}_j)$$
$$\text{subject to } \sum_{i=1}^{\ell} (\alpha_i - \hat{\alpha}_i) = 0$$
$$0 \le \hat{\alpha}_i, \alpha_i \le C, i = 1, ..., \ell$$

with corresponding KKT complementary conditions:

$$\alpha_i (\langle \mathbf{w}, \phi(\mathbf{x}_i) \rangle + b - y_i - \varepsilon - \xi) = 0 \qquad i = 1, ..., \ell$$
$$\hat{\alpha}_i (y_i - \langle \mathbf{w}, \phi(\mathbf{x}_i) \rangle - b - \varepsilon - \hat{\xi}_i) = 0 \qquad i = 1, ..., \ell$$
$$\xi_i \hat{\xi}_i = 0, \alpha_i \hat{\alpha}_i = 0 \qquad i = 1, ..., \ell$$
$$(\alpha_i - C) \xi_i = 0, (\hat{\alpha}_i - C) \hat{\xi}_i = 0 \qquad i = 1, ..., \ell.$$

If we consider a "tube" of $\pm \varepsilon$ around the function output by the above algorithm, the points that are on the edge of the tube and not strictly inside it are the support vectors. Those that are not touching the tube will have the absolute value of the corresponding α_i equal to C.

This completes our treatment of regression, and we have already seen two powerful algorithms that can be used in this domain, namely, kernel ridge regression and support-vector regression. Before moving on to look at kernel functions in more detail, we shall briefly discuss learning in an unsupervised setting.

Unsupervised Methods

Lack of space prevents us from giving a full account of unsupervised methods, but it suffices to say that kernel methods have also made a strong impact in the area of unsupervised learning. Many traditional linear methods such as clustering and principal components analysis can also be placed within the kernel framework and take advantage of the nonlinearity introduced by the use of kernels. In the following, we briefly review these two methods and then discuss how the use of kernel functions leads to a very flexible modular approach in the application of learning algorithms.

Principal Components Analysis

Detecting regularities in an unlabelled set $S = \{\mathbf{x}_1, ..., \mathbf{x}_\ell\}$ of points from $X \subseteq \mathbb{R}^n$ is referred to as unsupervised learning. One such task is finding a low-dimensional representation of the data such that the expected residual is as small as possible. Relations between features are important because they reduce the effective dimensionality of the data, causing it to lie on a lower dimensional surface. This may make it possible to recode the data in a more efficient way using fewer coordinates. The aim is to find a smaller set of variables defined by functions of the original features in such a way that the data can be approximately reconstructed from the new coordinates.

Despite the difficulties encountered if more general functions are considered, a good understanding exists of the special case when the relations are assumed to be linear. This subcase is attractive because it leads to analytical solutions and simple computations. For linear functions, the problem is equivalent to projecting the data onto a lower dimensional linear subspace in such a way that the distance between a vector and its projection is not too large. The problem of minimising the average squared distance between vectors and their projections is equivalent to projecting the data onto the space spanned by the first k eigenvectors of the matrix $\mathbf{X'X}$:

$$\mathbf{X'X}\mathbf{v}_i = \lambda_i \mathbf{v}_i,$$

and hence the coordinates of a new vector $\mathbf{x}$ in the new space can be obtained by considering its projection onto the eigenvectors $\langle \mathbf{x}, \mathbf{v}_i \rangle$, $i = 1, ..., k$. This technique is known as principal components analysis.

The algorithm can be rendered nonlinear by first embedding the data into a feature space and then considering projections in that space. Once again, we will see that kernels can be used to define the feature space since the algorithm can be rewritten in a form that only requires inner products between inputs. Hence, we can detect nonlinear relations between variables in the data by embedding the data into a kernel-induced feature space, where linear relations can be found by means of PCA in that space. This approach is known as *kernel PCA*.

Of course, some information about linear relations in the data is already implicit in the rank of the data matrix. The rank corresponds to the number of nonzero eigenvalues of the covariance matrix and is the dimensionality of the subspace in which the data lie. The rank can also be computed using only inner products since the eigenvalues of the inner product matrix are equal to those of the covariance matrix. We can think of PCA as finding a low-rank approximation, where the quality of the approximation depends on how close the data are to lying in a subspace of the given dimensionality.

Clustering

Finally, we mention finding clusters in a training set $S = \{\mathbf{x}_1, ..., \mathbf{x}_\ell\}$ of points from $X \subseteq \mathbb{R}^n$. One method of defining clusters is to identify a fixed number of centres or prototypes and assign points to the cluster defined by the closest centre. Identifying clusters by a set of prototypes divides the space into what is known as a Voronoi partitioning.

The aim is to minimise the expected squared distance of a point from its cluster centre. If we fix the number of centres to be k, a classic procedure is known as k-means and is a widely used heuristic for clustering data. The k-means procedure must have some method for measuring the distance between two points. Once again, this distance can always be computed using only inner product information through the equality:

$$\|\mathbf{x} - \mathbf{z}\|^2 = \langle \mathbf{x}, \mathbf{x} \rangle + \langle \mathbf{z}, \mathbf{z} \rangle - 2 \langle \mathbf{x}, \mathbf{z} \rangle.$$

This distance, together with a dual representation of the mean of a given set of points, implies the k-means procedure can be implemented in a kernel-defined feature space. This procedure is not, however, a typical example of a kernel method since it fails to produce what we termed earlier as an efficient algorithm. This is because the optimisation criterion is not convex and hence we cannot guarantee that the procedure will converge to the optimal arrangement. Clustering, however, is still a highly useful technique that has been applied in many application settings. A number of clustering methods that can be combined with kernels have been described in the literature, and we shall see more examples later on in this book.

The Modularity of Kernel Methods

The procedures outlined in the previous sections have several aspects in common: An algorithmic procedure is adapted to use only inner products between inputs. The method can then be combined with a kernel function that calculates the inner product between the images of two inputs in a feature space, hence making it possible to implement the algorithm in a high-dimensional space.

The modularity of kernel methods shows itself in the reusability of the learning algorithm. The same algorithm can work with any kernel and hence for any data domain. The kernel component is data specific, but can be combined with different algorithms to solve the full range of tasks that we will consider. All this leads to a very natural and elegant approach to learning systems design, where modules are combined together to obtain complex learning systems. Figure 5 shows the stages involved in the implementation of kernel pattern analysis. The data is processed using a kernel to create a kernel matrix, which in turn is processed by a pattern-analysis algorithm to produce a pattern function. This function is used to process unseen examples.

This approach will become more and more evident in later chapters, where the same kernel or algorithm is reused and adapted to very different real-world problems.

From a computational point of view, kernel methods have two important properties. First of all, they enable access to very high-dimensional and correspondingly flexible feature spaces at low computational cost both in space and time, and yet secondly, despite the complexity of the resulting function classes, a great many of the kernel techniques proposed and currently used solve convex optimisation problems that can be computed efficiently and hence do not suffer from local minima. Given the central nature of the kernel function to all kernel methods, we now give a more in-depth treatment of kernels in the next section.

Kernels

In this section, we focus on kernel functions, first showing how some basic manipulations and calculations can be performed in feature space, then following this, we provide some more detailed definitions and advanced discussions. This section provides the final link in our introductory chapter. We have introduced some of the elements of kernel methods through the example of linear regression. We then extended this to a fuller discussion of learning tasks and introduced the SVM algorithm for classification and regression. Finally, we now conclude with the properties of kernels.

Kernel Basics

We now give examples of how to perform some elementary and often-used calculations in feature space whilst only using the information provided via the kernel function (thus, once more reinforcing the idea that the feature mapping need not be explicit). We start by showing how means and distances can be calculated.

Means and Distances

Given a finite subset $S = \{\mathbf{x}_1, ..., \mathbf{x}_\ell\}$ of an input space X and a kernel $\kappa(\mathrm{x,z})$ satisfying:

$$\kappa(\mathbf{x}, \mathbf{z}) = \langle \phi(\mathbf{x}), \phi(\mathbf{z}) \rangle,$$

where ϕ is a feature map into a feature space F, let $\phi(S) = \{\phi(\mathbf{x}_1), ..., \phi(\mathbf{x}_\ell)\}$ be the image of S under the map ϕ. Hence $\phi(S)$ is a subset of the inner product space F. Significant information about the embedded data set $\phi(S)$ can be obtained by using only the inner product information contained in the kernel matrix K of kernel evaluations between all pairs of elements of S:

Figure 5. The stages involved in the application of kernel methods

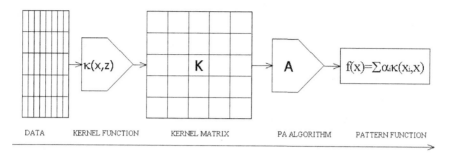

$$\mathbf{K}_{ij} = \kappa(\mathbf{x}_i, \mathbf{x}_j), \quad i, j = 1, ..., \ell.$$

Working in a kernel-defined feature space means that we are not able to explicitly represent points. For example, the image of an input point x is $\phi(\mathbf{x})$, but we do not have access to the components of this vector, only to the evaluation of inner products between this point and the images of other points. Despite this handicap, there is a surprising amount of useful information that can be gleaned about $\phi(S)$.

Norm of Feature Vectors

The simplest example of this is the evaluation of the norm of $\phi(x)$ that is given by:

$$\|\phi(\mathbf{x})\|_2 = \sqrt{\|\phi(\mathbf{x})\|^2} = \sqrt{\langle \phi(\mathbf{x}), \phi(\mathbf{x}) \rangle} = \sqrt{\kappa(\mathbf{x}, \mathbf{x})}.$$

We can also evaluate the norms of linear combinations of images in the feature space. For example, we have:

$$\left\| \sum_{i=1}^{\ell} \alpha_i \phi(\mathbf{x}_i) \right\|^2 = \left\langle \sum_{i=1}^{\ell} \alpha_i \phi(\mathbf{x}_i), \sum_{j=1}^{\ell} \alpha_j \phi(\mathbf{x}_j) \right\rangle$$

$$= \sum_{i=1}^{\ell} \alpha_i \sum_{j=1}^{\ell} \alpha_j \langle \phi(\mathbf{x}_i), \phi(\mathbf{x}_j) \rangle$$

$$= \sum_{i,j=1}^{\ell} \alpha_i \alpha_j \kappa(\mathbf{x}_i, \mathbf{x}_j).$$

Distance between Feature Vectors

A special case of the norm is the length of the line joining two images $\phi(\mathbf{x})$ and $\phi(\mathbf{z})$, which can be computed as:

$$\|\phi(\mathbf{x}) - \phi(\mathbf{z})\|^2 = \langle \phi(\mathbf{x}) - \phi(\mathbf{z}), \phi(\mathbf{x}) - \phi(\mathbf{z}) \rangle$$
$$= \langle \phi(\mathbf{x}), \phi(\mathbf{x}) \rangle - 2\langle \phi(\mathbf{x}), \phi(\mathbf{z}) \rangle + \langle \phi(\mathbf{z}), \phi(\mathbf{z}) \rangle$$
$$= \kappa(\mathbf{x}, \mathbf{x}) - 2\kappa(\mathbf{x}, \mathbf{z}) + \kappa(\mathbf{z}, \mathbf{z})$$

Norm and Distance from the Centre of Mass

As a more complex and useful example, consider the centre of mass of the set $\phi(S)$. This is the vector:

$$\phi_S = \frac{1}{\ell} \sum_{i=1}^{\ell} \phi(\mathbf{x}_i).$$

As with all points in the feature space, we will not have an explicit vector representation of this point. However, in this case, there may also not exist a point in X whose image under ϕ is ϕ_s. In other words, we are now considering points that potentially lie outside $\phi(X)$, that is, the image of the input space X under the feature map ϕ.

Despite this apparent inaccessibility of the point ϕ_s, we can compute its norm using only evaluations of the kernel on the inputs:

$$\|\phi_S\|_2^2 = \langle \phi_s, \phi_s \rangle = \left\langle \frac{1}{\ell} \sum_{i=1}^{\ell} \phi(\mathbf{x}_i), \frac{1}{\ell} \sum_{j=1}^{\ell} \phi(\mathbf{x}_j) \right\rangle$$
$$= \frac{1}{\ell^2} \sum_{i,j=1}^{\ell} \langle \phi(\mathbf{x}_i), \phi(\mathbf{x}_j) \rangle = \frac{1}{\ell^2} \sum_{i,j=1}^{\ell} \kappa(\mathbf{x}_i, \mathbf{x}_j).$$

Hence, the square of the norm of the centre of mass is equal to the average of the entries in the kernel matrix. Incidentally, this implies that this sum is greater than or equal to zero with equality if the centre of mass is at the origin of the coordinate system. Similarly, we can compute the distance of the image of a point x from the centre of mass ϕ_s:

$$\|\phi(\mathbf{x}) - \phi_S\|^2 = \langle \phi(\mathbf{x}), \phi(\mathbf{x}) \rangle + \langle \phi_S, \phi_S \rangle - 2\langle \phi(\mathbf{x}), \phi_S \rangle$$
$$= \kappa(\mathbf{x}, \mathbf{x}) + \frac{1}{\ell^2} \sum_{i,j=1}^{\ell} \kappa(\mathbf{x}_i, \mathbf{x}_j) - \frac{2}{\ell} \sum_{i=1}^{\ell} \kappa(\mathbf{x}, \mathbf{x}_i). \tag{14}$$

Expected Distance from the Centre of Mass

Following the same approach, it is also possible to express the expected squared distance of a point in a set from its mean:

$$\frac{1}{\ell}\sum_{s=1}^{\ell}\left|\phi(\mathbf{x}_s)-\phi_s\right|^2 = \frac{1}{\ell}\sum_{s=1}^{\ell}\kappa(\mathbf{x}_s,\mathbf{x}_s)+\frac{1}{\ell^2}\sum_{i,j=1}^{\ell}\kappa(\mathbf{x}_i,\mathbf{x}_j)$$

$$-\frac{2}{\ell^2}\sum_{i,s=1}^{\ell}\kappa(\mathbf{x}_s,\mathbf{x}_i) \tag{15}$$

$$= \frac{1}{\ell}\sum_{s=1}^{\ell}\kappa(\mathbf{x}_s,\mathbf{x}_s)-\frac{1}{\ell^2}\sum_{i,j=1}^{\ell}\kappa(\mathbf{x}_i,\mathbf{x}_j). \tag{16}$$

Hence, the average squared distance of points to their centre of mass is the average of the diagonal entries of the kernel matrix minus the average of all the entries.

We can design a whole range of kernel functions depending on the problem at hand. However, the general principles can be shown with a few examples. The approach we have outlined in this chapter shows how a number of useful tasks can be accomplished in high-dimensional feature spaces defined implicitly by a kernel function. So far we have only seen how to construct very simple polynomial kernels. Clearly, for the approach to be useful, we would like to have a range of potential kernels together with machinery to tailor their construction to the specifics of a given data domain. If the inputs are elements of a vector space such as $\mathbb{R}^n$, there is a natural inner product that is referred to as the *linear kernel* by analogy with the polynomial construction. Using this kernel corresponds to running the original algorithm in the input space. As we have seen above, at the cost of a few extra operations, the polynomial construction can convert the linear kernel into an inner product in a vastly expanded feature space. This example illustrates a general principle we will develop by showing how more complex kernels can be created from simpler ones in a number of different ways. Kernels can even be constructed that correspond to infinite-dimensional feature spaces at the cost of only a few extra operations in the kernel evaluations.

An example of creating a new kernel from an existing one is provided by normalising a kernel. Given a kernel $\kappa(\mathbf{x},\mathbf{z})$ that corresponds to the feature mapping ϕ, the *normalised kernel* $\kappa(\mathbf{x},\mathbf{z})$ corresponds to the feature map:

$$\mathbf{x} \mapsto \phi(\mathbf{x}) \mapsto \frac{\phi(\mathbf{x})}{\|\phi(\mathbf{x})\|}.$$

Hence, we can express the kernel $\hat{\kappa}$ in terms of κ as follows:

$$\hat{\kappa}(\mathbf{x},\mathbf{z}) = \left\langle \frac{\phi(\mathbf{x})}{\|\phi(\mathbf{x})\|}, \frac{\phi(\mathbf{z})}{\|\phi(\mathbf{z})\|} \right\rangle = \frac{\kappa(\mathbf{x},\mathbf{z})}{\sqrt{\kappa(\mathbf{x},\mathbf{x})\kappa(\mathbf{z},\mathbf{z})}}.$$

These constructions will not, however, in themselves extend the range of data types that can be processed. We will therefore also develop kernels that correspond to mapping inputs that are not vectors into an appropriate feature space. As an example, consider the input space consisting of all subsets of a fixed set D. Consider the kernel function of two subsets A_1 and A_2 of D defined by:

$$\kappa(A_1, A_2) = 2^{|A_1 \cap A_2|},$$

that is, the number of common subsets A_1 and A_2 share. This kernel corresponds to a feature map ϕ to the vector space of dimension $2^{|D|}$ indexed by all subsets of D, where the image of a set A is the vector with:

$$\phi(A)_U = \begin{cases} 1 \text{ if } U \subseteq A \\ 0, \text{ otherwise.} \end{cases}$$

This example is defined over a general set and yet we have seen that it fulfills the conditions for being a valid kernel, namely, that it corresponds to an inner product in a feature space. Developing this approach, we will show how kernels can be constructed from different types of input spaces in a way that reflects their structure even though they are not in themselves vector spaces. These kernels will be needed for many important applications such as text analysis and bioinformatics. In fact, the range of valid kernels is very large: some are given in closed form, and others can only be computed by means of a recursion or other algorithm; in some cases, the actual feature mapping corresponding to a given kernel function is not known, only a guarantee that the data can be embedded in some feature space that gives rise to the chosen kernel. In short, provided the function can be evaluated efficiently and it corresponds to computing the inner product of suitable images of its two arguments, it constitutes a potentially useful kernel.

Selecting the best kernel from among this extensive range of possibilities becomes the most critical stage in applying kernel-based algorithms in practice. The selection of the kernel can be shown to correspond in a very tight sense to the encoding of our prior knowledge about the data and the types of patterns we can expect to identify. It is possible to treat the kernel part of the algorithm in a modular fashion, constructing it from simple components and then modifying it by means of a set of well-defined operations.

A General Characterisation of Kernels

So far, we have only one way of verifying that the function is a kernel, that is, to construct a feature space for which the function corresponds to first performing the feature mapping and then computing the inner product between the two images. For example, we used this technique to show the polynomial function is a kernel and to show that the exponential of the cardinality of a set intersection is a kernel.

We will now introduce an alternative method of demonstrating that a candidate function is a kernel. This will provide one of the theoretical tools needed to create new kernels, and combine old kernels to form new ones.

One of the key observations is the relation with positive semidefinite matrices. The kernel matrix formed by evaluating a kernel on all pairs of any set of inputs is positive semidefinite. This forms the basis of the following definition.

Finitely Positive Semidefinite Functions

A function:

$$\kappa : X \times X \longrightarrow \mathbb{R}$$

satisfies the finitely positive semidefinite property if it is a symmetric function for which the matrices formed by restriction to any finite subset of the space X are positive semidefinite.

Note that this definition does not require the set X to be a vector space. We will now demonstrate that the finitely positive semidefinite property characterises kernels. We will do this by explicitly constructing the feature space assuming only this property. We first state the result in the form of a theorem.

Theorem 1 (Characterisation of Kernels).

A function:

$$\kappa : X \times X \longrightarrow \mathbb{R}$$

can be decomposed

$$\kappa(\mathbf{x},\mathbf{z}) = \langle \phi(\mathbf{x}), \phi(\mathbf{z}) \rangle$$

into a feature map ϕ into a Hilbert space F applied to both its arguments followed by the evaluation of the inner product in F if and only if it satisfies the finitely positive semidefinite property.

Mercer Kernel

We are now able to show Mercer's theorem as a consequence of the previous analysis. Mercer's theorem is usually used to construct a feature space for a valid kernel. Other methods for analysing feature spaces and the validity of a kernel exist (such as reproducing kernel Hilbert spaces); however, we do not have the space to cover them all. We include Mercer's theorem for completeness as it defines the feature space in terms of an explicit feature vector and reinforces the idea of a $\phi(\cdot)$ function mapping data points into a feature space.

Theorem 2 (Mercer).

Let X be a compact subset of $\mathbb{R}^n$. Suppose κ is a continuous symmetric function such that the integral operator:

$$T_\kappa : L_2(X) \to L_2(X),$$
$$(T_\kappa f)(\cdot) = \int_X \kappa(\cdot, \mathbf{x}) f(\mathbf{x}) d\mathbf{x}$$

is positive; that is

$$\int_{X \times X} \kappa(\mathbf{x}, \mathbf{z}) f(\mathbf{x}) f(\mathbf{z}) d\mathbf{x} d\mathbf{z} \geq 0$$

for all $f \in L_2(X)$. Then we can expand $\kappa(\mathbf{x},\mathbf{z})$ in a uniformly convergent series (on $X \times X$) in terms of functions ϕ_j, satisfying $\langle \phi_j, \phi_i \rangle = \delta_{ij}$:

$$\kappa(\mathbf{x}, \mathbf{z}) = \sum_{j=1}^{\infty} \phi_j(\mathbf{x}) \phi_j(\mathbf{z}).$$

Furthermore, the series $\sum_{i=1}^{\infty} \| \phi_i \|_{L_2(X)}^2$ is convergent.

Kernel Matrix as an Information Bottleneck

In view of our characterisation of kernels in terms of the finitely positive semidefinite property, it becomes clear why the kernel matrix is perhaps the core ingredient in the theory of kernel methods. It contains all the information available in order to perform the learning step, with the sole exception of the output labels in the case of supervised learning. It is worth bearing in mind that it is only through the kernel matrix that the learning algorithm obtains information about the choice of feature space or model, and indeed the training data itself.

The finitely positive semidefinite property can also be used to justify intermediate processing steps designed to improve the representation of the data and hence the overall performance of the system through manipulating the kernel matrix before it is passed to the learning machine. One simple example is the addition of a constant to the diagonal of the matrix. This has the effect of introducing a soft margin in classification or equivalently regularisation in regression, something that we have already seen in the ridge regression example. We will, however, describe more complex manipulations of the kernel matrix that correspond to more subtle tunings of the feature space.

In view of the fact that it is only through the kernel matrix that the learning algorithm receives information about the feature space and input data, it is perhaps not surprising that some properties of this matrix can be used to assess the generalisation performance of a learning system. The properties vary according to the type of learning task and the subtlety of the analysis, but once again, the kernel matrix plays a central role both in the derivation of generalisation bounds and in their evaluation in practical applications.

The kernel matrix is not only the central concept in the design and analysis of kernel machines, but it can also be regarded as the central data structure in their implementation. As we have seen, the kernel matrix acts as an interface between the data input module and the learning algorithms. Furthermore, many model adaptation and selection methods are implemented by manipulating the kernel matrix as it is passed between these two modules. Its properties affect every part of the learning system from the computation through the generalisation analysis to the implementation details.

Implementation Issues

One small word of caution is perhaps worth mentioning on the implementation side. Memory constraints mean that it may not be possible to store the full kernel matrix in memory for very large data sets. In such cases, it may be necessary to recompute the kernel function as entries are needed. This may have implications for both the choice of algorithm and the details of the implementation.

Another important aspect of our characterisation of valid kernels in terms of the finitely positive semidefinite property is that the same condition holds for kernels defined over any kind of inputs. We did not require that the inputs should be real vectors, so the characterisation applies whatever the type of the data, be it strings, discrete structures, images, time series, and so on. Provided the kernel matrices corresponding to any finite training set are positive semidefinite, the kernel computes the inner product after projecting pairs of inputs into some feature space. Figure 6 illustrates this point with an embedding showing objects being mapped to feature vectors by the mapping ϕ.

Kernels and Prior Knowledge

The kernel contains all of the information available to the learning machine about the relative positions of the inputs in the feature space. Naturally, if structure is to be discovered in the data set, the data must exhibit that structure through the kernel matrix. If the kernel is too general, it will not give enough importance to specific types of similarity. In the language of our prior discussion, this corresponds to giving weight to too many different classifications. The kernel therefore views with the same weight any pair of inputs as similar or dissimilar, and so the off-diagonal entries of the kernel matrix become very small, while the diagonal entries are close to one (assuming the kernel matrix is normalised). The kernel can therefore only represent the concept of identity. This leads to overfitting since we can easily classify a training set correctly, but the kernel has no way of generalising to new data. At the other extreme, if a kernel matrix is completely uniform, then every input is similar to every other input. This corresponds to every input being mapped to the same feature vector and leads to underfitting of the data since the only functions that can be represented easily are those that map all points to the same class. Geometrically, the first situation corresponds to inputs being mapped to orthogonal points in the feature space, while in the second situation, all points are merged into the same image. In both cases, there are no nontrivial natural classes in the data, and hence no real structure that can be exploited for generalisation.

Kernels as Oracles

It is possible to regard a kernel as defining a similarity measure between two data points. It can therefore be considered as an oracle, guessing the similarity of two inputs. If one uses normalised kernels, this can be thought of as the a priori probability of the inputs being in the same class minus the a priori probability of their being in different classes. In the case of a covariance kernel over a class of classification functions, this is precisely the meaning of the kernel function under the prior distribution $q(f)$ since:

$$\kappa_q(\mathbf{x}, \mathbf{z}) = \int_{calf} f(\mathbf{x}) f(\mathbf{z}) q(f) df = P_q \big(f(\mathbf{x}) = f(\mathbf{z}) \big) - P_q \big(f(\mathbf{x}) \neq f(\mathbf{z}) \big).$$

Kernel Construction

The characterisation of kernel functions and kernel matrices given in the previous sections is not only useful for deciding whether a given candidate is a valid kernel. One of its main consequences is that it can be used to justify a series of rules for manipulating and combining simple kernels to obtain more complex and useful ones. In other words, such operations on one or more kernels can be shown to preserve the finitely positive semidefinite kernel property. We will say that the class of kernel functions is closed under such operations. These will include operations on kernel functions and operations directly on the kernel matrix. As long as we can guarantee that the result of an operation will always be a positive semidefinite symmetric matrix, we will still be embedding the data in a feature space, albeit a feature space transformed by the chosen operation. We first consider the case of operations on the kernel function.

Figure 6. The use of kernels enables the application of the algorithms to nonvectorial data

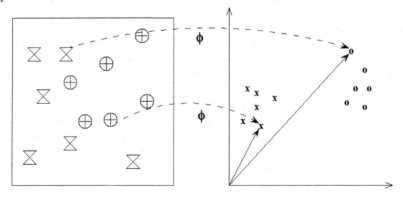

Operations on Kernel Functions

The following proposition can be viewed as showing that kernels satisfy a number of closure properties, allowing us to create more complicated kernels from simple building blocks.

Proposition 1 (Closure Properties).

Let κ_1 and κ_2 be kernels over $X \times X$, $X \subseteq \mathbb{R}^n$, $a \in \mathbb{R}^+$, $f(\cdot)$ a real-valued function on X, $\phi : X \longrightarrow \mathbb{R}^N$ with κ_3 a kernel over $\mathbb{R}^N \times \mathbb{R}^N$, and $\mathbf{B}$ a symmetric positive semidefinite $n \times n$ matrix. Then the following functions are kernels.

1. $\kappa(\mathbf{x},\mathbf{z}) = \kappa_1(\mathbf{x},\mathbf{z}) + \kappa_2(\mathbf{x},\mathbf{z})$

2. $\kappa(\mathbf{x},\mathbf{z}) = a\kappa_1(\mathbf{x},\mathbf{z})$

3. $\kappa(\mathbf{x},\mathbf{z}) = \kappa_1(\mathbf{x},\mathbf{z})\kappa_2(\mathbf{x},\mathbf{z})$

4. $\kappa(\mathbf{x},\mathbf{z}) = f(\mathbf{x})f(\mathbf{z})$

5. $\kappa(\mathbf{x},\mathbf{z}) = \kappa_3(\phi(\mathbf{x}),\phi(\mathbf{z}))$

6. $\kappa(\mathbf{x},\mathbf{z}) = \mathbf{x}'\mathbf{B}\mathbf{z}$

Proposition 2.

Let $\kappa_1(\mathbf{x},\mathbf{z})$ be a kernel over $X \times X$, where $\mathbf{x}$, $\mathbf{z} \in X$ and $p(\mathbf{x})$ is a polynomial with positive coefficients. Then the following functions are also kernels.

1. $\kappa(\mathbf{x},\mathbf{z}) = p(\kappa_1(\mathbf{x},\mathbf{z}))$

2. $\kappa(\mathbf{x},\mathbf{z}) = \exp(\kappa_1(\mathbf{x},\mathbf{z}))$

3. $\kappa(\mathbf{x},\mathbf{z}) = \exp(-\|\mathbf{x}-\mathbf{z}\|^2/(2\sigma^2))$

Embeddings Corresponding to Kernel Constructions

Proposition 1 shows that we can create new kernels from existing kernels using a number of simple operations. Our approach has demonstrated that new functions are kernels by showing that they are finitely positive semidefinite. This is sufficient to verify that the function is a kernel and hence demonstrates that there exists a feature space map for which the function computes the corresponding inner product. Often, this information provides sufficient insight for the user to sculpt an appropriate kernel for a particular application. It is, however, sometimes helpful to understand the effect of the kernel combination on the structure of the corresponding feature space.

The proof of Part 4 used a feature space construction, while Part 2 corresponds to a simple rescaling of the feature vector by $\sqrt{a}$. For the addition of two kernels in Part 1, the feature vector is the concatenation of the corresponding vectors:

$$\phi(\mathbf{x}) = [\phi_1(\mathbf{x}), \phi_2(\mathbf{x})]$$

since

$$\kappa(\mathbf{x}, \mathbf{z}) = \langle \phi(\mathbf{x}), \phi(\mathbf{z}) \rangle = \langle [\phi_1(\mathbf{x}), \phi_2(\mathbf{x})], [\phi_1(\mathbf{z}), \phi_2(\mathbf{z})] \rangle \qquad (17)$$

$$= \langle \phi_1(\mathbf{x}), \phi_1(\mathbf{z}) \rangle + \langle \phi_2(\mathbf{x}), \phi_2(\mathbf{z}) \rangle$$
$$= \kappa_1(\mathbf{x}, \mathbf{z}) + \kappa_2(\mathbf{x}, \mathbf{z}). \qquad (18)$$

For the Hadamard construction of Part 3, the corresponding features are the products of all pairs of features, one from the first feature space and one from the second. Thus, the (i, j) feature is given by:

$$\phi(\mathbf{x})_{ij} = \phi_1(\mathbf{x})_i \phi_2(\mathbf{x})_j \text{ for } i = 1, \ldots, N_1 \text{ and } j = 1, \ldots, N_2,$$

where N_i is the dimension of the feature space corresponding to ϕ_i, $i = 1,2$. The inner product is now given by:

$$\kappa(\mathbf{x}, \mathbf{z}) = \langle \phi(\mathbf{x}), \phi(\mathbf{z}) \rangle = \sum_{i=1}^{N_1} \sum_{j=1}^{N_2} \phi(\mathbf{x})_{ij} \phi(\mathbf{z})_{ij}$$

$$= \sum_{i=1}^{N_1} \phi_1(\mathbf{x})_i \phi_1(\mathbf{z})_i \sum_{j=1}^{N_2} \phi_2(\mathbf{x})_j \phi_2(\mathbf{z})_j \qquad (19)$$

$$= \kappa_1(\mathbf{x}, \mathbf{z}) \kappa_2(\mathbf{x}, \mathbf{z}). \qquad (20)$$

The definition of the feature space in this case appears to depend on the choice of coordinate system since it makes use of the specific embedding function. The fact that the new kernel can be expressed simply in terms of the base kernels shows that in fact it is invariant to this choice. For the case of an exponent of a single kernel:

$$\kappa(\mathbf{x}, \mathbf{z}) = \kappa_1(\mathbf{x}, \mathbf{z})^s,$$

we obtain by induction that the corresponding feature space is indexed by all monomials of degree s:

$$\phi_i(\mathbf{x}) = \phi_1(\mathbf{x})_1^{i_1} \phi_1(\mathbf{x})_2^{i_2} \ldots \phi_1(\mathbf{x})_N^{i_N}, \qquad (21)$$

where $\mathbf{i} = (i_1, ..., i_N) \in N^N$ satisfies

$$\sum_{j=1}^{N} i_j = s.$$

Feature Weightings

It is important to observe that the monomial features do not all receive an equal weighting in this embedding. This is due to the fact that in this case, there are repetitions in the expansion given in equation (21), that is, products of individual features that lead to the same function ϕ_i. For example, in the two-dimensional degree-2 case, the inner product can be written as:

$$\kappa(\mathbf{x}, \mathbf{z}) = 2x_1 x_2 z_1 z_2 + x_1^2 z_1^2 + x_2^2 z_2^2 \quad ,$$

$$= \left\langle \left(\sqrt{2}x_1 x_2, x_1^2, x_2^2 \right), \left(\sqrt{2}z_1 z_2, z_1^2, z_2^2 \right) \right\rangle$$

where the repetition of the cross-terms leads to a weighting factor of $\sqrt{2}$.

Polynomial Kernels

The above gives the properties and operations necessary to construct kernels. We have already seen polynomial-type kernels, but we are now in a position to give a formal definition of the polynomial kernel and describe its feature weightings in the general case.

The *derived polynomial kernel* for a kernel κ_1 is defined as:

$$\kappa(\mathbf{x}, \mathbf{z}) = p(\kappa_1(\mathbf{x}, \mathbf{z})),$$

where $p(\cdot)$ is any polynomial with positive coefficients. Frequently, it also refers to the special case:

$$\kappa_d(\mathbf{x}, \mathbf{z}) = (\langle \mathbf{x}, \mathbf{z} \rangle + R)^d$$

defined over a vector space X of dimension n, where R and d are parameters.

Expanding the polynomial kernel κ_d using the binomial theorem, we have:

$$\kappa_d(\mathbf{x}, \mathbf{z}) = \sum_{s=0}^{d} \binom{d}{s} R^{d-s} \langle \mathbf{x}, \mathbf{z} \rangle^s .$$

(22)

The features for each component in the sum together form the features of the whole kernel. Hence, we have a reweighting of the features of the polynomial kernels:

$$\hat{\kappa}_s(\mathbf{x}, \mathbf{z}) = \langle \mathbf{x}, \mathbf{z} \rangle^s, \text{ for } s = 0, ..., d.$$

Recall that the feature space corresponding to the kernel $\hat{\kappa}_s(\mathbf{x},\mathbf{z})$ has dimensions indexed by all monomials of degree s, for which we use the notation:

$$\phi_{\mathbf{i}}(\mathbf{x}) = \mathbf{x}^{\mathbf{i}} = x_1^{i_1} x_2^{i_2} ... x_n^{i_n},$$

where $\mathbf{i} = (i_1, ..., i_N) \in N^N$ satisfies

$$\sum_{j=1}^{n} i_j = s.$$

The features corresponding to the kernel $\kappa_d(\mathbf{x}, \mathbf{z})$ are therefore all functions of the form $\phi_{\mathbf{i}}(\mathbf{x})$ for i satisfying:

$$\sum_{j=1}^{n} i_j \leq d.$$

The dimension of the feature space for the polynomial kernel $\kappa_d(\mathbf{x}, \mathbf{z}) = (\langle \mathbf{x}, \mathbf{z} \rangle + R)^d$ is:

$$\binom{n+d}{d}.$$

Gaussian Kernels

Gaussian kernels are the most widely used kernels and have been extensively studied in neighbouring fields.

For $\sigma > 0$, the *Gaussian kernel* is defined by:

$$\kappa(\mathbf{x}, \mathbf{z}) = \exp\left(-\frac{\|\mathbf{x} - \mathbf{z}\|^2}{2\sigma^2}\right).$$

For the Gaussian kernel, the images of all points have norm 1 in the resulting feature space $\kappa(\mathbf{x}, \mathbf{x}) = \exp(0) = 1$. The feature space can be chosen so that the images all lie in a single orthant since all inner products between mapped points are positive.

Note that we are not restricted to using the Euclidean distance in the input space. If, for example, $\kappa(\mathbf{x}, \mathbf{z})$ is a kernel corresponding to a feature mapping ϕ_1 into a feature space F_1, we can create a Gaussian kernel in F_1 by observing that:

$$\|\phi_1(\mathbf{x}) - \phi_1(\mathbf{z})\|^2 = \kappa_1(\mathbf{x}, \mathbf{x}) - 2\kappa_1(\mathbf{x}, \mathbf{z}) + \kappa_1(\mathbf{z}, \mathbf{z})$$

giving the derived Gaussian kernel as

$$\kappa(\mathbf{x}, \mathbf{z}) = \exp\left(-\frac{\kappa_1(\mathbf{x}, \mathbf{x}) - 2\kappa_1(\mathbf{x}, \mathbf{z}) + \kappa_1(\mathbf{z}, \mathbf{z})}{2\sigma^2} \right).$$

The parameter σ controls the flexibility of the kernel in a similar way to the degree d in the polynomial kernel. Small values of σ correspond to large values of d since, for example, they allow classifiers to fit any labels, hence risking overfitting. In such cases, the kernel matrix becomes close to the identity matrix. On the other hand, large values of σ gradually reduce the kernel to a constant function, making it impossible to learn any nontrivial classifier. The feature space has infinite dimension for every value of σ, but for large values, the weight decays very fast on the higher order features. In other words, although the rank of the kernel matrix will be full, for all practical purposes, the points lie in a low-dimensional subspace of the feature space. Note that from the proofs of Parts ii and iii of Proposition 25, the Gaussian kernel is a polynomial kernel of infinite degree. Hence, its features are all possible monomials of input features with no restriction placed on the degrees. The Taylor expansion of the exponential function:

$$\exp(\mathbf{x}) = \sum_{i=0}^{\infty} \frac{1}{i!} x^i$$

shows that the weighting of individual monomials falls off as $i!$ with increasing degree.

Other Kernels

The polynomial and Gaussian kernels above are two of the simplest and most widely used kernels. In this short introduction, we do not have the space to go into some of the numerous other kernels that are in widespread use. As mentioned previously, one of the most powerful properties of kernel methods is their ability to operate on many formats of data, ranging from sequences to images, including graphs, vectors, and sets. This, and their modularity, makes it possible to apply any kernel-based algorithm to a vastly diverse range of problems. Indeed, kernel methods have been applied to biosequence analysis (Bresco, Turchi, De Bie, & Cristianini, in press; L. & Kuang, 2003), text categorization (Lodhi, Saunders, Shawe-Taylor, Cristianini, & Watkins, 2002; De Bie & Cristianini, 2004), trees (Collins & Duffy, 2002), graphs (Kashima & Inokuchi, 2002), general weighted transducers (Cortes, Haffner, & Mohri, 2002), and music data (Saunders, Hardoon, Shawe-Taylor, & Widmer, 2004), to name but a few. As one might expect, this is currently a very active area of research, and the reader will encounter many examples of these kernels being used and developed in the later chapters of this book.

In general, it has often proven possible and useful to translate domain knowledge into a kernel function, as in the case of text retrieval and remote protein homology detection (Jaakkola, Diekhaus, & Haussler, 2000; Joachims, 1998), where representations or models developed and refined within the application domain have been successfully turned into kernel functions. Finally, another key advantage to applications is the capability of kernel functions to fuse or integrate together various heterogeneous representations such as those methods presented in Lanckriet, Cristianini, Bartlett, Ghaoui, and Jordan (2004).

Discussion

The concepts outlined above show only the surface of a large and fast-expanding field of research in pattern analysis. Thousands of papers have already been published in this field, and accessing the primary literature is becoming increasingly a daunting task. Comprehensive introductions to the field have appeared, particularly the textbooks of Cristianini and Shawe-Taylor (2000), Schoelkopf and Smola (2002), Shawe-Taylor and Cristianini (2004), and Vapnik (1998). In this chapter, we will not have pointers to the primary literature, but will rather direct the readers to these textbooks, where extensive discussions of these ideas can be found. Many Web sites are also available with free software and pointers to recent publications in the field. In particular http://www.kernel-methods.net and http://www.support-vector.net contain free material, whereas http://www.kernel-machines.org contains updated pointers to all main events in the kernel methods community.

In this book, the reader will find many chapters that advance one or more of the key concepts highlighted above. As already has been outlined, kernel methods provide an advanced toolbox that the researcher or engineer can apply in a wide variety of application domains. However, as we shall see, the picture is not yet complete, and any application of these techniques to a specific problem provides opportunities to devise modifications and extensions to the linear methods and to design new kernels through the use of domain-specific knowledge. The three application areas discussed in the following chapters provide an excellent basis from which insight to all of these points can be gathered. The applications cover a wider variety of tasks ranging from classification and regression through clustering. The authors provide many applications of kernels and show how successful new kernels can be designed and applied. Finally, the focus on real-world applications gives rise to discussion on the choice of algorithm and the correct application of additional techniques such as feature selection.

References

Bresco, M., Turchi, M., De Bie, T., & Cristianini, N. (in press). *Modeling sequence evolution with kernel methods.* Computational Optimization and Applications.

Collins, M., & Duffy, N. (2002). *New ranking algorithms for parsing and tagging: Kernels over discrete structures.*

Cortes, C., Haffner, P., & Mohri, M. (2002). *Rational kernels.*

Cristianini, N., & Shawe-Taylor, J. (2000). *An introduction to support vector machines.* Cambridge, UK: Cambridge University Press.

De Bie, T., & Cristianini, N. (2004). Kernel methods for exploratory data analysis: A demonstration on text data. In *Proceedings of the Joint IAPR International Workshops on Syntactical and Structural Pattern Recognition (SSPR 2004) and Statistical Pattern Recognition (SPR 2004).*

De Bie, T., Cristianini, N., & Rosipal, R. (2004). Eigenproblems in pattern recognition. In E. Bayro-Corrochano (Ed.), *Handbook of computational geometry for pattern recognition, computer vision, neurocomputing and robotics.* Heidelberg, Germany: Springer-Verlag.

Jaakkola, T., Diekhaus, M., & Haussler, D. (2000). Using the fisher kernel method to detect remote protein homologies. *Journal of Computational Biology, 7*(1, 2), 95-114.

Joachims, T. (1998). Text categorization with support vector machines. In *Proceedings of the European Conference on Machine Learning (ECML).*

Kashima, H., & Inokuchi, A. (2002). *Kernels for graph classification.*

L., C., & Kuang, R. (2003). Fast kernels for inexact string matching. In *Proceedings of the 16th Conference on Learning Theory (COLT).*

Lanckriet, G., Cristianini, N., Bartlett, P., Ghaoui, L. E., & Jordan, M. I. (2004). Learning the kernel matrix with semidefinite programming. *Journal of Machine Learning Research, 5,* 27-72.

Lodhi, H., Saunders, C., Shawe-Taylor, J., Cristianini, N., & Watkins, C. (2002). Text classification using string kernels. *Journal of Machine Learning Research, 2,* 419-444.

Saunders, C., Hardoon, D., Shawe-Taylor, J., & Widmer, G. (2004). Using string kernels to identify famous performers from their playing style. In *Proceedings of the 15th European Conference on Machine Learning (ECML) and the 8th European Conference on Principles and Practice of Knowledge Discovery in Databases (PKDD),* 3201 (pp. 384-399).

Schoelkopf, B., & Smola, A. (2002). *Learning with kernels.* Cambridge, MA: MIT Press.

Shawe-Taylor, J., & Cristianini, N. (2004). *Kernel methods for pattern analysis.* Cambridge University Press.

Vapnik, V. (1998). *Statistical learning theory.* New York: Wiley.

List of notational symbols

N	dimension of feature space	L	primal Lagrangian
$y \in Y$	output and output space	W	dual Lagrangian
$\mathbf{x} \in X$	input and input space	$\|\cdot\|_p$	p-norm, default is 2-norm
$\|\mathbf{A}\|_F$	Frobenius norm of a matrix	$\|\mathbf{A}\|$	spectral/2-norm of a matrix
F	feature space	ln	natural logarithm
F	class of real-valued functions	e	base of the natural log
L	class of linear functions	log	log to the base 2
$\langle \mathbf{x}, \mathbf{z} \rangle$	inner product of $\mathbf{x}$ and $\mathbf{z}$	$\mathbf{x}', \mathbf{X}'$	transpose of vector, matrix
ϕ	mapping to feature space	$N, \mathbb{R}$	natural, real numbers
$\kappa(\mathbf{x}, \mathbf{z})$	kernel $\langle \phi(\mathbf{x}), \phi(\mathbf{z}) \rangle$	S	training set
$f(\mathbf{x})$	real-valued function	ℓ	training set size
n	dimension of input space	$\phi(S)$	training set in feature space
R	radius containing the data	η	learning rate
H	Heaviside function	ε	error probability
$\mathbf{w}$	weight vector	δ	confidence
b	bias	γ	margin
α	dual variables	ξ	slack variables
$\mathbf{C}$	covariance matrix	$\mathbf{I}$	identity matrix
$(x)_+$	equals x, if $x \geq 0$ else 0	$\mathbf{K}$	kernel matrix
$sgn(x)$	equals 1, if $x \geq 0$ else -1	#	cardinality of a set

Section I

Bio-Medical Engineering

Chapter II

Kernel Methods in Genomics and Computational Biology

Jean-Philippe Vert, Ecole des Mines de Paris, France

Abstract

Support vector machines and kernel methods are increasingly popular in genomics and computational biology due to their good performance in real-world applications and strong modularity that makes them suitable to a wide range of problems, from the classification of tumors to the automatic annotation of proteins. Their ability to work in a high dimension and process nonvectorial data, and the natural framework they provide to integrate heterogeneous data are particularly relevant to various problems arising in computational biology. In this chapter, we survey some of the most prominent applications published so far, highlighting the particular developments in kernel methods triggered by problems in biology, and mention a few promising research directions likely to expand in the future.

Introduction

Recent years have witnessed a dramatic evolution in many fields of life science with the apparition and rapid spread of so-called high-throughput technologies, which generate huge amounts of data to characterize various aspects of biological samples or phenomena. To name just a few, DNA sequencing technologies have already provided the whole genome of several hundreds of species, including the human genome (International Human Genome Sequencing Consortium, 2001; Venter, 2001). DNA microarrays (Schena, Shalon, Davis, & Brown, 1995), that allow the monitoring of the expression level of tens of thousands of transcripts simultaneously, opened the door to functional genomics, the elucidation of the functions of the genes found in the genomes (DeRisi, Iyer, & Brown, 1997). Recent advances in ionization technology have boosted large-scale capabilities in mass spectrometry and the rapidly growing field of proteomics, focusing on the systematic, large-scale analysis of proteins (Aebersold & Mann, 2003). As biology suddenly entered this new era characterized by the relatively cheap and easy generation of huge amounts of data, the urgent need for efficient methods to represent, store, process, analyze, and finally make sense out of these data triggered the parallel development of numerous data-analysis algorithms in computational biology. Among them, kernel methods in general and support vector machines (SVMs) in particular have quickly gained popularity for problems involving the classification and analysis of high-dimensional or complex data. Half a decade after the first pioneering papers (Haussler, 1999; T. S. Jaakkola, Diekhans, & Haussler, 1999; Mukherjee, Tamayo, Mesirov, Slonim, Verri, & Poggio, 1998), these methods have been applied to a variety of problems in computational biology, with more than 100 research papers published in 2004 alone.[1] The main reasons behind this fast development involve, beyond the generally good performances of SVM on real-world problems and the ease of use provided by current implementations, (a) the particular capability of SVM to resist high-dimensional and noisy data, typically produced by various high-throughput technologies, (b) the possibility to model linear as well as nonlinear relationships between variables of interest, and (c) the possibility to process nonvectorial data, such as biological sequences, protein structures, or gene networks, and to easily fuse heterogeneous data thanks to the use of kernels. More than a mere application of well-established methods to new data sets, the use of kernel methods in computational biology has been accompanied by new developments to match the specificities and the needs of the field, such as methods for feature selection in combination with the classification of high-dimensional data, the invention of string kernels to process biological sequences, or the development of methods to learn from several kernels simultaneously. In order to illustrate some of the most prominent applications of kernel methods in computational biology and the specific developments they triggered, this chapter focuses on selected applications related to the manipulation of high-dimensional data, the classification of biological sequences, and a few less developed but promising applications. This chapter is therefore not intended to be an exhaustive survey, but rather to illustrate with some examples why and how kernel methods have invaded the field of computational biology so rapidly. The interested reader will find more references in the book by Schölkopf, Tsuda, and Vert (2004) dedicated to the topic. Several kernels for structured data, such as sequences or trees, widely developed and used in computational biology, are also presented in detail in the book by Shawe-Taylor and Cristianini (2004).

Classification of High-Dimensional Data

Several recent technologies, such as DNA microarrays, mass spectrometry, or various miniaturized assays, provide thousands of quantitative parameters to characterize biological samples or phenomena. Mathematically speaking, the results of such experiments can be represented by high-dimensional vectors, and many applications involve the supervised classification of such data. Classifying data in high dimension with a limited number of training examples is a challenging task that most statistical procedures have difficulties in dealing with, due in particular to the risk of overfitting the training data. The theoretical foundations of SVM and related methods, however, suggest that their use of regularization allows them to better resist to the curse of dimension than other methods. SVMs were therefore naturally tested on a variety of data sets involving the classification of high-dimensional data, in particular, for the analysis of tumor samples from gene expression data, and novel algorithms were developed in the framework of kernel methods to select a few relevant features for a given high-dimensional classification problem.

Tumor Classification from Gene Expression Data

The early detection of cancer and prediction of cancer types from gene expression data have been among the first applications of kernel methods in computational biology (Furey, Cristianini, Duffy, Bednarski, Schummer, & Haussler, 2000; Mukherjee et al., 1998) and remain prominent. These applications indeed have potentially important impacts on the treatment of cancers, providing clinicians with objective and possibly highly accurate information to choose the most appropriate form of treatment. In this context, SVMs were widely applied and compared with other algorithms for the supervised classification of tumor samples from expression data of typically several thousands of genes for each tumor. Examples include the discrimination between acute myeloid and acute lymphoblastic leukemia (Mukherjee et al.); colon cancer and normal colon tissues (Moler, Chow, & Mian, 2000); normal ovarian, normal nonovarian, and ovarian cancer tissues (Furey et al.); melanoma; soft-tissue sarcoma and clear-cell sarcoma (Segal, Pavlidis, Noble, et al., 2003); different types of soft-tissue sarcomas (Segal, Pavlidis, Antonescu, et al., 2003); and normal and gastric tumor tissues (Meireles et al., 2003), to name just a few. Another typical application is the prediction of the future evolution of a tumor, such as the discrimination between relapsing and nonrelapsing Wilms tumors (Williams et al., 2004), the prediction of metastatic or nonmetastatic squamous cell carcinoma of the oral cavity (O'Donnell et al., 2005), or the discrimination between diffuse large B-cell lymphoma with positive or negative treatment outcome (Shipp et al., 2002).

The SVMs used in these studies are usually linear hard-margin SVMs, or linear soft-margin SVMs with a default C parameter value. Concerning the choice of the kernel, several studies observe that nonlinear kernels tend to decrease performance (Ben-Dor, Bruhn, Friedman, Nachman, Schummer, & Yakhini, 2000; Valentini, 2002) compared to the simplest linear kernel. In spite of contradictory opinions (Pochet, De Smet, Suykens, & De Moor, 2004), this is coherent with the intuition that the complexity of learning nonlinear functions in very high dimension does not play in their favor. On the other hand, the choice of hard-margin

SVM, sometimes advocated as a default method when data are linearly separable, is certainly worth questioning in more detail. Indeed, the theoretical foundations of SVM suggest that in order to learn in high dimension, one should rather increase the importance of regularization as opposed to fitting the data, which corresponds to decreasing the C parameter of the soft-margin formulation. A few recent papers highlight indeed the fact that the choice of C has an important effect on the generalization performance of SVM for the classification of gene expression data (Huang & Kecman, 2005).

A general conclusion of these numerous studies is that SVMs generally provide good classification accuracy in spite of the large dimension of the data. For example, in a comparative study of several algorithms for multiclass supervised classification, including naive Bayes, k-nearest neighbors, and decision trees, Li, Zhang, and Ogihara (2004, p. 2434) note that "[SVMs] achieve better performance than any other classifiers on almost all the datasets." However, it is fair to mention that other studies conclude that most algorithms that take into account the problem of large dimension either through regularization or through feature selection reach roughly similar accuracy on most data sets (Ben-Dor et al.). From a practical point of view, the use of the simplest linear kernel and the soft-margin formulation of SVM seems to be a reasonable default strategy for this application.

Feature Selection

In the classification of microarray data, it is often important, for classification performance, biomarker identification, and the interpretation of results, to select only a few discriminative genes among the thousands of candidates available on a typical microarray. While the literature on feature selection is older and goes beyond the field of kernel methods, several interesting developments with kernel methods have been proposed in the recent years, explicitly motivated by the problem of gene selection from microarray data.

For example, Su, Murali, Pavlovic, Schaffer, and Kasif (2003) propose to evaluate the predictive power of each single gene for a given classification task by the value of the functional minimized by a one-dimensional SVM, trained to classify samples from the expression of only the single gene of interest. This criterion can then be used to rank genes and select only a few with important predictive power. This procedure therefore belongs to the so-called filter approach to feature selection, where a criterion (here using SVM) to measure the relevance of each feature is defined, and only relevant features according to this criterion are kept.

A second general strategy for feature selection is the so-called wrapper approach, where feature selection alternates with the training of a classifier. The now widely used recursive feature elimination (RFE) procedure of Guyon, Weston, Bamhill, and Vapnik (2002), which iteratively selects smaller and smaller sets of genes and trains SVMs, follows this strategy. RFE can only be applied with linear SVMs, which is nevertheless not a limitation as long as many features remain, and works as follows. Starting from the full set of genes, a linear SVM is trained and the genes with the smallest weights in the resulting linear discrimination function are eliminated. The procedure is then repeated iteratively starting from the set of remaining genes and stops when a desired number of genes is reached.

Finally, a third strategy for feature selection, called the embedded approach, combines the learning of a classifier and the selection of features in a single step. A kernel method following this strategy has been implemented in the joint classifier and feature optimization (JCFO) procedure of Krishnapuram, Carin, and Hartemink (2004). JCFO is, roughly speaking, a variant of SVM with a Bayesian formulation, in which sparseness is obtained both for the features and the classifier expansion in terms of a kernel by appropriate choices of prior probabilities. The precise description of the complete procedure to train this algorithm, involving an expectation-maximization (EM) iteration, would go beyond the scope of this chapter, and the interested reader is referred to the original publication for further practical details.

Generally speaking, and in spite of these efforts to develop clever algorithms, the effect of feature selection on the classification accuracy of SVM is still debated. Although very good results are sometimes reported, for example, for the JCFO procedure (Krishnapuram et al., 2004), several studies conclude that feature selection, for example, with procedures like RFE, do not actually improve the accuracy of SVM trained on all genes (Ambroise & McLachlan, 2002; Ramaswamy et al., 2001). The relevance of feature-selection algorithms for gene expression data is therefore currently still a research topic that practitioners should test and assess case by case.

Other High-Dimensional Data in Computational Biology

While early applications of kernel methods to high-dimensional data in genomics and bioinformatics mainly focused on gene expression data, a number of other applications have flourished more recently, some being likely to expand quickly as major applications of machine learning algorithms. For example, studies focusing on tissue classification from data obtained by other technologies, such as methylation assays to monitor the patterns of cytosine methylation in the upstream regions of genes (Model, Adorjan, Olek, & Piepenbrock, 2001), or array comparative genomic hybridization (CGH) to measure gene copy number changes in hundreds of genes simultaneously (Aliferis, Hardin, & Massion, 2002), are starting to accumulate. A huge field of application that barely caught the interest of the machine learning community is proteomics, that is, the quantitative study of the protein content of cells and tissues. Technologies such as tandem mass spectrometry to monitor the protein content (proteins or characteristic fragments of proteins) of a biological sample are now well developed, and the classification of tissues from these data is a future potential application of SVM (Wagner, Naik, & Pothen, 2003; Wu et al., 2003). Applications in toxicogenomics (Steiner et al., 2004), chemogenomics (Bao & Sun, 2002; Bock & Gough, 2002), and the analysis of single-nucleotide polymorphisms (Listgarten et al., 2004; Yoon, Song, Hong, & Kim, 2003) are also promising applications for which the capacity of SVM to classify high-dimensional data has only started to be exploited.

Sequence Classification

The various genome sequencing projects have produced huge amounts of sequence data that need to be analyzed. In particular, the urgent need for methods to automatically process, segment, annotate, and classify various sequence data has triggered the fast development of numerous algorithms for strings. In this context, the possibility offered by kernel methods to process any type of data as soon as a kernel for the data to be processed is available has been quickly exploited to offer the power of state-of-the-art machine learning algorithms to sequence processing.

Problems that arise in computational biology consist of processing either sets of sequences of a fixed length, or sets of sequences with variable lengths. From a technical point of view, the two problems differ significantly: While there are natural ways to encode fixed-length sequences as fixed-length vectors, making them amenable to processing by most learning algorithms, manipulating variable-length sequences is less obvious. In both cases, many successful applications of SVM have been reported, combining ingenious developments of string kernels, sometimes specifically adapted to a given classification task, with the power of SVM.

Kernels for Fixed-Length Sequences

Problems involving the classification of fixed-length sequences appear typically when one wants to predict a property along a sequence, such as the local structure or solvent accessibility along a protein sequence. In that case, indeed, a common approach is to use a moving window, that is, to predict the property at each position independently from the others, and to base the prediction only on the nearby sequence contained in a small window around the site of interest. More formally, this requires the construction of predictive models that take a sequence of fixed length as input to predict the property of interest, the length of the sequences being exactly the width of the window.

To fix notations, let us denote by p the common length of the sequences, and by $\mathbf{x} = x_1 \ldots x_p$ a typical sequence, where each x_i is a letter from the alphabet, for example, an amino acid. The most natural way to transform such a sequence into a vector of fixed length is to first encode each letter itself into a vector of fixed length l, and then to concatenate the codes of the successive letters to obtain a vector of size $n = pl$ for the whole sequence. A simple code for letters is the following so-called sparse encoding: The size of the alphabet is denoted by α, and the i the letter of the alphabet is encoded as a vector of dimension α containing only zeros, except for the i the dimension that is set to l. For example, in the case of nucleotide sequences with alphabet (A,C,G,T), the codes for A, C, G, and T would respectively be (1,0,0,0), (0,1,0,0), (0,0,1,0), and (0,0,0,1), while the code for the sequence of length 3 AGT would be (1,0,0,0,0,0,1,0,0,0,0,1). Several more evolved codes for single letters have also been proposed. For example, if one has a prior matrix of pairwise similarities between letters, such as widely used similarity matrices between amino acids, it is possible to replace the 0/1 sparse encoding of a given letter by the vector of similarity with other letters; hence, the A in the previous example could, for instance, be represented by the vector (1,0,0.5,0) to emphasize one's belief that A and G share some similarity. This is particularly relevant for biological sequences where mutations of single letters to similar letters are very common. Alternatively, instead of using a prior matrix of similarity, one can automatically align the sequence of interest to similar sequences in a large sequence database, and encode each position by the frequency of each letter in the alignment. As a trivial example, if our previous sequence AGT was found to be aligned to the following sequences, AGA, AGC, CGT, and ATT, then it could be encoded by the vector (0.8,0.2,0,0,0,0,0.8,0.2,0.2,0.2,0,0.6), corresponding to the respective frequencies of each letter at each position.

In terms of a kernel, it is easy to see that the inner product between sparsely encoded sequences is the number of positions with identical letters. In this representation, any linear classifier, such as that learned by a linear SVM, associates a weight to each feature, that is, to each letter at each position, and the score of a sequence is the sum of the scores of its letters. Such a classifier is usually referred to as a position-specific score matrix in bioinformatics. Similar interpretations can be given for other letter encodings. An interesting extension of these linear kernels for sequences is to raise them to some small power d; in that case, the dimension of the feature space used by kernel methods increases, and the new features correspond to all products of d original features. This is particularly appealing for sparse encoding because a product of d binary factors is a binary variable equal to 1 if and only if all factors are 1, meaning that the features created by the sparse encoding to the power d exactly indicate the simultaneous presence of up to d particular letters at d particular positions. The trick to take a linear kernel to some power is therefore a convenient way to create a classifier for problems that involve the presence of several particular letters at particular positions.

A first limitation of these kernels is that they do not contain any information about the order of the letters: They are, for example, left unchanged if the letters in all sequences are shuffled according to any given permutation. Several attempts to include ordering information have been proposed. For example, Rätsch, Sonnenburg, and Schölkopf (2005) replace the local encoding of single letters by a local encoding of several consecutive letters; Zien, Rätsch, Mika, Schölkopf, Lengauer, and Müller (2000) propose an ingenious variant to the polynomial kernel in order to restrict the feature space to products of features at nearby positions only.

A second limitation of these kernels is that the comparison of two sequences only involves the comparison of features at identical positions. This can be problematic in the case of biological sequences where the insertion of deletions of letters is common, resulting in possible shifts within a window. This problem led Meinicke, Tech, Morgenstem, and Merkl (2004) to propose a kernel that incorporates a comparison of features at nearby positions using the following trick: If a feature f (e.g., binary or continuous) appears at position i in the first sequence, and a feature g appears at position j in the second sequence, then the kernel between the two sequences is increased by $\kappa_0(f,g)\exp(-(i-j)^2/\sigma^2)$, where $\kappa_0(f,g)$ is a basic kernel between the features f and g such as the simple product, and σ is a parameter that controls the range at which features are compared. When σ is chosen very large, then one recovers the classical kernels obtained by comparing only identical positions ($i=j$); the important point here is that for smaller values of σ, features can contribute positively even though they might be located at different positions on the sequences.

The applications of kernels for fixed-length sequences to solve problems in computational biology are already numerous. For example, they have been widely used to predict local properties along protein sequences using a moving window, such as secondary structure (Guermeur, Lifschitz, & Vert, 2004; Hua & Sun, 2001a), disulfide bridges involving cysteines (Chen, in, Lin, & Hwang, 2004; Passerini & Frasconi, 2004), phosphorylation sites (Kim, Lee, oh, Kimm, & Koh, 2004), interface residues (Res, Mihalek, & Lichtarge, 2005; Yan, Dobbs, & Honavar, 2004), and solvent accessibility (Yuan, Burrage, & Mattick, 2002). Another important field of application is the annotation of DNA using fixed-length windows centered on a candidate point of interest as an input to a classifier to detect translation initiation sites (Meinicke et al., 2004; Zien et al., 2000), splice sites (Degroeve, Saeys, De Baets, Rouze, & Van de Peer, 2005; Rätsch et al., 2005), or binding sites of transcription factors (O'Flanagan, Paillard, Lavery, & Sengupta, 2005; Sharan & Myers, 2005). The recent interest in short RNA such as antisense oligonucleotides or small interfering RNAs for the sequence-specific knockdown of messenger RNAs has also resulted in several works involving the classification of such sequences, which typically have a fixed length by nature (Camps-Valls, Chalk, Serrano-López, Martin-Guerrero, & Sonnhammer, 2004; Teramoto, Aoki, Kimura, & Kanaoka, 2005). Another important application field for these methods is immunoinformatics, including the prediction of peptides that can elicit an immune response (Bhasin & Raghava, 2004; Dönnes & Elofsson, 2002), or the classification of immunoglobulins collected from ill patients (Yu, Zavaljevski, Stevens, Yackovich, & Reifman, 2005; Zavaljevski, Stevens, & Reifman, 2002). In most of these applications, SVM lead to comparable if not better prediction accuracy than competing state-of-the-art methods such as neural networks.

Kernels for Variable-Length Sequences

Many problems in computational biology involve sequences of different lengths. For example, the automatic functional or structural annotation of genes found in sequenced genomes requires the processing of amino-acid sequences with no fixed length. Learning from variable-length sequences is a more challenging problem than learning from fixed-length sequences because there is no natural way to transform a variable-length string into a vector. For kernel methods, this issue boils down to the problem of defining kernels for variable-length strings, a topic that has deserved a lot of attention in the last few years and has given rise to a variety of ingenious solutions. As summarized in Table 1, three main approaches have been followed in the process of kernel design from strings: (a) computing an inner product in an explicitly defined feature space, (b) deriving a kernel from probabilistic models on strings,

Table 1. A typology of kernels for variable-length biological sequences

Strategy	Example
Define a (possibly high-dimensional) feature space of interest	- Physico-chemical kernels (Wang et al., 2004 ; Zhang et al., 2003a) - Spectrum, mismatch kernels (Leslie et al., 2002, 2004) - Pairwise, motif kernels (Logan et al., 2001; Liao & Noble, 2003; Ben-Hur & Brutlag, 2003)
Derive a kernel from a generative model	- Fisher kernel (Jaakkola et al., 2000) - Pair HMM kernel (Watkins, 2000 ; Haussler, 1999) - Mutual information kernels (Cuturi & Vert, 2005) - Marginalized kernels (Tsuda et al., 2002; Kin et al., 2002; Kashima et al., 2004 ; Vert et al., 2006)
Derive a kernel from a measure of similarity	- Local alignment kernels (Saigo et al., 2004 ; Vert et al., 2004)

and (c) adapting widely used measures of similarity. These general strategies, surveyed in more detail in this section, are relevant beyond the specific problem of designing kernels for biological sequences. For example, we point out below strong similarities between some of these kernels and kernels developed for speech-recognition applications (surveyed in more detail in the chapters by Picone, Ganapathiraju, and Hamaker; and Wan).

The most common approach to make a kernel for strings, as for many other types of data, is to design explicitly a set of numerical features that can be extracted from strings, and then to form a kernel as a dot product between the resulting feature vectors. As an example, Leslie, Eskin, and Noble (2002) represent a sequence by the vector of counts of occurrences of all possible k-mers in the sequence for a given integer k, effectively resulting in a vector of dimension a^k, where a is the size of the alphabet. As an example, the sequence AACGTCACGAA over the alphabet (A,C,G,T) is represented by the 16-dimensional vector (2,2,0,0,1,0,2,0,1,0,0,1,0,1,0,0) for $k = 2$; here, the features are the counts of occurrences of each 2-mer AA, AC, ..., TG, TT lexicographically ordered. The resulting spectrum kernel between this sequence and the sequence ACGAAA, defined as the linear product between the two 16-dimensional representation vectors, is equal to 9. It should be noted that although the number of possible k-mers easily reaches the order of several thousands as soon as k is equal to 3 or 4, the classification of sequences by SVM in this high-dimensional space results in fairly good results. A major advantage of the spectrum kernel is its fast computation; indeed, the set of k-mers appearing in a given sequence can be indexed in linear time in a tree structure, and the inner product between two vectors is linear with respect to the nonzero coordinates, that is, at most linear in the total lengths of the sequences. Several variants to the basic spectrum kernel have also been proposed, including, for example, kernels based on counts of k-mers appearing with up to a few mismatches in the sequences (Leslie, Eskin, Cohen, Weston, & Noble, 2004).

Another natural approach to represent variable-length strings by fixed-length numerical vectors is to replace each letter by one or several numerical features, such as physicochemical properties of amino acids, and then to extract features from the resulting variable-length numerical time series using classical signal processing techniques such as Fourier transforms (Wang, Yang, Liu, Xu, & Chou, 2004) or autocorrelation analysis (S.-W. Zhang, Pan, Zhang, Zhang, & Wang, 2003). For example, if $f_1,...,f_p$ denote P numerical features associated with the successive letters of a sequence of length P, then the autocorrelation function r_j for a given $j > 0$ is defined by:

$$r_j = \frac{1}{n-j} \sum_{i=1}^{n-j} f_i f_{i+j}.$$

One can then keep a fixed number of these coefficients, for example $r_1,...,r_n$, and create an n-dimensional vector to represent each sequence.

Finally, another popular approach to design features and therefore kernels for biological sequences is to "project" them onto a fixed dictionary of sequences or motifs using classical similarity measures, and to use the resulting vector of similarities as a feature vector. For example, Logan, Moreno, Suzek, Weng, and Kasif (2001) represent each sequence by a 10,000-dimensional vector indicating the presence of 10,000 motifs of the BLOCKS database; similarly, Ben-Hur and Brutlag (2003) use a vector that indicates the presence or absence of about 500,000 motifs in the eMOTIF database, requiring the use of a tree structure to compute efficiently the kernel without explicitly storing the 500,000 features. Liao and Noble (2003) represent each sequence by a vector of sequence similarities with a fixed set of sequences.

A second general strategy that has been followed for kernel design is to derive kernel functions from probabilistic models. This strategy has been particularly motivated by the fact that, before the interest in string kernels grew, a number of ingenious probabilistic models had been defined to represent biological sequences or families of sequences, including, for example, Markov and hidden Markov models for protein sequences, and stochastic context-free grammars for RNA sequences (Durbin, Eddy, Krogh, & Mitchison, 1998). Several authors have therefore explored the possibility to use such models to make kernels, starting with the seminal work of T. Jaakkola, Diekhans, and Haussler (2000) that introduced the Fisher kernel. The Fisher kernel is a general method to extract a fixed number of features from any data $\mathbf{x}$ for which a parametric probabilistic model P_θ is defined. Here, θ represents a continuous n-dimensional vector of parameters for the probabilistic model, such as transition and emission probabilities for a hidden Markov model, and each P_θ is a probability distribution. Once a particular parameter θ_0 is chosen to fit a given set of objects, for example, by maximum likelihood, then an n-dimensional feature vector for each individual object $\mathbf{x}$ can be extracted by taking the gradient in the parameter space of the log likelihood of the point:

$$\phi(\mathbf{x}) = \nabla_\theta \log P_\theta(\mathbf{x}).$$

The intuitive interpretation of this feature vector, usually referred to as the Fisher score in statistics, is that it represents how changes in the n parameters affect the likelihood of the point $\mathbf{x}$. In other words, one feature is extracted for each parameter of the model; the particularities of the data point are seen from the eyes of the parameters of the probabilistic model. The Fisher kernel is then obtained as the dot product of these n-dimensional vectors, eventually multiplied by the inverse of the Fisher information matrix to render it independent of the parametrization of the model.

A second line of thought to make a kernel out of a parametric probabilistic model is to use the concept of mutual information kernels (Seeger, 2002), that is, kernels of the form:

$$\kappa(\mathbf{x}, \mathbf{z}) = \int P_\theta(\mathbf{x}) P_\theta(\mathbf{z}) d\mu(\theta),$$

where $d\mu$ is a prior distribution on the parameter space. Here, the features correspond to the likelihood of the objects under all distributions of the probabilistic model; objects are considered similar when they have large likelihood under similar distributions. An important difference between the kernels seen so far is that here, no explicit extraction of finite-dimensional vectors can be performed. Hence, for practical applications, one must chose probabilistic models that allow the computation of the integral above. This was carried out by Cuturi and Vert (2005) who present a family of variable-length Markov models for strings and an algorithm to perform the exact integral over parameters and models in the same time, resulting in a string kernel with linear complexity in time and memory with respect to the total length of the sequences.

Alternatively, many probabilistic models for biological sequences, such as hidden Markov models, involve a hidden variable that is marginalized over to obtain the probability of a sequence, which be written as:

$$P(\mathbf{x}) = \sum_h P(\mathbf{x}, \mathbf{h}).$$

For such distributions, Tsuda, Kin, and Asai (2002) introduced the notion of a marginalized kernel, obtained by marginalizing a kernel for the complete variable over the hidden variable. More precisely, assuming that a kernel κ_0 for objects of the form $(\mathbf{x}, \mathbf{h})$ is defined, the marginalized kernel for observed objects X is given by:

$$\kappa(\mathbf{x}_1, \mathbf{x}_2) = \sum_{\mathbf{h}_1, \mathbf{h}_2} \kappa_0((\mathbf{x}_1, \mathbf{h}_1), (\mathbf{x}_2, \mathbf{h}_2)) P(\mathbf{h}_1 \mid \mathbf{x}_1) P(\mathbf{h}_2 \mid \mathbf{x}_2).$$

In order to motivate this definition with a simple example, let us consider a hidden Markov model with two possible hidden states to model sequences with two possible regimes, such as introns and exons in eukaryotic genes. In that case, the hidden variable corresponding to a sequence $\mathbf{x}$ of length P is a binary sequence $\mathbf{h}$ of length P describing the states along the sequence. For two sequences $\mathbf{x}_1$ and $\mathbf{x}_2$, if the correct hidden states $\mathbf{h}_1$ and $\mathbf{h}_2$ were known, such as the correct decomposition into introns and exons, then it would make sense to define a kernel $\kappa_0((\mathbf{x}_1, \mathbf{h}_1), (\mathbf{x}_2, \mathbf{h}_2))$ taking into account the specific decomposition of the sequences into two regimes; for example, the kernel for complete data could be a spectrum kernel restricted to the exons, that is, to positions with a particular state. Because the actual hidden states are not known in practice, the marginalization over the hidden state of this kernel using an adequate probabilistic model can be interpreted as an attempt to apply the kernel for complete data by guessing the hidden variables. Similar to the mutual information kernel, marginalized kernels can often not be expressed as inner products between feature vectors, and they require computational tricks to be computed. Several beautiful examples of such kernels for various probabilistic models have been worked out, including hidden Markov models for sequences (Tsuda et al.; Vert, Thurman, & Noble, 2006), stochastic context-free grammars for RNA sequences (Kin, Tsuda, & Asai, 2002), and random walk models on graphs for molecular structures (Kashima, Tsuda, & Inokuchi, 2004).

Following a different line of thought, Haussler (1999) introduced the concept of convolution kernels for objects that can be decomposed into subparts, such as sequences or trees. For example, the concatenation of two strings $\mathbf{x}_1$ and $\mathbf{x}_2$ results in another string $\mathbf{x} = \mathbf{x}_1 \mathbf{x}_2$. If two initial string kernels κ_1 and κ_2 are chosen, then a new string kernel is obtained by the convolution of the initial kernels following the equation:

$$\kappa(\mathbf{x}, \mathbf{z}) = \sum_{\mathbf{x}_1 \mathbf{x}_2 = \mathbf{x}} \sum_{\mathbf{z}_1 \mathbf{z}_2 = \mathbf{z}} \kappa_1(\mathbf{x}_1, \mathbf{z}_1) \kappa_2(\mathbf{x}_2, \mathbf{z}_2).$$

Here, the sum is over all possible decompositions of **x** and **z** into two concatenated subsequences. The rationale behind this approach is that it allows the combination of different kernels adapted to different parts of the sequences, such as introns and exons or gaps and aligned residues in alignment, without knowing the exact segmentation of the sequences. Besides proving that the convolution of two kernels is a valid kernel, Haussler (1999) gives several examples of convolution kernels relevant for biological sequences; for example, he shows that the joint probability $P(\mathbf{x},\mathbf{z})$ of two sequences under a pair hidden Markov model (HMM) is a valid kernel under mild assumptions, a property that was also proved independently by Watkins (2000).

Finally, a third general strategy to design kernels for strings is to start from classical measures of similarity between strings and turn them into kernels. In the case of biological sequences, for example, a scheme known as Smith-Waterman local alignment score (Smith & Waterman, 1981) is widely used to compare sequences. Saigo, Vert, Ueda, and Akutsu (2004) show that a slight modification of this measure of similarity is a valid kernel, called the local alignment kernel. In fact, the proof of the positive definiteness of the new kernels builds on the study of convolution kernels presented above (Vert, Saigo, & Akutsu, 2004). Interestingly, the Smith-Waterman alignment score between biological sequences optimizes an alignment between sequences by dynamic programming, just like dynamic time warping (DTW) algorithms compare variable-length sequences in speech recognition. DTW kernels that violate the positive semidefiniteness assumption (surveyed in the chapter by Wan) have been proposed for speaker-recognition applications; adapting the local alignment kernel to this context, that is, replacing a Viterbi optimization with a forward summation in the dynamic programming algorithm, would result in a valid DTW kernel for speech applications. The local alignment kernel gives excellent results on the problem of detecting remote homologs of proteins, suggesting that combining domain knowledge (in the form of a relevant measure of similarity turned into a kernel) with kernel methods is a promising research direction.

These kernels for variable-length sequences have been widely applied, often in combination with SVM, to various classification tasks in computational biology. Examples include the prediction of protein structural or functional classes from their primary sequence (Cai, Wang, Sun, & Chen, 2003; Ding & Dubchak, 2001; T. Jaakkola et al., 2000; Karchin, Karplus, & Haussler, 2002; Vert et al., 2004), the prediction of the subcellular localization of proteins (Hua & Sun, 2001b; Matsuda, Vert, Saigo, Ueda, Toh, & Akutsu, 2005; Park & Kanehisa, 2003), the classification of transfer RNA (Kin et al., 2002) and noncoding RNA (Karklin, Meraz, & Holbrook, 2005), the prediction of pseudoexons and alternatively spliced exons (Dror, Sorek, & Shamir, 2005; X. H.-F. Zhang, Heller, Hefter, Leslie, & Chasin, 2003b), the separation of mixed plant-pathogen expressed sequence tag (EST) collections (Friedel, Jahn, Sommer, Rudd, Mewes, & Tetko, 2005), the classification of mammalian viral genomes (Rose, Turkett, Oroian, Laegreid, & Keele, 2005), and the prediction of ribosomal proteins (Lin, Kuang, Joseph, & Kolatkar, 2002).

This short review of kernels developed for the purpose of biological sequence classification, besides highlighting the dynamism of research in kernel methods resulting from practical needs in computational biology, naturally raises the practical question of which kernel to use for a given application. Although no clear answer has emerged yet, some lessons can be learned from early studies. First, there is certainly no kernel universally better than others, and the choice of kernel should depend on the targeted application. Intuitively, a kernel for a classification task is likely to work well if it is based on features relevant to the task; for example, a kernel based on sequence alignments, such as the local alignment kernel, gives excellent results on remote homology detection problems, while a kernel based on the global content of sequences in short subsequences, such as the spectrum kernel, works well for the prediction of subcellular localization. Although some methods for the systematic selection and combination of kernels are starting to emerge (see the next section), an empirical evaluation of different kernels on a given problem seems to be the most common way to chose a kernel. Another important point to notice, besides the classification accuracy obtained with a kernel, is its computational cost. Indeed, practical applications often involve data sets of thousands or tens of thousands of sequences, and the computational cost of a method can become a critical factor in this context, in particular in an online setting. The kernels presented above differ a lot in their computational cost, ranging from fast linear-time kernels like the spectrum kernel to slower kernels like the quadratic-time local alignment kernel. The final choice of kernel for a given application often results from a trade-off between classification performance and computational burden.

Other Applications and Future Trends

Besides the important applications mentioned in the previous sections, several other attempts to import ideas of kernel methods in computational biology have emerged recently. In this section, we highlight three promising directions that are likely to develop quickly in the near future: the engineering of new kernels, the development of methods to handle multiple kernels, and the use of kernel methods for graphs in systems biology.

More Kernels

The power of kernel methods to process virtually any sort of data as soon as a valid kernel is defined has recently been exploited for a variety of data, besides high-dimensional data and sequences. For example, Vert (2002) derives a kernel for phylogenetic profiles, that is, a signature indicating the presence or absence of each gene in all sequenced genomes. Several recent works have investigated kernels for protein 3-D structures, a topic that is likely to expand quickly with the foreseeable availability of predicted or solved structures for whole genomes (Borgwardt, Ong, Schönauer, Vishwanathan, Smola, & Kreigel, 2005; Dobson & Doig, 2003). For smaller molecules, several kernels based on planar or 3-D structures have emerged, with many potential applications in computational chemistry (Kashima et al., 2004; Mahé, Ueda, Akutsu, Perret, & Vert, 2005; Swamidass, Chen, Bruand, Phung, Ralaivola, & Baldi, 2005). This trend to develop more and more kernels, often designed for specific data and applications, is likely to continue in the future because it has proved to be a good approach to obtain efficient algorithms for real-world applications. A nice by-product of these efforts, which is still barely exploited, is the fact that any kernel can be used by any kernel method, paving the way to a multitude of applications such as clustering (Qin, Lewis, & Noble, 2003; see also the chapter by Pochet, Ojeda, De Smet, De Bie, Suykens, & De Moor) or data visualization (Komura, Nakamura, Tsutsumi, Aburatani, & Ihara, 2005).

Integration of Heterogeneous Data

Operations on kernels provide simple and powerful tools to integrate heterogeneous data or multiple kernels; this is particularly relevant in computational biology, where biological objects can typically be described by heterogeneous representations, and the availability of a large number of possible kernels for even a single representation raises the question of choice or combination of kernels. Suppose, for instance, that one wants to perform a functional classification of genes based on their sequences, expression over a series of experiments, evolutionary conservation, and position in an interaction network. A natural approach with kernel methods is to start by defining one or several kernels for each sort of data, that is, string kernels for the gene sequences, vector kernels to process the expression profiles, and so forth. The apparent heterogeneity of data types then vanishes as one simply obtains a family of kernel functions $\kappa_1, \ldots, \kappa_p$. In order to learn from all data simultaneously, the simplest approach is to define an integrated kernel as the sum of the initial kernels:

$$\kappa = \sum_{i=1}^{p} \kappa_i.$$

The rationale behind this sum is that if each kernel is a simple dot product, then the sum of dot products is equal to the dot product of the concatenated vectors. In other words, taking a sum of kernels amounts to putting all features of each individual kernel together; if different features in different kernels are relevant for a given problem, then one expects the kernel method trained on the integrated kernel to pick those relevant features. This idea was pioneered by the authors of Pavlidis, Weston, Cai, and Noble (2002), in which gene expression profiles and gene phylogenetic profiles are integrated to predict the functional classes of genes, effectively integrating evolutionary and transcriptional information.

An interesting generalization of this approach is to form a convex combination of kernels of the form:

$$\kappa = \sum_{i=1}^{p} w_i \kappa_i,$$

where the w_i are nonnegative weights. Lanckriet, De Bie, Cristianini, Jordan and Noble (2004) propose a general framework based on semidefinite programming to optimize the weights and learn a discrimination function for a given classification task simultaneously. Promising empirical results on gene functional classification show that by integrating several kernels, better results can be obtained than with each individual kernel.

Finally, other kernel methods can be used to compare and search for correlations between heterogeneous data. For example, Vert and Kanehisa (2003) propose to use a kernelized version of canonical correlation analysis (CCA) to compare gene expression data on the one hand with the position of genes in the metabolic network on the other hand. Each type of data is first converted into a kernel for genes, the information about gene positions in the metabolic network being encoded with the so-called diffusion kernel (Kondor & Vert, 2004). These two kernels define embeddings of the set of genes into two Euclidean spaces, in which correlated directions are detected by CCA. It is then shown that the directions detected in the feature space of the diffusion kernel can be interpreted as clusters in the metabolic network, resulting in a method to monitor the expression patterns of metabolic pathways.

Kernel Methods in Systems Biology

Another promising field of research where kernel methods can certainly contribute is systems biology, which roughly speaking focuses on the analysis of biological systems of interacting molecules, in particular, biological networks.

A first avenue of research is the reconstruction of biological networks from high-through-put data. For example, the prediction of interacting proteins to reconstruct the interaction network can be posed as a binary classification problem—given a pair of proteins, do they interact or not?—and can therefore be tackled with SVM as soon as a kernel between pairs of proteins is defined. However, the primary data available are about individual proteins. In order to use SVM in this context, it is therefore natural to try to derive kernels for pairs of proteins from kernels for single proteins. This has been carried out, for example, by Bock and Gough (2001) who characterize each protein by a vector and concatenate two such individual vectors to represent a protein pair. Observing that there is usually no order in a protein pair, Martin, Roe, and Faulon (2005) and Ben-Hur and Noble (2005) propose to define a kernel between pairs (A,B) and (C,D) by the equation:

$$\kappa((A,B),(C,D)) = \kappa_0(A,C)\kappa_0(B,D) + \kappa_0(A,D)\kappa_0(B,C),$$

where κ_0 denotes a kernel for an individual protein and κ is the resulting kernel for pairs of proteins. The rationale behind this definition is that in order to match the pair (A,B) with the pair (C,D), one can either try to match A with C and B with D, or to match A with D and B with C. Reported accuracies on the problem of protein-interaction prediction are very high, confirming the potential of kernel methods in this fast-moving field.

A parallel approach to network inference from genomic data has been investigated by Yamanishi, Vert, and Kanehisa (2004), who show that learning the edges of a network can be carried out by first mapping the vertices, for example, the genes, onto a Euclidean space, and then connecting the pairs of points that are close to each other in this embedding. The problem then becomes that of learning an optimal embedding of the vertices, a problem known as distance metric learning that recently caught the attention of the machine learning community and for which several kernel methods exist (Vert & Yamanishi, 2005).

Finally, several other emerging applications in systems biology, such as inference on networks (Tsuda & Noble, 2004) or the classification of networks (Middendorf et al., 2004), are likely to be subject to increasing attention in the future due to the growing interest and amount of data related to biological networks.

Conclusion

This brief survey, although far from being complete, highlights the impressive advances in the applications of kernel methods in computational biology in the last 5 years. More than just importing well-established algorithms to a new application domain, biology has triggered the development of new algorithms and methods, ranging from the engineering of various kernels to the development of new methods for learning from multiple kernels and for feature selection. The widespread diffusion of easy-to-use SVM software and the ongoing integration of various kernels and kernel methods in major computing environments for bioinformatics are likely to foster again the use of kernel methods in computational biology as long as they will provide state-of-the-art methods for practical problems. Many questions remain open regarding, for example, the automatic choice and integration of kernels, the possibility to incorporate prior knowledge in kernel methods, and the extension of kernel methods to more general kernels that are positive definite, suggesting that theoretical developments are also likely to progress quickly in the near future.

References

Aebersold, R., & Mann, M. (2003). Mass spectrometry-based proteomics. *Nature, 422*(6928), 198-207.

Aliferis, C., Hardin, D., & Massion, P. (2002). Machine learning models for lung cancer classification using array comparative genomic hybridization. In *Proceedings of the 2002 American Medical Informatics Association (AMIA) Annual Symposium* (pp. 7-11).

Ambroise, C., & McLachlan, G. (2002). Selection bias in gene extraction on the basis of microarray gene-expression data. In *Proceedings of the National Academy of Science USA, 99*(10), 6562-6566.

Bao, L., & Sun, Z. (2002). Identifying genes related to drug anticancer mechanisms using support vector machine. *FEBS Letters, 521*, 109-114.

Ben-Dor, A., Bruhn, L., Friedman, N., Nachman, I., Schummer, M., & Yakhini, Z. (2000). Tissue classification with gene expression profiles. *Journal of Computational Biology, 7*(3-4), 559-583.

Ben-Hur, A., & Brutlag, D. (2003). Remote homology detection: A motif based approach. *Bioinformatics, 19*(Suppl. 1), i26-i33.

Ben-Hur, A., & Noble, W. S. (2005). Kernel methods for predicting protein-protein interactions. *Bioinformatics, 21*(Suppl. 1), i38-i46.

Bhasin, M., & Raghava, G. P. S. (2004). Prediction of CTL epitopes using QM, SVM, and ANN techniques. *Vaccine, 22*(23-24), 3195-3204.

Bock, J. R., & Gough, D. A. (2001). Predicting protein-protein interactions from primary structure. *Bioinformatics, 17*(5), 455-460.

Bock, J. R., & Gough, D. A. (2002). A new method to estimate ligand-receptor energetics. *Mol Cell Proteomics, 1*(11), 904-910.

Borgwardt, K. M., Ong, C. S., Schönauer, S., Vishwanathan, S. V. N., Smola, A. J., & Kriegel, H.-P. (2005). Protein function prediction via graph kernels. *Bioinformatics, 21*(Suppl. 1), i47-i56.

Cai, C., Wang, W., Sun, L., & Chen, Y. (2003). Protein function classification via support vector machine approach. *Mathematical Biosciences, 185*(2), 111-122.

Camps-Valls, G., Chalk, A., Serrano-Lopez, A., Martin-Guerrero, J., & Sonnhammer, E. (2004). Profiled support vector machines for antisense oligonucleotide efficacy prediction. *BMC Bioinformatics, 5*(135), 135.

Chen, Y., Lin, Y., Lin, C., & Hwang, J. (2004). Prediction of the bonding states of cysteines using the support vector machines based on multiple feature vectors and cysteine state sequences. *Proteins, 55*(4), 1036-1042.

Cuturi, M., & Vert, J.-P. (2005). The context-tree kernel for strings. *Neural Networks, 18*(4), 1111-1123.

Degroeve, S., Saeys, Y., De Baets, B., Rouze, P., & Van de Peer, Y. (2005). SpliceMachine: Predicting splice sites from high-dimensional local context representations. *Bioinformatics, 21*, 1332-1338.

DeRisi, J. L., Iyer, V. R., & Brown, P. O. (1997). Exploring the metabolic and genetic control of gene expression on a genomic scale. *Science, 278*(5338), 680-686.

Ding, C., & Dubchak, I. (2001). Multi-class protein fold recognition using support vector machines and neural networks. *Bioinformatics, 17*, 349-358.

Dobson, P., & Doig, A. (2003). Distinguishing enzyme structures from non-enzymes without alignments. *Journal of Molecular Biology, 330*(4), 771-783.

Dönnes, P., & Elofsson, A. (2002). Prediction of MHC class I binding peptides, using SVMHC. *BMC Bioinformatics, 3*(1), 25.

Dror, G., Sorek, R., & Shamir, R. (2005). Accurate identification of alternatively spliced exons using support vector machine. *Bioinformatics, 21*(7), 897-901.

Durbin, R., Eddy, S., Krogh, A., & Mitchison, G. (1998). *Biological sequence analysis: Probabilistic models of proteins and nucleic acids.* Cambridge University Press.

Friedel, C. C., Jahn, K. H. V., Sommer, S., Rudd, S., Mewes, H. W., & Tetko, I. V. (2005). Support vector machines for separation of mixed plant-pathogen EST collections based on codon usage. *Bioinformatics, 21*, 1383-1388.

Furey, T. S., Cristianini, N., Duffy, N., Bednarski, D. W., Schummer, M., & Haussler, D. (2000). Support vector machine classification and validation of cancer tissue samples using microarray expression data. *Bioinformatics, 16*(10), 906-914.

Guermeur, Y., Lifschitz, A., & Vert, R. (2004). A kernel for protein secondary structure prediction. In B. Schölkopf, K. Tsuda, & J. Vert (Eds.), *Kernel methods in computational biology* (pp. 193-206). MIT Press.

Guyon, I., Weston, J., Barnhill, S., & Vapnik, V. (2002). Gene selection for cancer classification using support vector machines. *Machine Learning, 46*(1/3), 389-422.

Haussler, D. (1999). *Convolution kernels on discrete structures* (Tech. Rep. No. UCSC-CRL-99-10). Santa Cruz: University of California.

Hua, S., & Sun, Z. (2001a). A novel method of protein secondary structure prediction with high segment overlap measure: Support vector machine approach. *Journal of Molecular Biology, 308*(2), 397-407.

Hua, S., & Sun, Z. (2001b). Support vector machine approach for protein subcellular localization prediction. *Bioinformatics, 17*(8), 721-728.

Huang, T. M., & Kecman, V. (2005). Gene extraction for cancer diagnosis by support vector machines: An improvement. *Artificial Intelligence in Medicine (Special Issue on Computational Intelligence Techniques in Bioinformatics), 35*, 185-194.

International Human Genome Sequencing Consortium. (2001). Initial sequencing and analysis of the human genome. *Nature, 409*(6822), 860-921.

Jaakkola, T., Diekhans, M., & Haussler, D. (2000). A discriminative framework for detecting remote protein homologies. *Journal of Computational Biology, 7*(1,2), 95-114.

Jaakkola, T. S., Diekhans, M., & Haussler, D. (1999). Using the Fisher kernel method to detect remote protein homologies. In *Proceedings of the Seventh International Conference on Intelligent Systems for Molecular Biology*, 149-158.

Karchin, R., Karplus, K., & Haussler, D. (2002). Classifying G-protein coupled receptors with support vector machines. *Bioinformatics, 18*, 147-159.

Karklin, Y., Meraz, R. F., & Holbrook, S. R. (2005). Classification of non-coding RNA using graph representations of secondary structure. In *Pacific Symposium on Biocomputing* (pp. 4-15).

Kashima, H., Tsuda, K., & Inokuchi, A. (2004). Kernels for graphs. In B. Schölkopf, K. Tsuda, & J. Vert (Eds.), *Kernel methods in computational biology* (pp. 155-170). MIT Press.

Kim, J. H., Lee, J., Oh, B., Kimm, K., & Koh, I. (2004). Prediction of phosphorylation sites using SVMs. *Bioinformatics, 20*(17), 3179-3184.

Kin, T., Tsuda, K., & Asai, K. (2002). Marginalized kernels for RNA sequence data analysis. In R. Lathtop, K. Nakai, S. Miyano, T. Takagi, & M. Kanehisa (Eds.), *Genome informatics 2002* (pp. 112-122). Universal Academic Press.

Komura, D., Nakamura, H., Tsutsumi, S., Aburatani, H., & Ihara, S. (2005). Multidimensional support vector machines for visualization of gene expression data. *Bioinformatics, 21*(4), 439-444.

Kondor, R., & Vert, J.-P. (2004). Diffusion kernels. In B. Schölkopf, K. Tsuda, & J. Vert, (Eds.), *Kernel methods in computational biology* (pp. 171-192). MIT Press.

Krishnapuram, B., Carin, L., & Hartemink, A. (2004). Joint classifier and feature optimization for comprehensive cancer diagnosis using gene expression data. *Journal of Computational Biology, 11*(2-3), 227-242.

Lanckriet, G. R. G., De Bie, T., Cristianini, N., Jordan, M. I., & Noble, W. S. (2004). A statistical framework for genomic data fusion. *Bioinformatics, 20*(16), 2626-2635.

Leslie, C., Eskin, E., & Noble, W. (2002). The spectrum kernel: A string kernel for SVM protein classification. In *Proceedings of the Pacific Symposium on Biocomputing 2002* (pp. 564-575).

Leslie, C. S., Eskin, E., Cohen, A., Weston, J., & Noble, W. S. (2004). Mismatch string kernels for discriminative protein classification. *Bioinformatics, 20*(4), 467-476.

Li, T., Zhang, C., & Ogihara, M. (2004). A comparative study of feature selection and multiclass classification methods for tissue classification based on gene expression. *Bioinformatics, 20*(15), 2429-2437.

Liao, L., & Noble, W. (2003). Combining pairwise sequence similarity and support vector machines for detecting remote protein evolutionary and structural relationships. *Journal of Computational Biology, 10*(6), 857-868.

Lin, K., Kuang, Y., Joseph, J. S., & Kolatkar, P. R. (2002). Conserved codon composition of ribosomal protein coding genes in Escherichia coli, mycobacterium tuberculosis and saccharomyces cerevisiae: Lessons from supervised machine learning in functional genomics. *Nucleic Acids Research, 30*(11), 2599-2607.

Listgarten, J., Damaraju, S., Poulin, B., Cook, L., Dufour, J., Driga, A., et al. (2004). Predictive models for breast cancer susceptibility from multiple single nucleotide polymorphisms. *Clinical Cancer Research, 10*(8), 2725-2737.

Logan, B., Moreno, P., Suzek, B., Weng, Z., & Kasif, S. (2001). *A study of remote homology detection* (Tech. Rep. No. CRL 2001/05). Compaq Cambridge Research laboratory.

Mahé, P., Ueda, N., Akutsu, T., Perret, J.-L., & Vert, J.-P. (2005). Graph kernels for molecular structure-activity relationship analysis with support vector machines. *Journal of Chemical Information and Modeling, 45*(4), 939-951.

Martin, S., Roe, D., & Faulon, J.-L. (2005). Predicting protein-protein interactions using signature products. *Bioinformatics, 21*(2), 218-226.

Matsuda, A., Vert, J.-P., Saigo, H., Ueda, N., Toh, H., & Akutsu, T. (2005). A novel representation of protein sequences for prediction of subcellular location using support vector machines. *Protein Science, 14*(11), 2804-2813.

Meinicke, P., Tech, M., Morgenstern, B., & Merkl, R. (2004). Oligo kernels for datamining on biological sequences: A case study on prokaryotic translation initiation sites. *BMC Bioinformatics, 5*, 169.

Meireles, S., Carvalho, A., Hirata, R., Montagnini, A., Martins, W., Runza, F., et al. (2003). Differentially expressed genes in gastric tumors identified by cDNA array. *Cancer Letters, 190*(2), 199-211.

Middendorf, M., Ziv, E., Adams, C., Hom, J., Koytcheff, R., Levovitz, C., et al. (2004). Discriminative topological features reveal biological network mechanisms. *BMC Bioinformatics, 5*, 181.

Model, F., Adorjan, P., Olek, A., & Piepenbrock, C. (2001). Feature selection for DNA methylation based cancer classification. *Bioinformatics, 17*(Supp. 1), S157-S164.

Moler, E. J., Chow, M. L., & Mian, I. S. (2000). Analysis of molecular profile data using generative and discriminative methods. *Physiological Genomics, 4*(2), 109-126.

Mukherjee, S., Tamayo, P., Mesirov, J. P., Slonim, D., Verri, A., & Poggio, T. (1998). *Support vector machine classification of microarray data* (Tech. Rep. No. 182).

O'Donnell, R. K., Kupferman, M., Wei, S. J., Singhal, S., Weber, R., O'Malley, B., et al. (2005). Gene expression signature predicts lymphatic metastasis in squamous cell carcinoma of the oral cavity. *Oncogene, 24*(7), 1244-1251.

O'Flanagan, R. A., Paillard, G., Lavery, R., & Sengupta, A. M. (2005). Non-additivity in protein-DNA binding. *Bioinformatics, 21*(10), 2254-2263.

Park, K.-J., & Kanehisa, M. (2003). Prediction of protein subcellular locations by support vector machines using compositions of amino acids and amino acid pairs. *Bioinformatics, 19*(13), 1656-1663.

Passerini, A., & Frasconi, P. (2004). Learning to discriminate between ligand-bound and disulfide-bound cysteines. *Protein Engineering Design and Selection, 17*(4), 367-373.

Pavlidis, P., Weston, J., Cai, J., & Noble, W. (2002). Learning gene functional classifications from multiple data types. *Journal of Computational Biology, 9*(2), 401-411.

Pochet, N., De Smet, F., Suykens, J. A. K., & De Moor, B. L. R. (2004). Systematic benchmarking of microarray data classification: Assessing the role of non-linearity and dimensionality reduction. *Bioinformatics, 20*(17), 3185-3195.

Qin, J., Lewis, D. P., & Noble, W. S. (2003). Kernel hierarchical gene clustering from microarray expression data. *Bioinformatics, 19*(16), 2097-2104.

Ramaswamy, S., Tamayo, P., Rifkin, R., Mukherjee, S., Yeang, C., Angelo, M., et al. (2001). Multiclass cancer diagnosis using tumor gene expression signatures. In *Proceedings of the National Academy of Science USA, 98*(26), 15149-15154.

Rätsch, G., Sonnenburg, S., & Schölkopf, B. (2005). RASE: Recognition of alternatively spliced exons in c. elegans. *Bioinformatics, 21*(Suppl. 1), i369-i377.

Res, I., Mihalek, I., & Lichtarge, O. (2005). An evolution based classifier for prediction of protein interfaces without using protein structures. *Bioinformatics, 21*(10), 2496-2501.

Rose, J. R., Turkett, W. H. J., Oroian, I. C., Laegreid, W. W., & Keele, J. (2005). Correlation of amino acid preference and mammalian viral genome type. *Bioinformatics, 21*(8), 1349-1357.

Saigo, H., Vert, J.-P., Ueda, N., & Akutsu, T. (2004). Protein homology detection using string alignment kernels. *Bioinformatics, 20*(11), 1682-1689.

Schena, M., Shalon, D., Davis, R., & Brown, P. (1995). Quantitative monitoring of gene expression patterns with a complimentary DNA microarray. *Science, 270*, 467-470.

Schölkopf, B., Tsuda, K., & Vert, J.-P. (2004). *Kernel methods in computational biology.* MIT Press.

Seeger, M. (2002). Covariance kernels from Bayesian generative models. *Advances in Neural Information Processing Systems, 14*, 905-912.

Segal, N. H., Pavlidis, P., Antonescu, C. R., Maki, R. G., Noble, W. S., DeSantis, D., et al. (2003). Classification and subtype prediction of adult soft tissue sarcoma by functional genomics. *American Journal of Pathology, 163*(2), 691-700.

Segal, N. H., Pavlidis, P., Noble, W. S., Antonescu, C. R., Viale, A., Wesley, U. V., et al. (2003). Classification of clear-cell sarcoma as a subtype of melanoma by genomic profiling. *Journal of Clinical Oncology, 21*(9), 1775-1781.

Sharan, R., & Myers, E. W. (2005). A motif-based framework for recognizing sequence families. *Bioinformatics, 21*(Suppl. 1), i387-i393.

Shawe-Taylor, J., & Cristianini, N. (2004). *Kernel methods for pattern analysis.* Cambridge University Press.

Shipp, M. A., Ross, K. N., Tamayo, P., Weng, A. P., Kutok, J. L., Aguiar, R. C. T., et al. (2002). Diffuse large B-cell lymphoma outcome prediction by gene-expression profiling and supervised machine learning. *Nature Medicine, 8*(1), 68-74.

Smith, T., & Waterman, M. (1981). Identification of common molecular subsequences. *Journal of Molecular Biology, 147*, 195-197.

Steiner, G., Suter, L., Boess, F., Gasser, R., de Vera, M. C., Albertini, S., et al. (2004). Discriminating different classes of toxicants by transcript profiling. *Environmental Health Perspectives, 112*(12), 1236-1248.

Su, Y., Murali, T., Pavlovic, V., Schaffer, M., & Kasif, S. (2003). RankGene: Identification of diagnostic genes based on expression data. *Bioinformatics, 19*(12), 1578-1579.

Swamidass, S. J., Chen, J., Bruand, J., Phung, P., Ralaivola, L., & Baldi, P. (2005). Kernels for small molecules and the prediction of mutagenicity, toxicity and anti-cancer activity. *Bioinformatics, 21*(Suppl. 1), i359-i368.

Teramoto, R., Aoki, M., Kimura, T., & Kanaoka, M. (2005). Prediction of siRNA functionality using generalized string kernel and support vector machine. *FEBS Letters, 579*(13), 2878-2882.

Tsuda, K., Kin, T., & Asai, K. (2002). Marginalized kernels for biological sequences. *Bioinformatics, 18*, S268-S275.

Tsuda, K., & Noble, W. (2004). Learning kernels from biological networks by maximizing entropy. *Bioinformatics, 20*, i326-i333.

Valentini, G. (2002). Gene expression data analysis of human lymphoma using support vector machines and output coding ensembles. *Artificial Intelligence in Medicine, 26*(3), 281-304.

Venter, J. C. e. a. (2001). The sequence of the human genome. *Science, 291*(5507), 1304-1351.

Vert, J.-P. (2002). A tree kernel to analyze phylogenetic profiles. *Bioinformatics, 18*, S276-S284.

Vert, J.-P., & Kanehisa, M. (2003). Extracting active pathways from gene expression data. *Bioinformatics, 19*, 238ii-234ii.

Vert, J.-P., Saigo, H., & Akutsu, T. (2004). Local alignment kernels for biological sequences. In B. Schölkopf, K. Tsuda, & J. Vert, (Eds.), *Kernel methods in computational biology* (pp. 131-154). Cambridge, MA: MIT Press.

Vert, J.-P., Thurman, R., & Noble, W. S. (2006). Kernels for gene regulatory regions. In Y. Weiss, B. Schölkopf, & J. Platt (Eds.), *Advances in Neural Information Processing Systems 18* (pp. 1401-1408). Cambridge, MA: MIT Press.

Vert, J.-P., & Yamanishi, Y. (2005). Supervised graph inference. *Advances in Neural Information Processing Systems, 17*, 1433-1440.

Wagner, M., Naik, D., & Pothen, A. (2003). Protocols for disease classification from mass spectrometry data. *Proteomics, 3*(9), 1692-1698.

Wang, M., Yang, J., Liu, G.-P., Xu, Z.-J., & Chou, K.-C. (2004). Weighted-support vector machines for predicting membrane protein types based on pseudo-amino acid composition. *Protein Engineering Design and Selection, 17*(6), 509-516.

Watkins, C. (2000). Dynamic alignment kernels. In A. J. Smola, P. L. Bartlett, B. Schölkopf, & D. Schuurmans (Eds.), *Advances in large margin classifiers* (pp. 39-50). Cambridge, MA: MIT Press.

Williams, R., Hing, S., Greer, B., Whiteford, C., Wei, J., Natrajan, R., et al. (2004). Prognostic classification of relapsing favorable histology Wilms tumor using cDNA microarray expression profiling and support vector machines. *Genes Chromosomes Cancer, 41*(1), 65-79.

Wu, B., Abbott, T., Fishman, D., McMurray, W., Mor, G., Stone, K., et al. (2003). Comparison of statistical methods for classification of ovarian cancer using mass spectrometry data. *Bioinformatics, 19*(13), 1636-1643.

Yamanishi, Y., Vert, J.-P., & Kanehisa, M. (2004). Protein network inference from multiple genomic data: A supervised approach. *Bioinformatics, 20*, i363-i370.

Yan, C., Dobbs, D., & Honavar, V. (2004). A two-stage classifier for identification of protein-protein interface residues. *Bioinformatics, 20*(Suppl. 1), i371-i378.

Yoon, Y., Song, J., Hong, S., & Kim, J. (2003). Analysis of multiple single nucleotide polymorphisms of candidate genes related to coronary heart disease susceptibility by using support vector machines. *Clinical Chemistry and Laboratory Medicine, 41*(4), 529-534.

Yu, C., Zavaljevski, N., Stevens, F. J., Yackovich, K., & Reifman, J. (2005). Classifying noisy protein sequence data: A case study of immunoglobulin light chains. *Bioinformatics, 21*(Suppl. 1), i495-i501.

Yuan, Z., Burrage, K., & Mattick, J. (2002). Prediction of protein solvent accessibility using support vector machines. *Proteins, 48*(3), 566-570.

Zavaljevski, N., Stevens, F., & Reifman, J. (2002). Support vector machines with selective kernel scaling for protein classification and identification of key amino acid positions. *Bioinformatics, 18*(5), 689-696.

Zhang, S.-W., Pan, Q., Zhang, H.-C., Zhang, Y.-L., & Wang, H.-Y. (2003). Classification of protein quaternary structure with support vector machine. *Bioinformatics, 19*(18), 2390-2396.

Zhang, X. H.-F., Heller, K. A., Hefter, I., Leslie, C. S., & Chasin, L. A. (2003). Sequence information for the splicing of human pre-mRNA identified by support vector machine classification. *Genome Research, 13*(12), 2637-2650.

Zien, A., Rätsch, G., Mika, S., Schölkopf, B., Lengauer, T., & Müller, K.-R. (2000). Engineering support vector machine kernels that recognize translation initiation sites. *Bioinformatics, 16*(9), 799-807.

Chapter III

Kernel Clustering for Knowledge Discovery in Clinical Microarray Data Analysis

Nathalie L. M. M. Pochet, Katholieke Universiteit Leuven, Belgium

Fabian Ojeda, Katholieke Universiteit Leuven, Belgium

Frank De Smet, Katholieke Universiteit Leuven, Belgium
& National Alliance of Christian Mutualities, Belgium

Tijl De Bie, Katholieke Universiteit Leuven, Belgium

Johan A. K. Suykens, Katholieke Universiteit Leuven, Belgium

Bart L. R. De Moor, Katholieke Universiteit Leuven, Belgium

Abstract

Clustering techniques like k-means and hierarchical clustering have shown to be useful when applied to microarray data for the identification of clinical classes, for example, in oncology. This chapter discusses the application of nonlinear techniques like kernel k-means and spectral clustering, which are based on kernel functions like linear and radial basis function (RBF) kernels. External validation techniques (e.g., the Rand index and the adjusted Rand index) can immediately be applied to these methods for the assessment of clustering results. Internal validation methods like the global silhouette index, the distortion score, and the Calinski-Harabasz index (F-statistic), which have been commonly used in the input space, are reformulated in this chapter for usage in a kernel-induced feature space.

Introduction

Microarrays are a recent technology that allows for determining the expression levels of thousands of genes simultaneously. One important application area of this technology is clinical oncology. Parallel measurements of these expression levels result in data vectors that contain thousands of values, which are called expression patterns. A microarray consists of a reproducible pattern of several DNA probes attached to a small solid support. Labeled cDNA, prepared from extracted mRNA, is hybridized with the complementary DNA probes attached to the microarray. The hybridizations are measured by means of a laser scanner and transformed quantitatively. Two important types of microarrays are cDNA microarrays and oligonucleotide arrays. cDNA microarrays consist of about 10,000 known cDNA (obtained after PCR amplification) that are spotted in an ordered matrix on a glass slide. Oligonucleotide arrays (or DNA chips) are constructed by the synthesis of oligonucleotides on silicium chips. Figure 1 gives a schematic overview of an experiment with the cDNA technology. Both technologies have specific characteristics that will not be discussed here. When studying, for example, tumor tissues with microarrays, the challenge mainly lies in the analysis of the experiments in order to obtain relevant clinical information. Most of the techniques that have been widely used for analyzing microarrays require some preprocessing stage such as gene selection, filtering, or dimensionality reduction, among others. These methods cannot directly deal with high-dimensional data vectors. Moreover, these are methods that are specifically designed to deal with the particular challenges posed by gene expression data and thus they do not provide a more general framework that can be easily extended to other kinds of data. For this purpose, methods and algorithms capable of handling high-dimensional data vectors and that are capable of working under a minimal set of assumptions are required. The chapter by Jean-Philippe Vert in this book focuses on the classification of high-dimensional data, while this chapter elaborates on the cluster analysis of these high-dimensional data.

Clustering techniques are generally applied to microarray data for the identification of clinical classes, which could allow for refining clinical management. Cluster analysis of entire microarray experiments (expression patterns from patients or tissues) allows for the discovery of possibly unknown diagnostic categories without knowing the properties of these classes in advance. These clusters could form the basis of new diagnostic schemes in which the different categories contain patients with less clinical variability.

Clustering microarray experiments have already shown to be useful in a large number of cancer studies. Alon et al. (1999), for example, separated cancerous colon tissues from noncancerous colon tissues by applying two-way clustering. The distinction between acute myeloid leukemia (AML) and acute lymphoblastic leukemia (ALL) has been rediscovered by using self-organizing maps (SOM) by Golub et al. (1999). By using hierarchical clustering, van 't Veer et al. (2002) were able to distinguish between the presence (poor prognosis) and the absence (good prognosis) of distant subclinical metastases in breast cancer patients where the histopathological examination did not show tumor cells in local lymph nodes at diagnosis (lymph node negative).

For this purpose, methods such as the classical k-means clustering and hierarchical clustering are commonly used (Bolshakova, Azuaje, & Cunningham, 2005; Handl, Knowles, & Kell, 2005). These methods are based on simple distance or similarity measures (e.g., the

Figure 1. Schematic overview of an experiment with a cDNA microarray: (1) Spotting of the presynthesized DNA probes (derived from the genes to be studied) on the glass slide. These probes are the purified products from PCR amplification of the associated DNA clones. (2) Labeling (via reverse transcriptase) of the total mRNA of the test sample (tumor in red) and reference sample (green). (3) Pooling of the two samples and hybridization. (4) Readout of the red and green intensities separately (measure for the hybridization by the test and reference sample) in each probe. (5) Calculation of the relative expression levels (intensity in the red channel and intensity in the green channel). (6) Storage of results in a database. (7) Data mining.

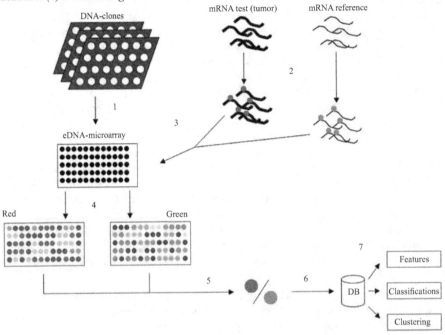

Euclidean distance). However, only linear relationships in the data can be discovered using these techniques. Recently, methods have emerged for clustering data in which the clusters are not linearly separable. Two important methods are kernel k-means clustering (Dhillon, Guan, & Kulis, 2004a, 2004b; Zhang & Rudnicky, 2002) and the related spectral clustering (Cristianini, Shawe-Taylor, & Kandola, 2002; Ng et al., 2001). Introducing these techniques in microarray data analysis allows for dealing with both high-dimensional data and nonlinear relationships in the data.

Validation techniques are used to assess and compare the performance of different clustering methods. These methods can also be employed for tuning the cluster settings, for example, optimizing the number of clusters or tuning the kernel parameters. A recent review of Handl et al. (2005) presents the state of the art in cluster validation on high-dimensional data, among others, on microarray data, referring to some previous important manuscripts in the field (Bolshakova & Azuaje, 2003; Halkidi, Batistakis, & Vazirgiannis, 2001). Two main kinds of validation techniques are internal and external validation. Internal validation assesses the quality of a clustering result based on statistical properties, for example, assessing the compactness of a cluster or maximizing the intercluster distances while minimizing the intracluster distances. External validation reflects the level of agreement of a clustering result with an external partition, for example, existing diagnostic classes generally used by experts in clinical practice. The global silhouette index, the distortion score, and the Calinski-Harabasz index (F-statistic) are commonly used for internal validation, and the Rand index and adjusted Rand index for external validation.

This chapter describes classical k-means, kernel k-means, and spectral clustering algorithms and discusses their advantages and disadvantages in the context of clinical microarray data analysis. Since classical k-means clustering cannot handle high-dimensional microarray experiments for computational reasons, principal component analysis (PCA) is used as a preceding dimensionality-reduction step. Kernel k-means and spectral clustering are capable of directly handling the high-dimensional microarray experiments since they make use of the kernel trick, which allows them to work implicitly in the feature space. Several internal and external cluster-validation criteria commonly used in the input data space are described and extended for usage in the feature space. The advantages of nonlinear clustering techniques in case of clinical microarray data analysis are further demonstrated by means of the clustering results on several microarray data sets related to cancer.

Preprocessing

This chapter uses standardization as a preceding preprocessing step for all clustering methods. However, classical k-means clustering should not be directly applied to the high-dimensional microarray data as such. In all practical cases, the number of genes (the dimensionality) is much larger than the number of arrays (the data points) such that only a small subspace of the data space is actually spanned by the data. Therefore, in case of classical k-means, standardization is followed by principal component analysis to obtain a representation of the data with a reduced dimensionality (without any selection of principal components). In this section, we describe these unsupervised preprocessing steps, as well as filtering, which is also commonly used for that purpose.

Filtering

A set of microarray experiments, generating gene expression profiles (measurements of a single gene under several conditions), frequently contains a considerable number of genes that do not really contribute to the clinical process that is being studied. The expression values of these profiles often show little variation over the different experiments (they are called "constitutive" with respect to the clinical process studied). Moreover, these constitutive genes will have seemingly random and meaningless profiles after standardization (division by a small standard deviation resulting in noise inflation), which is a very common preprocessing step. Another problem with microarray data sets is the fact that these regularly contain highly unreliable expression profiles with a considerable number of missing values. Due to their number, replacing these missing values in these expression profiles is not possible within the desired degree of accuracy.

If these data sets were passed to the clustering algorithms as such, the quality of the clustering results could significantly degrade. A simple solution (that can also be used in combination with other preprocessing steps) is to remove at least a fraction of the undesired genes from the data. This procedure is in general called filtering (Eisen, Spellman, Brown, & Botstein, 1998). Filtering involves removing gene expression profiles from the data set that do not satisfy one or possibly more criteria. Commonly used criteria include a minimum threshold for the standard deviation of the expression values in a profile (removal of constitutive genes) and a threshold on the maximum percentage of missing values. Another similar method for filtering takes a fixed number or fraction of genes best satisfying one criterion (like the criteria stated above).

Standardization or Rescaling

Biologists are mainly interested in the relative behavior instead of the absolute behavior of genes. Genes that are up- and down-regulated together should have the same weights in subsequent algorithms. Applying standardization or rescaling (sometimes also called normalization) to the gene expression profiles can largely achieve this (Quackenbush, 2001).Consider a gene expression profile, denoted by the column vector $\mathbf{g} = [g^1, g^2, ..., g^j, ..., g^\ell]$, measured for ℓ experiments. Rescaling is commonly done by replacing every expression level g^j in g by:

$$\frac{g^j - \mu}{\hat{\sigma}} \, ,$$

where μ is the average expression level of the gene expression profile and is given by

$$\mu = \frac{\sum_{j=1}^{\ell} g^j}{\ell} \, ,$$

and $\hat{\sigma}$ is the standard deviation given by

$$\hat{\sigma} = \sqrt{\frac{1}{\ell-1} \sum_{j=1}^{\ell} (g^j - \mu)^2} \, .$$

This is repeated for every gene expression profile in the data set and results in a collection of expression profiles all having an average of zero and standard deviation of one (i.e., the absolute differences in expression behavior have been largely removed). The division by the standard deviation is sometimes omitted (rescaling is then called mean centering).

Principal Component Analysis

PCA looks for linear combinations of gene expression levels in order to obtain a maximal variance over a set of patients. In fact, those combinations are most informative for this set of patients and are called the principal components. One can either use all principal components or select only a subset for usage in subsequent analyses.

One formulation (Joliffe, 1986) to characterize PCA problems is to consider a given set of centered (zero mean) input data $\{\mathbf{x}_j\}_{j=1}^{\ell}$ as a cloud of points for which one tries to find projected variables $\mathbf{w}^T \mathbf{x}$ with maximal variance. This means:

$$\max_{\mathbf{w}} \ \mathrm{Var}(\mathbf{w}^T \mathbf{x}) = \mathbf{w}^T \mathbf{C} \mathbf{w},$$

where the covariance matrix $\mathbf{C}$ is estimated as

$$\mathbf{C} \cong \frac{1}{\ell - 1} \sum_{j=1}^{\ell} \mathbf{x}_j \mathbf{x}_j^T.$$

One optimizes this objective function under the constraint that $\mathbf{w}^T \mathbf{w} = 1$. Solving the constrained optimization problem gives the eigenvalue problem:

$$\mathbf{C}\mathbf{w} = \lambda \mathbf{w}.$$

The matrix $\mathbf{C}$ is symmetric and positive semidefinite. The eigenvector $\mathbf{w}$ corresponding to the largest eigenvalue determines the projected variable having maximal variance.

Kernel versions of principal component analysis and canonical correlation analysis among others have been formulated by Schölkopf, Smola, and Müller (1998). Primal-dual formulations of these methods are introduced by Suykens, Van Gestel, De Brabanter, De Moor, and Vandewalle (2002). This formulation for kernel principal component analysis has already extensively been tested as a dimensionality-reduction technique on microarray data by Pochet, De Smet, Suykens, and De Moor (2004).

Classical Clustering Methods

In a recent review, Handl et al. (2005) state that although there have recently been numerous advances in the development of improved clustering techniques for (biological and clinical) microarray data analysis (e.g., biclustering techniques [Madeira & Oliveira, 2004; Sheng, Moreau, & De Moor, 2003], adaptive quality-based clustering [De Smet, Mathys, Marchal, Thijs, De Moor, & Moreau, 2002], and gene shaving [Hastie et al., 2000]), traditional clustering techniques such as k-means (Rosen et al., 2005; Tavazoie, Hughes, Campbell, Cho, & Church, 1999) and hierarchical clustering algorithms (Eisen et al., 1998) remain the predominant methods. According to this review, this fact is arguably more owing to their conceptual simplicity and their wide availability in standard software packages than to their intrinsic merits. In this context, this chapter focuses on a class of linear and nonlinear clustering techniques based on the traditional k-means clustering.

k-Means

The k-means clustering algorithm aims at partitioning the data set, consisting of ℓ expression patterns $\{\mathbf{x}_1, ..., \mathbf{x}_\ell\}$ in an n-dimensional space, into k disjoint clusters $\{C_i\}_{i=1}^{k}$, such that the expression patterns in each cluster are more similar to each other than to the expression patterns in other clusters (Dubes & Jain, 1988). The centers or centroids (i.e., prototypes) of all clusters $\mathbf{m}_1, ..., \mathbf{m}_k$ are returned as representatives of the data set, together with the cluster assignments of all expression patterns. The general objective of k-means is to obtain a partition that minimizes the mean squared error for a fixed number of clusters, where the mean squared error is the sum of the Euclidean distances between each expression pattern and its cluster center.

Suppose a set of expression patterns $\mathbf{x}_j, j = 1,...,\ell$. The objective function, that is, the mean squared error criterion, is then defined as:

$$se = \sum_{i=1}^{k}\sum_{j=1}^{\ell} z_{C_k,\mathbf{x}_j} \left\| \mathbf{x}_j - \mathbf{m}_i \right\|^2,$$

where $z_{C_k,\mathbf{x}_j}$ is an indicator function defined as

$$z_{C_i,\mathbf{x}_j} = \begin{cases} 1 & \text{if } \mathbf{x}_j \in C_i \\ 0 & \text{otherwise}, \end{cases}$$

with

$$\sum_{i=1}^{k} z_{C_i,\mathbf{x}_j} = 1 \quad \forall j,$$

and m_i is the center of cluster C_i defined as

$$\mathbf{m}_i = \frac{1}{|C_i|}\sum_{j=1}^{\ell} z_{C_i,\mathbf{x}_j} \mathbf{x}_j,$$

where $|C_i|$ is the cardinality (number of elements) of the set C_i. The Euclidean distance is often used as dissimilarity function $D(\mathbf{x}_j, \mathbf{m}_i)$ in the indicator function. The iterative k-means clustering algorithm first proposed by MacQueen (1967) optimizes this nonconvex objective function as follows.

k-Means Clustering Algorithm

1.   Select k initial centroids $\mathbf{m}_1, ..., \mathbf{m}_k$.

2.   Assign each expression pattern $\mathbf{x}_j, 1 \leq j \leq \ell$, to cluster C_i with the closest centroid m_i based on the indicator function:

$$z_{C_i, x_j} = \begin{cases} 1 & D(\mathbf{x}_j, \mathbf{m}_i) < D(\mathbf{x}_j, \mathbf{m}_h), \forall h \neq i, i, h = 1, ..., k \\ 0 & \text{otherwise} \end{cases}$$

3.   Calculate the new centers m_i of all clusters C_i as:

$$\mathbf{m}_i = \frac{1}{|C_i|} \sum_{j=1}^{\ell} z_{C_i, x_j} \mathbf{x}_j.$$

4.   Repeat Steps 2 and 3 until convergence (no change).

5.   Return $\mathbf{m}i$, $1 \leq i \leq k$.

This algorithm can easily be implemented and works very well for compact and hyperspherically shaped clusters. Although convergence is always reached, k-means does not necessarily find the most optimal clustering (i.e., the global minimum for the objective function). The result of the algorithm is highly dependent on the number of clusters k and the initial selection of the k cluster centroids. Cluster-validation criteria are required in order to choose the optimal settings for k and the initialization. Finally, remember that one disadvantage of this classical k-means algorithm is that preprocessing is required in order to allow clustering.

Kernel Clustering Methods

Kernel clustering methods have already shown to be useful in text-mining applications (De Bie, Cristianini, & Rosipal, 2004; Dhillon et al., 2004) and image data analysis (Zhang & Rudnicky, 2002), among others. For example, Qin, Lewis, and Noble (2003) proposed a kernel hierarchical clustering algorithm on microarray data for identifying groups of genes that share similar expression profiles. Support vector clustering (Ben-Hur, Horn, Siegelmann, & Vapnik, 2001) is another clustering method based on the approach of support vector machines. These kernel clustering methods have recently emerged for clustering data in which the clusters are not linearly separable in order to find nonlinear relationships in the data. Moreover, these techniques allow for dealing with high-dimensional data, which makes it specifically interesting for application on microarray data. In this section, we focus on kernel k-means and spectral clustering.

Kernel k-Means

Kernel k-means clustering is an extension of the linear k-means clustering algorithm in order to find nonlinear structures in the data. Consider a nonlinear mapping $\phi(\cdot)$ from the input space to the feature space. No explicit construction of the nonlinear mapping $\phi(\cdot)$ is required since in this feature space inner products can easily be computed by using the kernel trick $\kappa(\mathbf{x}, \mathbf{y}) = \phi(\mathbf{x})^T \phi(\mathbf{y})$. Mercer's condition (Vapnik, 1998) guaranties that each kernel function $\kappa(\mathbf{x}, \mathbf{y})$, that is, a positive semidefinite symmetric function, corresponds to an inner product in the feature space. This allows for the construction of an $\ell \times \ell$ symmetric and positive definite kernel matrix K holding all pairwise inner products of the input data $\mathbf{K}_{ij} = \kappa(\mathbf{x}_i, \mathbf{x}_j), \forall i, j = 1, \dots, \ell$. This kernel trick can be applied to each algorithm that can be expressed in terms of inner products. The kernel functions used in this chapter are thelinear kernel, $\kappa(\mathbf{x}_i, \mathbf{x}_j) = \mathbf{x}_j^T \mathbf{x}_i$, and the RBF kernel:

$$\kappa(\mathbf{x}_i, \mathbf{x}_j) = \exp(-\left\| \mathbf{x}_i - \mathbf{x}_j \right\|^2 / \sigma^2).$$

The polynomial kernel of degree d, $\kappa(\mathbf{x}_i, \mathbf{x}_j) = (\tau + \mathbf{x}_j^T \mathbf{x}_i)^d$, with $\tau > 0$, is another commonly used kernel function.

The objective function of kernel k-means clustering is exactly the same as the objective function of the classical k-means clustering stated earlier except for the fact that it is now rewritten in terms of inner products that can be replaced by a kernel function $\kappa(\mathbf{x}, \mathbf{y})$(Dhillon et al., 2004; Zhang & Rudnicky, 2002). By introducing the feature map $\phi(\cdot)$, the mean squared error function can be expressed in the feature space by:

$$\mathrm{se}^\phi = \sum_{i=1}^{k} \sum_{j=1}^{\ell} z_{C_i, \mathbf{x}_j} \left\| \phi(\mathbf{x}_j) - \mathbf{m}_i^\phi \right\|^2$$

with $\mathbf{m}_i^\phi$, the cluster center of cluster C_i, defined by

$$\mathbf{m}_i^\phi = \frac{1}{|C_i|} \sum_{j=1}^{\ell} z_{C_i, \mathbf{x}_j} \phi(\mathbf{x}_j)$$

The Euclidean distance between $\phi(\mathbf{x}_i)$ and $\phi(\mathbf{x}_j)$ can be written as:

$$\begin{aligned}
D^2(\phi(\mathbf{x}_i), \phi(\mathbf{x}_j)) &= \left\| \phi(\mathbf{x}_i) - \phi(\mathbf{x}_j) \right\|^2 \\
&= \phi(\mathbf{x}_i)^T \phi(\mathbf{x}_i) - 2\phi(\mathbf{x}_i)^T \phi(\mathbf{x}_j) + \phi(\mathbf{x}_j)^T \phi(\mathbf{x}_j) \\
&= \kappa(\mathbf{x}_i, \mathbf{x}_i) - 2\kappa(\mathbf{x}_i, \mathbf{x}_j) + \kappa(\mathbf{x}_j, \mathbf{x}_j)
\end{aligned}$$

The computation of distances in this feature space can then be carried out by:

$$D^2(\phi(\mathbf{x}_j),\mathbf{m}_i^\phi) = \left\| \phi(\mathbf{x}_j) - \mathbf{m}_i^\phi \right\|^2$$

$$= \left\| \phi(\mathbf{x}_j) - \frac{1}{|C_i|} \sum_{l=1}^{\ell} z_{C_i,\mathbf{x}_l} \phi(\mathbf{x}_l) \right\|^2$$

$$= \phi(\mathbf{x}_j)^T \phi(\mathbf{x}_j) - \frac{2}{|C_i|} \sum_{l=1}^{\ell} z_{C_i,\mathbf{x}_l} \phi(\mathbf{x}_j)^T \phi(\mathbf{x}_l) + \frac{1}{|C_i|^2} \sum_{l=1}^{\ell} \sum_{p=1}^{\ell} z_{C_i,\mathbf{x}_l} z_{C_i,\mathbf{x}_p} \phi(\mathbf{x}_l)' \phi(\mathbf{x}_p)$$

Application of the kernel trick results in:

$$D^2(\phi(\mathbf{x}_j),\mathbf{m}_i^\phi) = \mathbf{K}_{jj} + f(C_i,\mathbf{x}_j) + g(C_i),$$

with

$$f(C_i,\mathbf{x}_j) = -\frac{2}{|C_i|} \sum_{l=1}^{\ell} z_{C_i,\mathbf{x}_l} \mathbf{K}_{jl}$$

$$g(C_i) = \frac{1}{|C_i|^2} \sum_{l=1}^{\ell} \sum_{p=1}^{\ell} z_{C_i,\mathbf{x}_l} z_{C_i,\mathbf{x}_p} \mathbf{K}_{lp}.$$

This gives the following formulation of the mean squared error criterion in the feature space:

$$se^\phi = \sum_{i=1}^{k} \sum_{j=1}^{\ell} z_{C_i,\mathbf{x}_j} (\mathbf{K}_{jj} + f(C_i,\mathbf{x}_j) + g(C_i)).$$

The kernel-based k-means algorithm solving the nonconvex optimization problem is then as follows.

Kernel k-Means Clustering Algorithm

1. Assign an initial clustering value to each sample, $z_{C_i,\mathbf{x}_j}, 1 \le i \le k, 1 \le j \le \ell$, forming k initial clusters $C_1, ..., C_k$.
2. For each cluster C_i, compute $|C_i|$ and $g(C_i)$.
3. For each training sample $\mathbf{x}_j$ and cluster C_i compute $f(C_i, \mathbf{x}_j)$.
4. Assign $\mathbf{x}_j$ to the closest cluster by computing the value of the indicator function

$$z_{C_i,\mathbf{x}_j} = \begin{cases} 1 & f(C_i,\mathbf{x}_j)+g(C_i) < f(C_h,\mathbf{x}_j)+g(C_h), \forall h \ne i, i, h = 1,\ldots,k \\ 0 & \text{otherwise} \end{cases}.$$

5. Repeat Steps 2, 3, and 4 until convergence is reached.

6. For each cluster C_i select the sample that is closest to the center as the representative centroid of cluster C_i by computing:

$$\mathbf{m}_i = \min_{\mathbf{x}_j \text{ s.t. } z_{C_i,\mathbf{x}_j}=1} D(\phi(\mathbf{x}_j), \mathbf{m}_i^\phi), \ 1 \leq i \leq k.$$

Note also that in this algorithm, the factor $\mathbf{K}_{jj}$ is ignored because it does not contribute to determine the closest cluster. Remember that the term $g(C_i)$ needs to be computed only once for each cluster in each iteration, while the term $f(C_i, \mathbf{x}_j)$ is calculated once per data point.

The objective function of the kernel k-means algorithm (see distortion score in the feature space) monotonically decreases in each iteration, which also holds for the classical k-means algorithm. The general structure of the traditional algorithm is thus preserved in its nonlinear version. Nevertheless, there are two main differences between both algorithms, namely, the nonlinear mapping via the kernel trick and the lack of an explicit centroid in the feature space. The mapping from the feature space back to the input space is called the pre-image problem and is nontrivial. Typically, the exact pre-image does not exist and can therefore only be approximated, which is typically considered with respect to kernel principal component analysis (Schölkopf et al., 1998). In this algorithm, a pseudocentroid is calculated instead. However, there exist iterative nonlinear optimization methods that attempt to solve this problem (Mika, Schölkopf, Smola, Müller, Scholz, & Rätsch, 1999).

This algorithm, unfortunately, is prone to local minima since the optimization problem is not convex. Considerable effort has been devoted to finding good initial guesses or inserting additional constraints in order to limit the effect of this fact on the quality of the solution obtained. The spectral clustering algorithm is a relaxation of this problem for which it is possible to find the global solution.

Spectral Clustering

Spectral clustering techniques have emerged as promising unsupervised learning methods to group data points that are similar. These methods have been successfully applied to machine learning, data analysis, image processing, pattern recognition, and very large-scale integration (VLSI) design. These methods can be regarded as relaxations of graph-cut problems on a fully connected graph. In this graph, each node represents a data point, and the edges between the data points are assigned weights that are equal to the affinities. Clustering then corresponds to partitioning the nodes in the graph into groups. Such a division of the graph nodes in two disjoint sets is called a graph cut.

In order to achieve a good clustering, one can see that it is undesirable to separate two nodes into different clusters if they are connected by an edge with a large weight (meaning that they have a large affinity). To cast this into an optimization problem, several graph-cut cost functions for clustering have been proposed in the literature, among which are the cut cost, the average cut cost, and the normalized cut cost (Shi & Malik, 2000). The cut cost is immediately computationally tractable (Blum & Chawla, 2001), but it often leads to degenerate results (where all but one of the clusters is trivially small; see Figure 2 (right) and Joachims,

2003, for an instructive artificially constructed example). This problem can largely be solved by using the average or normalized cut-cost functions, of which the average cut cost seems to be more vulnerable to outliers (distant samples, meaning that they have low affinity to all other points). Unfortunately, both optimizing the average and normalized cut costs are NP-complete problems. To get around this, spectral relaxations of these optimization problems have been proposed (Cristianini et al., 2002; Ng, Jordan, & Weiss, 2002; Shi & Malik, 2000). These spectral relaxations are known as spectral clustering algorithms.

Given an undirected graph $G = (V, E)$ where V is the set of ℓ nodes and E is the set of edges, the problem of graph partitioning consists of separating the graph into two sets A and B by eliminating edges connecting the two sets. The sets should be disjoint such that $A \cup B = V$ and $A \cap B = \varnothing$. The total weight of the edges that have to be eliminated is called the cut

$$cut(\mathcal{A}, \mathcal{B}) = \sum_{a \in A, b \in B} w(a, b) = \sum_{i,j} w(i, j)(q_i - q_j)^2,$$

where $w(a,b)$ is the associating weight between nodes a and b, and q_i is a cluster membership indicator of the form:

$$q_i = \begin{cases} 1, & \text{if } i \in A \\ -1, & \text{if } i \in B. \end{cases}$$

Minimizing the cut cost is equivalent to the following problem:

$$\min_{q} q^T (D - W) q$$

such that $\mathbf{q} \in \{-1, 1\}^\ell$,

where $\mathbf{D}$ is an $\ell \times \ell$ diagonal matrix with

$$d_i = \sum_j w(i, j)$$

on its diagonal, that is, the total connection from node i to all other nodes, and $\mathbf{W}$ is an $\ell \times \ell$ symmetric with ijth entry equal to $w(i,j)$. This problem, however, is NP hard due to the constraint on $\mathbf{q}$. A suboptimal solution can be found by relaxing the constraint and allowing real values for $\mathbf{q}$. The solution to the relaxed problem with constraint $\tilde{\mathbf{q}}^T \tilde{\mathbf{q}} = 1$ is given by the following eigenvalue problem:

$$\mathbf{L}\tilde{\mathbf{q}} = \lambda \tilde{\mathbf{q}}.$$

The matrix $\mathbf{L}$ is the Laplacian of the graph, and it is defined as $\mathbf{L} = \mathbf{D} - \mathbf{W}$, though other definitions may be found in the literature. The suboptimal solution $\tilde{\mathbf{q}}$ is the eigenvector corresponding to the second smallest eigenvalue (also called the Fiedler vector). The cut-cost criterion, however, has a bias for separating small sets of points. This is due to the fact that there are no restrictions related to the size or the balance of the clusters.

The normalized-cut criterion (Shi & Malik, 2000), defined as:

$$ncut(\mathcal{A},\mathcal{B}) = \frac{cut(\mathcal{A},\mathcal{B})}{d_{\mathcal{A}}} + \frac{cut(\mathcal{A},\mathcal{B})}{d_{\mathcal{B}}}$$

with $d_{\mathcal{A}} = \sum_{i \in \mathcal{A}} d_i$,

penalizes small sets or isolated points by taking into account the total weight of each cluster. Minimizing the normalized cut is equivalent to:

$$\min_{\mathbf{q}} \frac{\mathbf{q}^T \mathbf{L} \mathbf{q}}{\mathbf{q}^T \mathbf{D} \mathbf{q}}$$

such that $\mathbf{q} \in \{-1,1\}^{\ell}, \mathbf{q}^T \mathbf{D} \mathbf{1} = 0$,

where $\mathbf{1}$ is a $\ell \times 1$ vector of ones. However, this problem is NP complete in the same manner as the cut cost; an approximate solution can be found efficiently by relaxing the discrete constraint on $\mathbf{q}$. If $\mathbf{q}$ can take real values, then the normalized cut corresponds to the Rayleigh quotient of the following generalized eigenvalue problem:

$$\mathbf{L}\widetilde{\mathbf{q}} = \lambda \mathbf{D}\widetilde{\mathbf{q}}.$$

The constraint $\widetilde{\mathbf{q}}^T \mathbf{D} \mathbf{1} = 0$ is automatically satisfied in the generalized eigenproblem. The relaxed solution to the normalized cut is the Fiedler vector. Figure 2 illustrates a comparison between the normalized-cut and cut costs.

A different spectral algorithm was proposed in Ng et al. (2002), where the affinity matrix is first normalized using symmetric divisive normalization. The resulting eigenvalue problem is:

$$\mathbf{D}^{-1/2} \mathbf{W} \mathbf{D}^{-1/2} \widetilde{\mathbf{q}} = \lambda \widetilde{\mathbf{q}}.$$

Whereas standard clustering methods often assume Gaussian class distributions, spectral clustering methods do not. In order to achieve this goal, one avoids the use of the Euclidean distance (as a dissimilarity measure) or the inner product (as a similarity or affinity measure). Instead, often an affinity measure based on an RBF kernel is used:

$$\mathbf{A}(\mathbf{x}_i, \mathbf{x}_j) = \exp(-\|\mathbf{x}_i - \mathbf{x}_j\|^2 / 2\sigma^2).$$

Figure 2. Partitioning for two different fully connected graphs. (Left) Normalized-cut cost of the graph attempts to produce balanced (similar-sized) clusters, while the cut cost (number of edges) is minimized. (Right) Cut cost favors cutting small sets of isolated nodes in the graph as the cut increases with the number of edges going across the two partitioned parts.

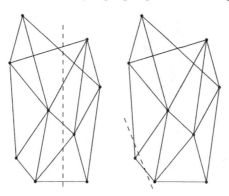

The width σ^2 of the kernel function controls how rapidly the affinity matrix $\mathbf{A}_{ij}$ falls off with the distance between x_i and x_j. Even though in spectral clustering often (though not exclusively) an RBF kernel is used, the positive definiteness of the RBF kernel is in fact not a requirement. On the other hand, affinities should be symmetric and all entries must be positive (which is the case indeed for the RBF kernel). The matrix containing the affinities between all pairs of samples should therefore be referred to as the affinity matrix in a spectral clustering context (and not as the kernel matrix).

Suppose a data set that contains samples $\mathbf{x}_1, ..., \mathbf{x}_\ell$. A well-known instance of spectral clustering, proposed by Ng et al. (2002), finds k clusters in the data as follows.

Spectral Clustering Algorithm

1. Form the affinity matrix A (with dimensions $\ell \times \ell$) defined by $\mathbf{A}_{ij} = \exp(-\left\| \mathbf{x}_i - \mathbf{x}_j \right\|^2 / 2\sigma^2)$ if $i \neq j$, and $\mathbf{A}_{ii} = 0$.

2. Define $\mathbf{D}$ to be the diagonal matrix of which the element (i, i) is the sum of row i of $\mathbf{A}$, and construct the matrix $\mathbf{L} = \mathbf{D}^{-1/2}\mathbf{A}\mathbf{D}^{-1/2}$.

3. Find $\mathbf{u}_1, ..., \mathbf{u}_k$ the k largest eigenvectors of $\mathbf{L}$ (chosen to be orthogonal to each other in the case of repeated eigenvalues), and form the matrix $\mathbf{U} = [\mathbf{u}_1, \mathbf{u}_2, ..., \mathbf{u}_k]$ (with dimensions $\ell \times k$) by stacking the eigenvectors in columns.

4. Form the matrix $\mathbf{V}$ from $\mathbf{U}$ by renormalizing each row of $\mathbf{U}$ to have unit length, that is, $\mathbf{V}_{ij} = \mathbf{U}_{ij} / ((\sum_j \mathbf{U}_{ij}^2)^{1/2})$.

5. Treating each row of $\mathbf{V}$ as a sample with dimension k, cluster these into k clusters via k-means or any other algorithm (that attempts to minimize the distortion).

6. Finally, assign the original sample $\mathbf{x}_i$ to cluster C_j if and only if row i of the matrix $\mathbf{V}$ is assigned to cluster C_j.

Figure 3. (Left) The block diagonal structure of the affinity matrix clearly shows that two dense clusters with sparse connections between them are present. (Right) Eigenvector $\widetilde{q}_2$ holds the information of the true partition of the data.

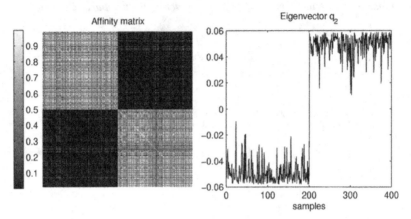

Conditions in which the algorithm is expected to do well are described by Ng et al. (2002). Once the samples are represented by rows of **V** (with dimension k), tight clusters are formed. An artificial example is illustrated in Figure 3.

Cluster-Validation Methods

Validation of the clustering results can be done internally, that is, by assessing the quality of a clustering result based on statistical properties, and externally, that is, reflecting the level of agreement of a clustering result with an external partition, for example, existing diagnostic classes generally used in clinical practice (Bolshakova et al., 2005; Halkidi & Vazirgiannis, 2005; Handl et al., 2005; Jain & Dubes, 1988; Milligan & Cooper, 1985). Moreover, internal cluster-validation techniques can also be used for selecting the best clustering result when comparing different clustering methods, several random initializations, a different number of clusters, a range of kernel parameters (e.g., the width σ^2 of the RBF kernel), and so forth. In this section, a formulation of three well-known internal validation methods in the input space (global silhouette index, Calinski-Harabasz index [F-statistic], and distortion score) and two external validation methods (Rand index and adjusted Rand index) are given first (applied in the input space) for reason of completeness. However, in order to be useful for kernel k-means clustering (and eventually other kernel clustering methods as well), we also derive the internal validation criteria for usage in the feature space.

Internal Validation

Global Silhouette Index

An expression pattern from a patient can be considered to be well clustered if its distance to the other expression patterns of the same cluster is small and the distance to the expression patterns of other clusters is larger. This criterion can be formalized by using the silhouette index (Kaufman & Rousseeuw, 1990), that is, for testing the cluster coherence. This measure validates the cluster result on statistical grounds only (statistical validation). Clinical information is not used here.

Suppose $\mathbf{x}_j$ is an expression pattern that belongs to cluster C_i. Call $v(\mathbf{x}_j)$ (also called the within dissimilarity) the average distance of x_j to all other expression patterns from C_i. Suppose C_h is a cluster different from C_i. Define $w(\mathbf{x}_j)$ (also called the between dissimilarity) as the minimum over all clusters C_h different from C_i of the average distance from $\mathbf{x}_j$ to all expression patterns of C_h. The silhouette width $s(\mathbf{x}_j)$ of expression patterns $\mathbf{x}_j$ is now defined as follows:

$$s(\mathbf{x}_j) = \frac{w(\mathbf{x}_j) - v(\mathbf{x}_j)}{\max(v(\mathbf{x}_j), w(\mathbf{x}_j))},$$

with $\mathbf{x}_j \in C_i$, and

$$v(\mathbf{x}_j) = \frac{1}{|C_i| - 1} \sum_{\substack{\mathbf{x}_l \in C_i \\ \mathbf{x}_l \neq \mathbf{x}_j}} \left\| \mathbf{x}_j - \mathbf{x}_l \right\|^2$$

$$w(\mathbf{x}_j) = \min_{h=1,\ldots,i-1,i+1,\ldots,k} \left(\frac{1}{|C_h|} \sum_{\mathbf{x}_l \in C_h} \left\| \mathbf{x}_j - \mathbf{x}_l \right\|^2 \right).$$

Note that $-1 \leq s(\mathbf{x}_j) \leq 1$. Consider two extreme situations now. First, suppose that the within dissimilarity $v(\mathbf{x}_j)$ is significantly smaller than the between dissimilarity $w(\mathbf{x}_j)$. This is the ideal case and $s(\mathbf{x}_j)$ will be approximately equal to one. This occurs when $\mathbf{x}_j$ is well clustered and there is little doubt that $\mathbf{x}_j$ is assigned to an appropriate cluster. Second, suppose that $v(\mathbf{x}_j)$ is significantly larger than $w(\mathbf{x}_j)$. Now $s(\mathbf{x}_j)$ will be approximately -1 and $\mathbf{x}_j$ has in fact been assigned to the wrong cluster (worst-case scenario).

Two other measures can now be defined: the average silhouette width of a cluster and the average silhouette width of the entire data set. The first is defined as the average of $s(\mathbf{x}_j)$ for all expression patterns of a cluster, and the second is defined as the average of $s(\mathbf{x}_j)$ for all expression patterns in the data set. This last value can be used to mutually compare different cluster results and can be used as an inherent part of clustering algorithms if its value is optimized during the clustering process.

When using this validation measure in combination with kernel clustering methods performing the actual clustering in the feature space, for example, kernel k-means clustering, using this definition of the silhouette index leads to wrong results since the distances between the expression patterns are computed in the input space. We therefore derive the definition of the silhouette index for computation in the feature space.

By introducing the feature map $\phi(\cdot)$, $v(\mathbf{x}_j)$ and $w(\mathbf{x}_j)$ can be expressed in the feature space as:

$$v^{\phi}(\mathbf{x}_j) = \frac{1}{(|C_i|-1)} \sum_{\substack{\mathbf{x}_l \in C_i \\ \mathbf{x}_l \neq \mathbf{x}_j}} \left\| \phi(\mathbf{x}_j) - \phi(\mathbf{x}_l) \right\|^2$$

$$w^{\phi}(\mathbf{x}_j) = \min_{h=1,\ldots,i-1,i+1,\ldots,k} \left(\frac{1}{|C_h|} \sum_{\mathbf{x}_j \in C_h} \left\| \phi(\mathbf{x}_j) - \phi(\mathbf{x}_l) \right\|^2 \right), \text{ for } \mathbf{x}_j \in C_i.$$

Replacing all the dot products by a kernel function $\kappa(\cdot,\cdot)$ results in:

$$v^{\phi}(\mathbf{x}_j) = \frac{1}{(|C_i|-1)} \kappa(\mathbf{x}_j, \mathbf{x}_j) - \frac{2}{(|C_i|-1)} \sum_{\substack{\mathbf{x}_l \in C_i \\ \mathbf{x}_l \neq \mathbf{x}_j}} \kappa(\mathbf{x}_j, \mathbf{x}_l) + \frac{1}{(|C_i|-1)} \sum_{\substack{\mathbf{x}_l \in C_i \\ \mathbf{x}_l \neq \mathbf{x}_j}} \kappa(\mathbf{x}_l, \mathbf{x}_l)$$

$$w^{\phi}(\mathbf{x}_j) = \min_{h=1,\ldots,i-1,i+1,\ldots,k} \left(\frac{1}{|C_h|} \kappa(\mathbf{x}_j, \mathbf{x}_j) - \frac{2}{|C_h|} \sum_{\mathbf{x}_l \in C_h} \kappa(\mathbf{x}_j, \mathbf{x}_l) + \frac{1}{|C_h|} \sum_{\mathbf{x}_l \in C_h} \kappa(\mathbf{x}_l, \mathbf{x}_l) \right), \text{ for } \mathbf{x}_j \in C_i.$$

Consequently, the silhouette index can be computed in the feature space as:

$$s^{\phi}(\mathbf{x}_j) = \frac{w^{\phi}(\mathbf{x}_j) - v^{\phi}(\mathbf{x}_j)}{\max(v^{\phi}(\mathbf{x}_j), w^{\phi}(\mathbf{x}_j))}.$$

Calinski-Harabasz Index

The Calinski-Harabasz index (Calinski & Harabasz, 1974; Milligan & Cooper, 1985), also called F-statistic, is a measure of intercluster dissimilarity over intracluster dissimilarity. For ℓ expression patterns and k clusters, the Calinski-Harabasz index CH is defined as:

$$CH = \frac{trB/(k-1)}{trW/(\ell-k)},$$

with B and W the between- and within-cluster scatter matrices (measures of dissimilarity), respectively. A larger value for CH indicates a better clustering since the between-cluster dissimilarity is then supposed to be large, while the within-cluster dissimilarity is then supposed to be small. Maximum values of the CH index are often used to indicate the correct number of partitions in the data. The trace of the between-cluster scatter matrix B can be written as:

$$trB = \sum_{i=1}^{k} |C_i| \, \|\mathbf{m}_i - \mathbf{m}\|^2 = \sum_{i=1}^{k} |C_i| \left\| \frac{1}{|C_i|} \sum_{\mathbf{x}_j \in C_i} \mathbf{x}_j - \frac{1}{\ell} \sum_{\mathbf{x}_l \in S} \mathbf{x}_l \right\|^2,$$

where $|C_i|$ denotes the number of elements in cluster C_i with centroid m_i, and m the centroid of the entire data set S. The trace of the within-cluster scatter matrix W can be written as:

$$trW = \sum_{i=1}^{k} \sum_{\mathbf{x}_j \in C_i} \|\mathbf{x}_j - \mathbf{m}_i\|^2 = \sum_{i=1}^{k} \sum_{\mathbf{x}_j \in C_i} \left\| \mathbf{x}_j - \frac{1}{|C_i|} \sum_{\mathbf{x}_l \in C_i} \mathbf{x}_l \right\|^2.$$

Therefore, the CH index can be written as:

$$CH = \frac{\displaystyle\sum_{i=1}^{k} |C_i| \left\| \frac{1}{|C_i|} \sum_{\mathbf{x}_j \in C_i} \mathbf{x}_j - \frac{1}{\ell} \sum_{\mathbf{x}_l \in S} \mathbf{x}_l \right\|^2 \Big/ k - 1}{\displaystyle\sum_{i=1}^{k} \sum_{\mathbf{x}_j \in Ci} \left\| \mathbf{x}_j - \frac{1}{|C_i|} \sum_{\mathbf{x}_l \in C_k} \mathbf{x}_l \right\|^2 \Big/ \ell - k}.$$

By introducing the feature map $\phi(\cdot)$, the traces of the between-cluster scatter matrix B and of the within-cluster scatter matrix W can be expressed as:

$$trB^{\phi} = \sum_{i=1}^{k} |C_i| \left\| \frac{1}{|C_i|} \sum_{\mathbf{x}_j \in C_i} \phi(\mathbf{x}_j) - \frac{1}{\ell} \sum_{\mathbf{x}_l \in S} \phi(\mathbf{x}_l) \right\|^2$$

and

$$trW^{\phi} = \sum_{i=1}^{k} \sum_{\mathbf{x}_j \in C_i} \left\| \phi(\mathbf{x}_j) - \frac{1}{|C_i|} \sum_{\mathbf{x}_l \in C_i} \phi(\mathbf{x}_l) \right\|^2.$$

After applying the kernel trick (as done for the global silhouette index), the CH index can be calculated in feature space by:

$$CH^{\phi} = \frac{trB^{\phi}/(k-1)}{trW^{\phi}/(\ell-k)}.$$

Distortion Score

The mean squared error criterion, which is the objective function in both classical and kernel *k*-means clustering, can be used for internal validation. In this context, the mean squared error criterion is called the distortion score.

For a set of expression patterns $\mathbf{x}_j, j = 1, ..., \ell$, the distortion score is formulated as:

$$se = \sum_{i=1}^{k} \sum_{j=1}^{\ell} z_{C_i, \mathbf{x}_j} \left\| \mathbf{x}_j - \mathbf{m}_i \right\|^2,$$

with the indicator function $z_{C_i, \mathbf{x}_j}$ defined as

$$z_{C_i, \mathbf{x}_j} = \begin{cases} 1 & \text{if } \mathbf{x}_j \in C_i \\ 0 & \text{otherwise} \end{cases}$$

with

$$\sum_{i=1}^{k} z_{C_i, \mathbf{x}_j} = 1 \qquad \forall j$$

and the centroid (or prototype) $\mathbf{m}_i$ of cluster C_i defined as

$$\mathbf{m}_i = \frac{1}{|C_i|} \sum_{j=1}^{\ell} z_{C_i \mathbf{x}_j} \mathbf{x}_j.$$

In the feature space, the distortion score can be expressed by:

$$se^{\phi} = \sum_{i=1}^{k} \sum_{j=1}^{\ell} z_{C_i, \mathbf{x}_j} \left\| \phi(\mathbf{x}_j) - \mathbf{m}_i^{\phi} \right\|^2$$

$$= \sum_{i=1}^{k} \sum_{j=1}^{\ell} z_{C_i, \mathbf{x}_j} (\mathbf{K}_{jj} + f(C_i, \mathbf{x}_j) + g(C_i)),$$

with $f(C_i, \mathbf{x}_j)$, $g(C_i)$, and $\mathbf{m}_i^{\phi}$ defined as in the kernel *k*-means algorithm.

External Validation

Rand Index

The Rand index (Rand, 1971; Yeung, Fraley, Murua, Raftery, & Ruzzo, 2001; Yeung, Haynor, & Ruzzo, 2001) is a measure that reflects the level of agreement of a cluster result with an external partition, that is, an existing partition of a known cluster structure of the data. This external criterion could, for example, be the existing diagnostic classes generally used by experts in clinical practice (e.g., groups of patients with a similar type of cancer, groups of patients responding to therapy in a similar way, or groups of patients with a similar kind of diagnosis), a predefined cluster structure if one is clustering synthetic data where the clusters are known in advance, or another cluster result obtained using other parameter settings for a specific clustering algorithm or obtained using other clustering algorithms. Note that the latter could be used to investigate how sensitive a cluster result is to the choice of the algorithm or parameter setting. If this result proves to be relatively stable, one could assume that pronounced structures are present in the data possibly reflecting subcategories that are clinically relevant.

Suppose one wants to compare two partitions (the cluster result at hand and the external criterion) of a set of ℓ expression patterns. Suppose that a is the number of expression pattern pairs that are placed in the same subset (or cluster) in both partitions. Suppose that d is the number of expression pattern pairs that are placed in different subsets in both partitions. The Rand index is then defined as the fraction of agreement between both partitions:

$$r = \frac{a+d}{M}$$

with M as the maximum number of all expression pattern pairs in the data set, that is, $M = \ell(\ell - 1)/2$. This can also be rewritten by $M = a + b + c + d$, with b as the number of expression pattern pairs that are placed in the same cluster according to the external criterion but in different clusters according to the cluster result, and c as the number of expression pattern pairs that are placed in the same cluster according to the cluster result but in different clusters according to the external criterion. The Rand index lies between zero and one (one if both partitions are identical), and can be viewed as the proportion of agreeing expression pattern pairs between two partitions.

Adjusted Rand Index

One disadvantage of the Rand index is that the expected value of two random partitions is not a constant value (Yeung, Haynor, et al., 2001) and depends on the number of clusters k. In order to compare clustering results with different numbers of clusters k, the adjusted Rand index was proposed by Hubert and Arabie (1985).

The general form of an index with a constant expected value is:

$$\frac{\text{index} - \text{expected index}}{\text{maximum index} - \text{expected index}},$$

which is bounded above by 1 and below by -1, and has an expected value of 0 for random clustering.

Let n_{ij} be the number of expression patterns that are in both cluster u_i (according to the external criterion) and cluster v_j (according to the cluster result). Let n_i and n_j be the number of expression patterns in cluster u_i and cluster v_j, respectively. According to Hubert and Arabie (1985), the adjusted Rand index can be expressed in a simple form by:

$$ar = \frac{\sum_{i,j}\binom{n_{ij}}{2} - \left(\sum_{i}\binom{n_{i\cdot}}{2}\sum_{j}\binom{n_{\cdot j}}{2}\right)/\binom{n}{2}}{\frac{1}{2}\left(\sum_{i}\binom{n_{i\cdot}}{2} + \sum_{j}\binom{n_{\cdot j}}{2}\right) - \left(\sum_{i}\binom{n_{i\cdot}}{2}\sum_{j}\binom{n_{\cdot j}}{2}\right)/\binom{n}{2}}.$$

Experiments

In this section, the clustering and cluster-validation methods described are demonstrated on acute leukemia data (Golub et al., 1999) and colon cancer data (Alon et al., 1999). Golub et al. studied microarray data obtained from the bone marrow or peripheral blood of 72 patients with ALL or AML using an Affymetrix chip. Although the structure of this data set is simple and the separation between the two conditions is more pronounced than in most other cases, it can still be considered as a frequently used benchmark. The data set contains 47 patients with ALL and 25 patients with AML. The expression matrix contains 7,129 genes. Alon et al. studied 40 tumor and 22 normal colon tissue samples using an Affymetrix chip. The array contained probes for more than 6,500 genes, but the data that can be downloaded includes only the 2,000 genes with the highest minimal intensity across the 62 tissues.

Preprocessing of the acute leukemia data set is done by thresholding and log transformation, similar to how it was done in the original publication. Thresholding is achieved by restricting gene expression levels to be larger than 20; that is, expression levels that are smaller than 20 will be set to 20. Concerning the log transformation, the natural logarithm of the expression levels is taken. For the colon cancer data set, only log transformation is done, as in the original publication. Further preprocessing of both data sets is done by standardization (normalization). For classical k-means, this is followed by principal component analysis (without the selection of principal components). Although kernel clustering techniques are capable of handling high-dimensional data, one should not forget the possible benefits of performing preprocessing steps that remove noise before using any clustering technique.

Tuning of the hyperparameters is an important issue, discussed previously in a large number of publications. We therefore only refer to some of these studies (Halkidi & Vazirgiannis, 2005; Handl et al., 2005). However, since kernel clustering methods require tuning of the kernel parameters as well, some research effort still needs to be performed on this subject.

Note that classical k-means clustering and kernel k-means clustering with a linear kernel require the optimization of a number of clusters and the random initialization. Kernel k-means with an RBF kernel and spectral clustering, however, also require the additional optimization of the kernel parameter σ^2. Tuning these hyperparameters needs to be performed based on internal validation criteria.

Results

Since both data sets contain two given diagnostic categories, we restrict the number of clusters k to be equal to two. The initialization is optimized by repeating each k-means or kernel k-means algorithm 100 times, selecting the best result based on the distortion score within these algorithms (note that this is done for each value of σ^2). Optimization of this kernel parameter σ^2 is done based on the global silhouette index. Note that only intervals for σ^2 with meaningful cluster results are considered. For the optimal value of σ^2, both external validation indices (i.e., the Rand and adjusted Rand index) are reported as well.

Silhouette plots (representing for each cluster the sorted silhouette indices for all samples) and tuning curves (tuning the kernel parameter σ^2 based on the global silhouette index), followed by a table presenting global silhouette, Rand, and adjusted Rand indices for the optimal kernel parameter σ^2, are first shown for the acute leukemia data and then for the colon cancer data.

From these results, we can conclude that spectral clustering, unlike the other clustering algorithms, gives very good and consistent clustering results in terms of the global silhouette index (internal validation) for both data sets. Note that the results obtained by any optimally tuned clustering algorithm (classical k-means, kernel k-means with linear or RBF kernel, and spectral clustering) are not correlated to the given diagnostic categories (external partitions). However, this does not mean that these clustering results are clinically or biologically irrelevant; that is, these could correspond to other known or unknown diagnostic categories.

Figure 4. Silhouette plots of classical k-means (left) and kernel k-means clustering (right) on the acute leukemia data. These plots show the sorted silhouette indices (x-axis) for all samples in each cluster (y-axis).

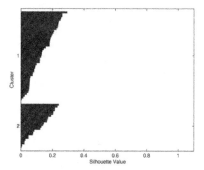 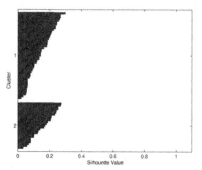

Figure 5. Tuning curve (left) and silhouette plot (right) of kernel k-means clustering on the acute leukemia data. The tuning curve shows the global silhouette index (y-axis) for a range of values for kernel parameter σ^2 (x-axis). The silhouette plot shows the sorted silhouette indices (x-axis) for all samples in each cluster (y-axis).

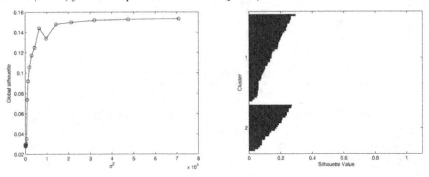

Figure 6. Tuning curve (left) and silhouette plot (right) of spectral clustering on the acute leukemia data. See Figure 5 for more detailed information on the tuning curve and silhouette plot.

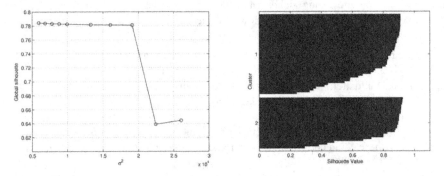

Table 1. Global silhouette, Rand, and adjusted Rand indices for the optimal kernel parameter σ^2 are given for all clustering methods on the acute leukemia data. There are two conclusions: (a) Spectral clustering clearly gives the best results in terms of internal validation, and (2) external validation shows that the clustering results are not correlated to the given diagnostic categories. However, these results could correspond to other known or unknown diagnostic categories.

	Kernel parameter σ^2	Global silhouette index	Adjusted Rand index	Rand index
k-means clustering	-	0.12988	-0.021418	0.49335
Kernel k-means clustering with linear kernel	-	0.15456	-0.017564	0.49452
Kernel k-means clustering with RBF kernel	709220.0	0.15337	-0.017564	0.49452
Spectral clustering	5913.0	0.78436	0.00258	0.49656

Figure 7. Silhouette plots of classical k-means (left) and kernel k-means clustering (right) on the colon cancer data. See Figure 4 for more detailed information on the silhouette plot.

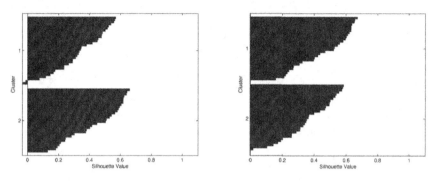

Figure 8. Tuning curve (left) and silhouette plot (right) of kernel k-means clustering on the colon cancer data. See Figure 5 for more detailed information on the tuning curve and silhouette plot.

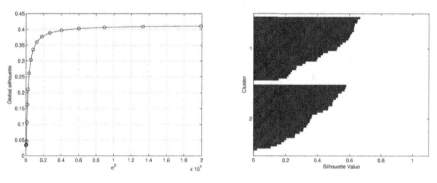

Figure 9. Tuning curve (left) and silhouette plot (right) of spectral clustering on the colon cancer data. See Figure 5 for more detailed information on the tuning curve and silhouette plot.

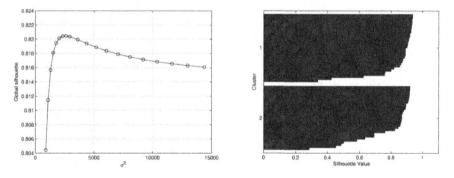

Table 2. Global silhouette, Rand, and adjusted Rand indices for the optimal kernel parameter σ^2 are given for all clustering methods on the colon cancer data. There are two conclusions: (a) Spectral clustering clearly gives the best results in terms of internal validation, and (b) external validation shows that the clustering results are not correlated to the given diagnostic categories. However, these results could correspond to other known or unknown diagnostic categories.

	Kernel parameter σ^2	Global silhouette index	Adjusted Rand index	Rand index
k-means clustering	-	0.3948	-0.0058061	0.49656
Kernel k-means clustering with linear kernel	-	0.41423	-0.0058	0.49656
Kernel k-means clustering with RBF kernel	198970.0	0.41073	-0.0058061	0.49656
Spectral clustering	2596.4	0.82046	-0.0058	0.49656

Conclusion

Most of the classical techniques that have previously been applied to analyze microarrays rely on specifically designed procedures in order to deal with the particular challenges posed by the gene expression data at hand (Alon et al., 1999; Golub et al., 1999). Therefore, these procedures are not guaranteed to perform well on other microarray data sets and cannot be considered as a general approach. In most publications, some way of input selection of a subset of relevant genes is performed first instead of systematically analyzing thousands of genes simultaneously. Although performing gene selection before clustering may improve the discrimination between the known groups, the choice for the best gene-selection method is highly dependent on the data set considered. The techniques presented here do not make any assumptions neither on the distribution of the data nor on the relevance on the input variables (genes), providing a more general approach that can be systematically extended to other microarray data sets. The model-selection step, that is, the choice of the kernel width and the choice of the optimal number of clusters, is often skipped for both kernel k-means and spectral clustering in most of the related publications. In this chapter, at least three variants for tuning this parameter based on different internal quality measures of the clusters have been proposed. Since these are internal measures, however, high correlations with external partitions are not ensured. Consequently, more sophisticated methods rather than the silhouette index (e.g., kernel alignment [Cristianini et al., 2002] and bounds derived from the formulation [Shi & Malik, 2000]) need to be considered or even defined for model selection. This way, the results and correlation with external partitions could be further improved.

In summary, kernel clustering methods like kernel k-means and spectral clustering are especially designed for clustering data that contain clusters that are not linearly separable in order to handle nonlinear relationships in the data. Moreover, these techniques allow for dealing with high-dimensional data. It was shown in this chapter that these properties make kernel clustering methods specifically interesting for application on the high-dimensional microarray data (with or without preprocessing steps). Using these techniques for knowledge discovery in clinical microarray data analysis may therefore allow the discovery of new clinically relevant groups in the future.

Acknowledgments

Nathalie Pochet is a research assistant of the IWT at the Katholieke Universiteit Leuven, Belgium. Fabian Ojeda is a research assistant at the Katholieke Universiteit Leuven, Belgium. Frank De Smet is a postdoctoral research assistant at the Katholieke Universiteit Leuven, Belgium, and a medical advisor at the National Alliance of Christian Mutualities, Belgium. Tijl De Bie is a postdoctoral research assistant at the Katholieke Universiteit Leuven, Belgium. Johan Suykens is an associate professor at the Katholieke Universiteit Leuven, Belgium. Bart De Moor is a full professor at the Katholieke Universiteit Leuven, Belgium. Research was supported by GOA-Mefisto 666, GOA-Ambiorics, IDO (IOTA), and several PhD, postdoc, and fellow grants of the Research Council KUL; PhD and postdoc Grants and Projects G.0240.99, G.0115.01, G.0407.02, G.0197.02, G.0141.03, G.0491.03, G.0120.03, G.0413.03, G.0388.03, G.0229.03, G.0241.04, G.0452.04, and G.0499.04, and research communities ICCoS, ANMMM, and MLDM of the Flemish government (FWO); Bil. Int. Collaboration Hungary/Poland (AWI); PhD Grants STWW-Genprom, GBOU-Mc-Know, GBOU-SQUAD, and GBOU-ANA of IWT; DWTC: IUAP V-22 (2002-2006) and PODO-II (CP/01/40) of the Belgian federal government; FP5 CAGE of the European Union; ERNSI; NoE Biopattern; NoE E-tumours; Eureka 2063-IMPACT; Eureka 2419-FliTE; and contracts and research agreements with ISMC/IPCOS, Data4s, TML, Elia, LMS, IPCOS, and Mastercard.

References

Alon, A., Barkai, N., Notterman, D. A., Gish, K., Ybarra, S., Mack, D., et al. (1999). Broad patterns of gene expression revealed by clustering analysis of tumor and normal colon tissues probed by oligonucleotide arrays. In *Proceedings of the National Academy of Science USA, 96*, (pp. 6745-6750).

Ben-Hur, A., Horn, D., Siegelmann, H. T., & Vapnik, V. (2001). Support vector clustering. *Journal of Machine Learning Research, 2*, 125-137.

Blum, A., & Chawla, S. (2001). Learning from labeled and unlabeled data using graph mincuts. In *Proceedings of the 18th International Conference on Machine Learning* (pp. 19-26).

Bolshakova, N., & Azuaje, F. (2003). Cluster validation techniques for genome expression data. *Signal Processing, 83*, 825-833.

Bolshakova, N., Azuaje, F., & Cunningham, P. (2005). An integrated tool for microarray data clustering and cluster validity assessment. *Bioinformatics, 21*(4), 451-455.

Calinski, T., & Harabasz, J. (1974). A dendrite method for cluster analysis. *Communications in Statistics, 3*(1), 1-27.

Cristianini, N., Shawe-Taylor, J., & Kandola, J. (2002). Spectral kernel methods for clustering. *Advances in Neural Information Processing Systems, 14*.

De Bie, T., Cristianini, N., & Rosipal R. (2004). Eigenproblems in pattern recognition. In E. Bayro-Corrochano (Ed.), *Handbook of computational geometry for pattern recognition, computer vision, neurocomputing and robotics*. Springer-Verlag.

De Smet, F., Mathys, J., Marchal, K., Thijs, G., De Moor, B., & Moreau, Y. (2002). Adaptive quality based clustering of gene expression profiles. *Bioinformatics, 18*(5), 735-746.

Dhillon, I. S., Guan, Y., & Kulis, B. (2004a). Kernel k-means, spectral clustering and normalized cuts. In *Proceedings of the 10th ACM SIGKDD International Conference on Knowledge Discovery and Data Mining* (pp. 551-556).

Dhillon, I. S., Guan, Y., & Kulis, B. (2004b). *A unified view of kernel k-means: Spectral clustering and graph partitioning* (Tech. Rep. No. TR-04-25). UTCS.

Dubes, R., & Jain, A. K. (1979). Validity studies in clustering methodologies. *Pattern Recognition Letters, 11*, 235-254.

Eisen, M. B., Spellman, P. T., Brown, P. O., & Botstein, D. (1998). Cluster analysis and display of genome-wide expression patterns. In *Proceedings of the National Academy of Science USA, 95* (pp. 14863-14868).

Golub, T. R., Slonim, D. K., Tamayo, P., Huard, C., Gassenbeck, M., Mesirov, J. P., et al. (1999). Molecular classification of cancer: Class discovery and class prediction by gene expression monitoring. *Science, 286*, 531-537.

Halkidi, M., Batistakis, Y., & Vazirgiannis, M. (2001). On clustering validation techniques. *Journal of Intelligent Information Systems, 17*(2-3), 107-145.

Halkidi, M., & Vazirgiannis, M. (2005). Quality assessment approaches in data mining. In *The data mining and knowledge discovery handbook* (pp. 661-696).

Handl, J., Knowles, J., & Kell, D. B. (2005). Computational cluster validation in post-genomic data analysis. *Bioinformatics, 21*, 3201-3212.

Hastie, T., Tibshirani, R., Eisen, M. B., Alizadeh, A., Levy, R., Staudt, L., et al. (2000). Gene shaving as a method for identifying distinct sets of genes with similar expression patterns. *Genome Biology, 1*, 1-21.

Hubert, L., & Arabie, P. (1985). Comparing partitions. *Journal of Classification*, 193-218.

Jain, A. K., & Dubes, R. C. (1988). *Algorithms for clustering data*. Englewood Cliffs, NJ: Prentice Hall.

Joachims, T. (2003). Transductive learning via spectral graph partitioning. In *Proceedings of the International Conference on Machine Learning* (pp. 290-297).

Joliffe, I. T. (1986). *Principal component analysis*. Springer-Verlag.

Kannan, R., Vempala, S., & Vetta, A. (2004). On clusterings: Good, bad and spectral. *Journal of the ACM, 51*(3), 497-515.

MacQueen, J. (1967). Some methods for classification and analysis of multivariate observations. In *Proceedings of the 5th Berkeley Symposium on Mathematical Statistics and Probability* (Vol. 1, pp. 281-297).

Madeira, S. C., & Oliveira, A. L. (2004). Biclustering algorithms for biological data analysis: A survey. *IEEE Transactions on Computational Biology and Bioinformatics, 1*, 24-45.

Mika, S., Schölkopf, B., Smola, A. J., Müller, K. R., Scholz, M., & Rätsch, G. (1999). Kernel PCA and de–noising in feature spaces. *Advances in Neural Information Processing Systems, 11*.

Milligan, G. W., & Cooper, M. C. (1985). An examination of procedures for determining the number of clusters. *Psychometrika, 50*, 159-179.

Ng, A., Jordan, M. I., & Weiss, Y. (2002). On spectral clustering: Analysis and an algorithm. *Advances in Neural Information Processing Systems, 14*.

Pochet, N., De Smet, F., Suykens, J. A. K., & De Moor, B. L. R. (2004). Systematic benchmarking of microarray data classification: Assessing the role of nonlinearity and dimensionality reduction. *Bioinformatics, 20*, 3185-3195.

Qin, J., Lewis, D. P., & Noble, W. S. (2003). Kernel hierarchical gene clustering from microarray expression data. *Bioinformatics, 19*, 2097-2104.

Quackenbush, J. (2001). Computational analysis of microarray data. *Nature Reviews Genetics*, 418-427.

Rand, W. M. (1971). Objective criteria for the evaluation of clustering methods. *Journal of the American Statistical Association, 66*, 846-850.

Rosen, J. E., Costouros, N. G., Lorang, D., Burns, A. L., Alexander, H. R., Skarulis, M. C., et al. (2005). Gland size is associated with changes in gene expression profiles in sporadic parathyroid adenomas. *Annals of Surgical Oncology, 12*(5), 412-416.

Rousseeuw, P. J. (1987). Silhouettes: A graphical aid to the interpretation and validation of cluster analysis. *Journal of Computational and Applied Mathematics*, 53-65.

Schölkopf, B., Smola, A., & Müller, K. (1998). Nonlinear component analysis as a kernel eigenvalue problem. *Neural Computation, 10*, 1299-1319.

Sheng, Q., Moreau, Y., & De Moor, B. (2003). Biclustering microarray data by Gibbs sampling. *Bioinformatics, European Conference on Computational Biology Proceedings, 19*, ii196-ii205.

Shi, J., & Malik, J. (2000). Normalized cuts and image segmentation. *IEEE Transactions on Pattern Analysis and Machine Intelligence, 22*(8), 808-905.

Suykens, J. A. K., Van Gestel, T., De Brabanter, J., De Moor, B., & Vandewalle, J. (2002). *Least squares support vector machines*. Singapore: World Scientific Publishing.

Tavazoie, S., Hughes, J. D., Campbell, M. J., Cho, R. J., & Church, G. M. (1999). Systematic determination of genetic network architecture. *Nature Genetics, 22*, 281-285.

Van 't Veer, L. J., Dai, H., Van De Vijver, M. J., He, Y. D., Hart, A. A. M., Mao, M., et al. (2002). Gene expression profiling predicts clinical outcome of breast cancer. *Nature, 415*, 530-536.

Vapnik, V. N. (1998). *Statistical learning theory.* New York: Wiley-Interscience.

Yeung, K., Fraley, C., Murua, A., Raftery, A., & Ruzzo, W. (2001). Model-based clustering and data transformations for gene expression data. *Bioinformatics, 17*(10), 977-987.

Yeung, K., Haynor, D., & Ruzzo, W. (2001). Validating clustering for gene expression data. *Bioinformatics, 17*(4), 309-318.

Zhang, R., & Rudnicky, A. I. (2002). A large scale clustering scheme for kernel *k*-means. In *Proceedings of the International Conference on Pattern Recognition.*

Chapter IV

Support Vector Machine for Recognition of White Blood Cells of Leukaemia

Stanislaw Osowski, Warsaw University of Technology & Military University of Technology, Poland

Tomasz Markiewicz, Warsaw University of Technology, Poland

Abstract

This chapter presents an automatic system for white blood cell recognition in myelogenous leukaemia on the basis of the image of a bone-marrow smear. It addresses the following fundamental problems of this task: the extraction of the individual cell image of the smear, generation of different features of the cell, selection of the best features, and final recognition using an efficient classifier network based on support vector machines. The chapter proposes the complete system solving all these problems, beginning from cell extraction using the watershed algorithm; the generation of different features based on texture, geometry, morphology, and the statistical description of the intensity of the image; feature selection using linear support vector machines; and finally classification by applying Gaussian kernel support vector machines. The results of numerical experiments on the recognition of up to 17 classes of blood cells of myelogenous leukaemia have shown that the proposed system is quite accurate and may find practical application in hospitals in the diagnosis of patients suffering from leukaemia.

Introduction

Acute myelogenous leukaemia (AML) is a very serious illness caused by the abnormal growth and development of early nongranular *white blood cells*. It begins with abnormalities in the bone-marrow blast cells that develop to form granulocytes, the white blood cells that contain small particles, or granules. The ML cells do not mature, and they become too numerous in the blood and bone marrow. As the cells build up, they hamper the body's ability to fight infection and prevent bleeding. Therefore, it is necessary to treat this disease within a short time after making a diagnosis.

The recognition of the cells in the bone marrow of patients suffering from AML, and especially the relative counts of different classes of blood cells in bone marrow, is a very important step in the recognition of the development stage of the illness and proper treatment of the patients (Bennett et al., 1976; Lewandowski & Hellmann, 2001). The percentage contribution of different cells (the so-called myelogram) is a fundamental factor in defining various subtypes of ML (Bennet et al.) and the proper treatment of patients.

Specialists recognize different cell-lines developments in the bone marrow: the erythrocyte, monocyte, lymphocyte, plasma, and granulocytic series (Bennet et al., 1976; Lewandowski & Hellmann, 2001). A lot of different blood-cell types belonging to these lines have been defined up to now by specialists. They differ by the size, texture, shape, density, color, size of the nucleus and cytoplasm, and so forth. The difficulty of cell recognition follows from the fact that there are also large variations among the cells belonging to the same family.

In the numerical experiments concerning feature selection, we have considered up to 17 classes of *white blood cells*. The considered classes include (a) proerythroblast, (b) basophilic erythroblast, (c) polychromatic erythroblast, (d) ortochromatic (pyknotic) erythroblast, (e) megaloerythroblast, (f) myeloblast/monoblast, (g) promyelocyte, (h) neutrophilic myelocyte, (i) neutrophilic metamyelocyte, (j) neutrophilic band, (k) neutrophilic segmented, (l) eosinophils, (m) prolymphocyte, (n) lymphocyte, (o) proplasmocyte, and (p) plasmocyte. To cope with the cells not classified to any of the mentioned above classes, for example, the red blood corpuscles, the scarce cells not belonging to any already defined class, the so-called shadows of the cells deprived of the nucleus, parts of the cut blasts, and so forth, we have created the heterogeneous class denoted as the 17th.

The classes presented above represent different cell lines in the bone marrow as well as different stages of development within the same line. The cell types from 1 to 4 represent the erythrocyte development line. The classes from 6 to 11 form the succeeding stages of the granulocytic line. The classes 13 and 14 are members of the lymphocyte line, while 15 and 16 belong to the plasma line of development.

Table 1 presents four samples of these 17 blood-cell types extracted from the bone marrow. The considered classes represent different cell lines in the bone marrow as well as different stages of development within the same line. There is visible a well-defined *nucleus* in each cell, and the brighter irregular shape of the *cytoplasm*. All these images have been obtained as the result of an automatic extraction of the cells from the images of the bone marrow. Observe that the differences among classes are not well defined and it is not easy to recognize between them. Moreover, if we consider the representatives of separate classes, we can observe large differences with regard to the shape, size, and granulites (see, for example, the neutrophilic segmented or neutrophilic band).

Table 1. Representatives of the considered 17 blood-cell types

Proerythroblast				
Basophilic erythroblast				
Polychromatic erythroblast				
Pycnotic erythroblast				
Megaloerythroblast				
Myeloblast/ monoblast				
Promyelocyte				
Neutrophilic myelocyte				
Neutrophilic metamyelocyte				
Neutrophilic band				

Table 1. continued

Neutrophilic segmented				
Eosinophil				
Prolymphocyte				
Lymphocyte				
Proplasmocyte				
Plasmocyte				
The mixed class (not-classified cells)				

There is no public database available for these cells. Up to now, no automatic system exists that could recognize and classify the blood cells. Everything is done manually by the human expert and relies on the subjective assessment of him or her. The estimated accuracy of the human expert is around 85% (Theera-Umpon & Gader, 2002). This accuracy is understood as the difference of the results produced by two independent human experts.

The number of published or online works on automatic recognizing systems of blood cells is very scarce (below 10), and it is difficult to find the appropriate solution satisfying the basic requirement for accuracy. One of the first was the paper by Beksac, Beksac, Tippi, Duru, Karakas, and Nurcakar (1997), presenting a half-automatic system of blood recognition applying multilayer perceptron (MLP). However, its accuracy is far from good (39% misclassification rate) with the recognition of 16 types of cells. Sohn (1999) has presented his MLP-based solution, allowing one to reduce the error rate to 22%, but the number of cell types has been limited to 6 only. He has proved that multilayer perceptron leads to better results than the method of learning vector quantization (LVQ). Also, the paper by Theera-Umpon and Gader (2002) has reported the recognition of 6 types of cells by using multilayer perceptron with a 42% misclassification rate. The paper by Osowski, Markiewicz, Mariańska, and Moszczyński (2004) has presented a systematic procedure for the automatic recognition of cells, including the extraction of individual cells, the generation of the statistical, geometrical, and textural diagnostic features, and a SVM (support vector machine) -based classifying system. The reported average misclassification ratio for 12 classes was on the level of 12%. The more advanced cell-recognizing system created by authors Markiewicz, Osowski, Mariańska, and Moszczyński (2005) has applied also SVM as the classifier and the systematic method of feature generation, assessment, and selection. The results have been presented for the recognition of 17 classes, and the reported average misclassification rate was equal to 18.7%. It is evident that the results are still not satisfactory from the accuracy point of view. It is a common opinion that a lot of research should be done, especially in feature generation and selection, to achieve efficiency comparable to the human expert.

The problem is really very complex since the cells belonging to the same class differ a lot and at the same time are similar to the cells belonging to different classes. Another problem follows from the chemical treatment of the bone-marrow samples. Its results depend on many human-dependent factors that are difficult to control. As a result, the same cells may differ in color, background, and even granulites. At the same time, the image processing leading to the extraction of individual cells is very complex and prone to errors in this phase as well.

The most important problem of cell recognition is the generation of the diagnostic *features* of the blood cells that characterize them in a way suppressing the differences among the members of the same class and enhancing the differences between the cells belonging to different classes. Only the best features allow one to achieve the recognition of cells with the highest accuracy. Most recent solutions for feature generation rely on the texture, geometry, and analysis of the intensity distribution of the images of cells (Markiewicz et al., 2005; Theera-Umpon & Gader, 2002).

The aim of this chapter is to present an advanced approach to cell recognition that leads to the highest efficiency in recognizing and classifying cells. First, we have developed an extended set of features. We characterize the cells by applying additional families of features. To the existing geometrical, textural, and statistical descriptions, we have added morphological features. They are related to the geometry of cells after performing some morphological operations. The number of features generated in this way has grown to more than 100. However, not all of them are equally important for blood-cell recognition. Some of them may be regarded as noise from the point of view of cell recognition and should be removed from the list.

Hence, a very important step is the evaluation of the quality of features. After a careful study of different feature-selection methods, we have proposed here the application of the linear SVM approach for the selection of the best features. The final recognizing and classifying system applies only a limited number of the best features. It is built on the basis of Gaussian kernel SVM networks, working in a one-against-one mode. The results of the recognition of up to 17 different blast-cell types are given and discussed here. The results confirm good efficiency of the proposed system. With the recognition of 17 types of cells, we have achieved accuracy close to 85%, comparable to the human expert and acceptable from the practical point of view. The proposed system has been also checked positively on the basis of additional data corresponding to many patients in the form of the so-called myelogram, prepared independently by our system and by a human expert.

Extraction of the Individual Cells from the Image

The introductory step in the automatic recognition of white blood cells is the extraction of the individual cells from the bone-marrow smear image. We have applied here the image-segmentation technique based on morphological operations and the watershed algorithm (Soille, 2003).

Image segmentation is the division of the image into different regions, each having common properties. In a segmented image, the picture elements are no longer pixels, but connected sets of pixels, all belonging to the same region. The task of segmentation of the image is focused on an automatic recognition of the separate blood-cell regions and the extraction of them for further processing.

In solving the image-segmentation problem, we have applied morphological operations, such as erosion, dilation, opening, and closing (Soille, 2003). They aim at extracting relevant structures of the image by probing the image with another set of a known shape called the structuring element S, chosen as the result of prior knowledge concerning the geometry of the relevant and irrelevant image structures. The erosion of the image X by a structuring element S will be denoted by $\varepsilon_S(X)$ and is defined as the locus of points $\mathbf{x}$ such that S is included in X when its origin is placed at $\mathbf{x}$, $\varepsilon_S(X) = \{\mathbf{x} | S_x \subseteq X\}$. The dilation of the image X by a structuring element S will be denoted by $\delta_S(X)$ and is defined as the locus of points $\mathbf{x}$ such that S hits X when its origin coincides with $\mathbf{x}$, $\delta_S(X) = \{\mathbf{x} | S_x \cap X \neq 0\}$. The opening of an image X by a structuring element S is denoted by $\gamma_S(X)$ and is defined as the erosion of X by S followed by the dilation with the reflected structuring element $\breve{S}$, that is, $\gamma_S(X) = \delta_{\breve{S}}[\varepsilon_S(X)]$, where $\breve{S} = \{-s | s \subset S\}$. The closing of an image X by a structuring element S is denoted by $\phi_S(X)$ and is defined as the dilation of X with S followed by the erosion with the reflected structuring element $\breve{S}$, that is, $\phi_S(X) = \varepsilon_{\breve{S}}[\delta_S(X)]$.

The morphological approach to *image segmentation* combines region-growing and edge-detection techniques. It groups the pixels around the regional minima of the image. In our experiments, we have achieved this by applying the so-called watershed transformation. The watershed transformation (Soille, 2003) takes its origin from the topographic interpretation of the grey-scale image. According to the law of gravitation, the water dropped on such a surface will flow down until it reaches a minimum. The whole set of points of the surface whose steepest slope paths reach a given minimum constitutes the catchment's basin associated with this minimum. The watersheds are the zones dividing adjacent catchments' basins.

In the numerical implementation of the watershed algorithm, the original image is transformed so as to output an image whose minima mark relevant image objects (blood cells) and whose crest lines correspond to image object boundaries. In this way, the image is partitioned into meaningful regions that correspond to the individual blood cells. In our experiments, we have used the watershed algorithm implemented using the Matlab platform (*Matlab User Guide*, 1999). The applied procedure of the watershed image segmentation and cell separation consists of the following stages (Soille, 2003):

Figure 1. The illustration of the succeeding stages of extraction of the cells from the bone-marrow smear: (a) original image, (b) the differential image between the blue and green colors, (c) the black and white filtered image, (d) the map of distances, (e) contours of cells as a result of the watershed transformation, and (f) the final result of the segmentation of the image.

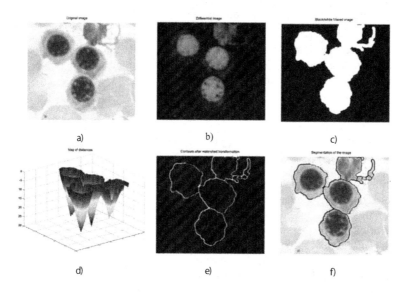

- transformation of the original image of the bone-marrow smears first into grey level and finally into binary scale;

- application of the morphological operations of closing and erosion to smooth the contours and to eliminate the distortions of the image;

- generation of the map of distances from the black pixel to the nearest white pixels of the image;

- application of the watershed algorithm based on these distances for the final division of the image into catchment basins, each corresponding to one cell; and

- extraction of the regions corresponding to the individual cells and a return to a color picture.

Figure 1 illustrates the succeeding stages of the procedure of the extraction of the separate cells from the image of the bone-marrow smear (Figure 1a). The image of Figure 1b corresponds to the differential image obtained by subtracting the blue and green colors. The black and white image is presented in Figure 1c. The map of distances from the black pixel to the nearest white pixels of the image is illustrated in Figure 1d. Figure 1e presents the contours of blood cells as a result of the applied watershed transformation. The final *image segmentation* with extracted cells is presented in Figure 1f. There were three white blood cells in the image and all of them have been well segmented and then extracted as individual cells. Observe that the blast cells are composed mostly of nuclei (the dark portion of cell). The cytoplasm (the light, narrow border around the nucleus) occupies only a very small area of the whole cell. Their separation is straightforward by applying the Otsu method of thresholding (Otsu, 1979). The shape of the cytoplasm is not regular due to some irregularities in the intensity of the colors and some imperfection of the automatic system of cell extraction (no human intervention in the extraction process).

The extraction procedure is not very time consuming. At the region of the bone-marrow smear covered by the microscope field, the process takes about 30 seconds on a personal computer with a speed of 2GHz and 512M of RAM.

Generation of Features Describing the Cell Images

The recognition of the cell images requires generating the numerical diagnostic **features** well characterizing different classes of cells. In generating features, we try to follow the human expert by stressing the details on the basis of which the recognition will be done. To such details belong the shape, size of the cells, granulation, distribution of intensity, color, and so forth. The efficient recognition of the images by an automatic system requires the preprocessing step in order to extract the features imitating the details the human expert takes into account. They should characterize the image in a way suppressing the differences within the same class and enhancing them for cells belonging to different classes. In our approach to this problem, we rely on the features belonging to four main groups of textural, geometrical, statistical, and morphological nature.

The texture refers to an arrangement of the basic constituents of the material and in the digital image is depicted by the interrelationships between spatial arrangements of the image pixels. They are seen as the changes in intensity patterns, or the grey tones. The rigorous description of the texture features may be found in the excellent paper of Wagner (1999). Among many existing techniques of texture preprocessing for the extraction of features, we have chosen two texture preprocessing methods: Unser and Markov random field (MRF). According to our experience, these two methods were the best suited for representation of the texture patterns of different cell images.

In the Unser approach, the sum and difference histograms of grey levels of the neighboring pixels are created for different directions, for example, $0°$, $45°$, $90°$, and $135°$. On the basis of this analysis, the mean value, angular second momentum, contrast, and entropy of the intensity of the neighboring pixels in one chosen direction have been selected as the features. These values have been determined for three colors, independently for the nucleus and *cytoplasm*. Up to 42 features have been generated in this way. For a detailed quantitative description of this set of features, refer to Wagner (1999).

In MRF method, the signal corresponding to each pixel location is regarded as a random variable. This random field texture model is characterized by the geometric structure and quantitative strength of interactions among the neighbors. The autoregressive model parameters of the probability distribution have been used as the features. For this particular application, only two carefully selected MRF parameters of highest stability for each class of cells have been selected as features generated for the cytoplasm and nucleus separately.

Additional sets of texture features have been generated by analyzing the cell images at the reduced resolution. The reduced resolution of the image gives an additional look at the properties of the particular regions of the image. After careful analysis of the cell images, we have reduced their resolution four times, and for these transformed images, 22 texture features for the nucleus only have been generated.

The next set of parameters corresponds to the geometrical shapes of the **nucleus** and to the whole cell. For this characterization of the blood cells, we have used the following geometrical parameters:

- Radius of the nucleus measured by averaging the length of the radial line segments defined by the centroid and border points.
- Perimeter of the nucleus, which is the total distance between consecutive points of the border.
- Area of the nucleus and the whole cell, which the number of pixels on the interior of the cell with the addition of one half of the pixels on the perimeter. It is defined separately for the nuclei and for the total cells. As the features, we take the area of the nucleus and the ratio of the areas of the nucleus to the whole cell.
- Area of the convex part of the nucleus.
- Circumference of the nucleus.
- Filled area, which is the number of pixels in the image of the same size as the bounding box of the region.
- Compactness, given by the formula $perimeter^2/area$.
- Concavity of the nucleus, which is the severity of the concavities or indentations in a cell (the extent to which the actual boundary of a cell lies on the inside of each chord between nonadjacent boundary points.
- Concavity points, which is the number of concavities irrespective of their amplitudes.
- Symmetry, which is the difference between lines perpendicular to the major axis to the cell boundary in both directions.
- Major and minor axis lengths of the nucleus—they are used as separate features, not combined together.
- The mean distance of pixels to the central pixel of the nucleus.

The meaning of all used parameters like concavity, convexity, symmetry, compactness, and so forth are compatible with the definitions used in Pratt (1991) and in the Matlab implementation (*Matlab User Guide*, 1999). Up to 19 geometrical features have been generated for each cell on the basis of the geometrical parameters. Most of these features are related to the nucleus. This is caused by the fact that the shape of the nucleus is much more stable and less susceptible to segmentation noise. Moreover, before measuring these parameters, we performed the smoothing of the cell shape by performing the opening operation of the image.

The next set of features has been generated on the basis of the analysis of the intensity distribution of the image. This refers to the color information taken into account by the human expert at the manual assessment of the cells. The histograms of the image and the gradient matrices of such intensity have been determined independently for three color components R, G, and B. On the basis of such analysis, the following features have been generated:

- The mean value and variance of the histogram of the image of the nucleus and cytoplasm (separately).
- The mean value and variance of the histogram of the gradient matrix of the image of the nucleus and cytoplasm (separately).
- The skewness and kurtosis of the histogram of the image of the whole cell.
- The skewness and kurtosis of the histogram of the gradient matrix of the image of the whole cell.

Up to 36 features have been generated in this way. Analyzing the correlations of the features related to different colors, we have decided to remove the whole set corresponding to one color. Only two colors (red and green) have been left for feature generation (a reduction from 36 to 24 statistical features) after such analysis.

The last set of features is related to the morphological transformations of the image. They characterize the smoothness and internal structure of the cells, very susceptible to the morphological operations. To such features belong the following:

- The area of the nucleus before and after erosion done by a structuring element in the form of the disc of the radius equal to 4 pixels.
- The number of separated regions in the nucleus after erosion.
- The smallest number of erosions needed to remove the whole nucleus.

The features have been generated for black and white images obtained by the bias defined in two different ways: 2/5 of the length of histogram and by applying the method of Otsu (Otsu, 1979). In this way, we have generated eight morphological features of the image.

Up to 117 features have been generated altogether in this way. All features have been normalized through dividing their values by their corresponding maximum value. The numerical experiments of feature generation have been implemented using the platform of Matlab (*Matlab User Guide*, 1999). The approximate time for generation of the whole set of features for one cell is around 8 seconds on a computer running at 2GHz with 512M of RAM.

Selection of the Most Important Features

It is well known that *features* have different impact on the process of pattern recognition. A good feature should be very stable for samples belonging to the same class (the smallest possible variance) and at the same time it should differ significantly for different classes. The feature assuming similar values for different classes has no discriminative power and may be treated as noise from the classifier point of view. Thus, the main problem in classification and machine learning is to find out the efficient methods of the *selection of features* according to their importance for the problem solution. Note that the elimination of some features leads to the reduction of the dimensionality of the feature space and the improvement of the performance of the classifier in the testing mode due to the data not taking part in learning.

There are many techniques of feature selection (Guyon & Elisseeff, 2003; Guyon, Weston, Barnhill, & Vapnik, 2002; Schurmann, 1996). To the most popular belong principal component analysis (PCA), projection pursuit, correlation existing among features, correlation between the features and the classes, analysis of mean and variance of the features belonging to different classes, application of linear SVM feature ranking, and so forth.

Figure 2. The image of the correlations of the features. The features from 1 to 66 are textural, from 67 to 95 are geometrical, from 96 to 109 are statistical, and from 110 to 117 are morphological.

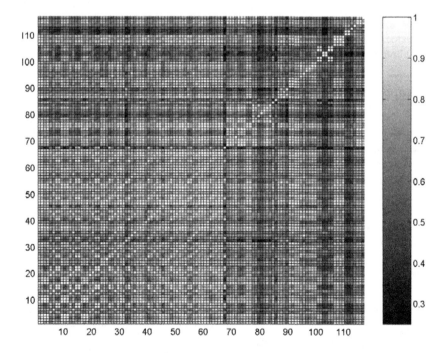

PCA, one of the most often-used feature-selection methods in the past, represents a classical statistical technique for analyzing the covariance structure of the feature set, enhancing the most important elements of information hidden in the data set. Linear PCA is described by the linear transformation $y=Wx$, mapping the N-dimensional original feature vector x into the K-dimensional output vector y, (K<N), through the PCA transformation matrix W. The vector y preserves all the most important elements of the original information. The reduced set of features described by the vector y is used as the input vector to the classifier. However, on the basis of our experiments, we have found that the transformed set of reduced features does not perform sufficiently well for the recognition of the cells. This is mainly due to the fact that the values of succeeding principal components are very close to each other, and it is very difficult to find the proper discrimination level. The application of nonlinear PCA did not improve their discrimination properties.

Correlation Analysis of the Features

It is a general opinion (Schurmann, 1996) that the reduction of the dimensionality of the feature space is possible by eliminating the features that are strongly correlated with the others. The correlated features usually dominate over others and reduce the discrimination ability of the whole set. Eliminating them should improve the performance of the whole system.

Figure 2 presents the pictorial view of the correlations existing among textural, geometrical, statistical, and morphological features. They take the form of the image matrices. The largest correlations can be observed among the texture features, and these features can be reduced at the highest rate. A relatively high number of correlated features is observed among the members of the geometrical group. The morphological and statistical features seem to be least correlated. On the basis of the correlation analysis, many features (up to one third) have been eliminated from the feature set.

The Selection Based on the Mean and Variance of the Data

The next criterion of *feature selection* very-often exploited in the practical classification systems is the analysis of the variance and means of the data samples belonging to each class. The variance of the features corresponding to cells being the members of one class should be as small as possible. Moreover, to distinguish between different classes, the positions of means of feature values for the data belonging to different classes should be separated as much as possible. The feature of the standard-deviation value being much higher than the distance between two neighboring class centers is useless for these two particular classes' recognition since it does not distinguish between them. Observe that the particular feature may be very good for recognition between some chosen classes and useless for some others. Therefore, the class-oriented features should be considered to get the optimal choice of features used for the separation of two particular classes.

A more systematic policy for feature selection is to combine both measures (variance and mean) together to form a single quality measure (Duda, Hart, & Stork, 2003; Schurmann,

Figure 3. The graph illustrating the changes of the value of $S_{AB}(f)$ for a single chosen feature and all combinations of classes .

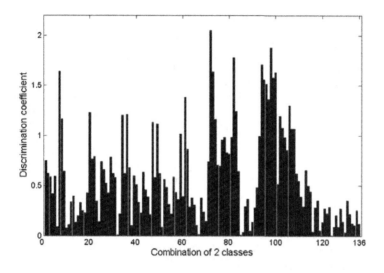

Figure 4. The values of the discriminating coefficient $S_{AB}(f)$ of all features for a chosen exemplary pair of classes A and B.

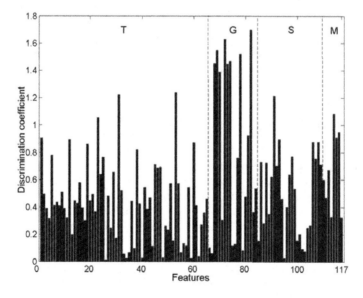

1996). This has been done by defining the so-called discrimination coefficient $S_{AB}(f)$. For two classes A and B, the discrimination coefficient of the feature f was defined as follows:

$$S_{AB}(f) = \frac{|c_A(f) - c_B(f)|}{\sigma_A(f) + \sigma_B(f)}. \tag{1}$$

In this definition, c_A and c_B are the mean values of the feature f in the classes A and B, respectively. The variables σ_A and σ_B represent the standard deviations determined for both classes. The large value of $S_{AB}(f)$ indicates a good potential separation ability of the feature f for these two classes. On the other hand, a small value of it means that this particular feature is not good for the recognition between classes A and B.

Usually, the importance of the feature f changes for different pairs of classes. The value of $S_{AB}(f)$ varies in a large range. Figure 3 shows the typical variation of the chosen geometrical feature (the convex area of the cell) for all class combinations among 17 classes.

As it can be seen, the value of $S_{AB}(f)$ changes from the minimal level equal to 0.04 (a lack of recognition ability) to the maximal level of 2.1 (the highest recognition ability).

The multiclass classification problem may be solved by separating the considered task into two-class recognition subproblems, as it is done in the one-against-one mode of operation of SVM classifiers. In such a case, the separate set of optimal features should be generated for each two-class recognition problem.

Figure 4 presents the typical distribution of values of the discriminating coefficient $S_{AB}(f)$ for all considered features through the recognition of two exemplary classes of the blood cells. The letter T denotes the textural features, G the geometrical features, S the statistical features, and M the morphological features. As it is seen, the features have different discrimination abilities. For this particular pair of classes, the smallest value of 0.01 possesses the textural feature 26. On the other hand, the best feature for these particular two-class recognition is the geometrical feature 83, for which the discrimination coefficient reached the value of 1.7. Summarizing Figure 4, it is evident that the best individual discrimination abilities are distributed among different types of features. However, it should be noted that for each pair of classes, the importance of the particular feature may be different.

Correlation of the Feature with the Class

The discriminative power of the candidate feature f for the recognition of a particular class among K classes **(feature selection)** can also be measured by the correlation of this feature with the class (Schurmann, 1996). Let us assume that the target class k is one among the classes forming the target vector of all classes, denoted by **d**. Let us assume that the feature f is described by its unconditional and conditional means $m_c = E\{f\}$ and $m_{ck} = E\{f|k\}$. Assume that the variance of f is known: $\text{vaf}(f) = E\{(f - m_c)^2\}$. The correlation between f and **d** is derived from the covariance vector $\mathbf{cov}(f, \mathbf{d})$, related by the respective variance. The discriminative power of the feature f is measured as the squared magnitude of the vector $\mathbf{corr}(f, \mathbf{d})$, that is:

Figure 5. The values of the discriminating coefficient $S_{AB}(f)$ of all features for the chosen exemplary pair of classes A and B.

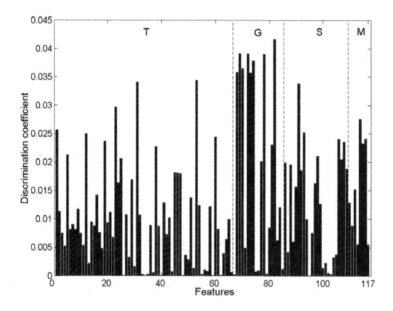

$$S(f) = |\mathbf{corr}(f, \mathbf{d})|^2 = \frac{|\mathbf{cov}(f, \mathbf{d})|^2}{\mathrm{var}(f)\,\mathrm{var}(\mathbf{d})}. \tag{2}$$

Denoting by P_k the probability of the kth class and taking into account $\mathrm{var}(\mathbf{d}) = \sum_{k=1}^{K} P_k(1 - P_k)$, we get $\mathbf{cov}(f, \mathbf{d}) = [P_1(m_{c1} - m_c), ..., P_K(m_{cK} - m_c)]^T$. The discriminative power of feature f is then given in the form (Schurmann, 1996):

$$S(f) = \frac{\sum_{k=1}^{K} P_k (m_{ck} - m_c)^2}{\mathrm{var}(f) \sum_{k=1}^{K} P_k (1 - P_k)}. \tag{3}$$

Figure 5 presents the distribution of the discriminative power of all features for the discrimination between two classes (K=2) of class A and B chosen identically as in the previous experiment (Figure 4). The best discriminative power possesses the feature of the highest value of $S(f)$. There is visible similarity in the distribution of the importance of the features to that presented in Figure 4.

The Feature Selection Based on the Application of Single-Input SVM

One way of applying the SVM network for feature selection is training the network using only one feature at a time. The predictive power of the single feature for a classification task is characterized by the value of the error function minimized by a one-dimensional linear SVM trained to classify learning samples on the basis of only one feature of interest. The smaller this error, the better the quality of the feature. This criterion may be used to rank features and select only those with an important predictive power.

The Feature Selection Based on the Application of Multiple-Input SVM

It should be stressed that all feature analyses described above are concerned with the importance of a single feature acting alone. However, it is intuitively understandable that this importance may change significantly when the feature is acting together with the other features. Recently, the authors of the papers Guyon and Elisseeff (2003) and Guyone et al. (2002) introduced the interesting common *feature selection* method based on the application of linear SVM. They proposed the ranking of the features working together as the whole set. The method is based on the idea that the absolute values of the weights of a linear classifier

Figure 6. Results of feature ranking for the recognition of the two exemplary classes of blood cells by using linear multiple-input SVM

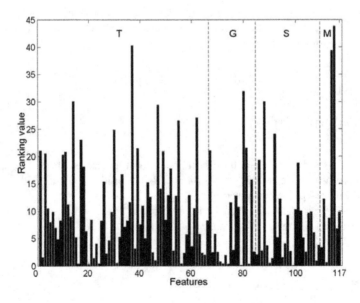

produce a feature ranking. The feature associated with the larger weight is more important than that associated with the small one. The method proposed in Guyon et al. (2002) is recursive in nature, and the elimination of features is done in many steps. The linear kernel SVM is used as the classifier because this kernel does not deform the original impact of the feature on the result of the classification.

Linear SVM is a particular linear discriminant classifier working on the principle of the maximum margin between two classes (Hsu & Lin, 2002; Schölkopf & Smola, 2002; Vapnik, 1998). The decision function of the N-dimensional input vector $\mathbf{x}$ is a linear function defined as $D(\mathbf{x})=\mathbf{w}^T\mathbf{x}+b$, with the weight vector $\mathbf{w}$ and bias b dependent of the linear combination of the training patterns $(\mathbf{x}_k, d_k)$ belonging to the support vectors, where:

$$\mathbf{w} = \sum_k \alpha_k d_k \mathbf{x}_k \tag{4}$$

and $b = d_k - \mathbf{w}^T\mathbf{x}_k$, and α_k is the nonzero Lagrange multiplier corresponding to the kth training data set.

In contrast to the general procedure of Guyon et al. (2002), we have applied a single training of linear SVM for each pair of classes because this strategy was found to be more efficient in our problem. The features connected with the output of SVM through the weights of highest absolute values are regarded as the most important for the recognition of these classes. All values of weights have been arranged in decreasing order and only the most important have been selected for each pair of classes. The significant problem is the determination of the number of selected features. Two approaches to this problem are possible: to keep the constant number of features for each two-class recognition problem or to determine the minimum value of weight below which the feature is cut. We have applied the first one since there is no reasonable premise as to how to choose the proper value of the discrimination level. Analyzing the distribution of feature ranking for all combinations of classes and after extensive experiments on the validation data set, we have left only 30 features applied for the recognition of each pair of classes. The corresponding features have been used in the final classification system.

Figure 6 illustrates the importance of all features for the recognition of the two chosen classes. The ranking value of the feature is simply the absolute value of the appropriate weight connecting this feature (component of the vector $\mathbf{x}$) with the output of the SVM network. The ranking presented in Figure 6 has been provided for the same two classes as in figures 4 and 5. The significant differences in the importance of the features with respect to previous methods can be observed now. This is due to the fact that each selection procedure explores a different mathematical formulation of the importance of the feature. Moreover, most of the presented ranking methods were based on the assessment of the feature acting alone; only the multiple-input SVM ranking has been determined for all features cooperating together. So, in the last case, some form of mutual dependency among the features has been also explored. Hence, such ranking is expected to be more efficient and able of producing a more realistic assessment of the importance of the individual feature. The results of the verification of these selection methods embedded in the full classification system will be presented in the next section.

Gaussian Kernel Support Vector Machine Classifier System

For the recognition and classification of the cells, we have applied the support vector machine, the universal feed-forward network, known as the excellent tool of good generalization ability for classification problems (Schölkopf & Smola, 2002; Vapnik, 1998). This choice was made after a series of experiments with other neural network solutions, such as MLP (Haykin, 1999) and the neuro-fuzzy networks (Osowski & Tran Hoai, 2003). The Gaussian kernel SVM-based classifiers have been found the best. The relative superiority of SVM over other solutions in terms of accuracy was on the level of 25% in the introductory experiments. So, in further numerical experiments, only the Gaussian kernel SVM classifier has been investigated. The principle of the operation of such a classifier and the review of the learning algorithms can be found in Chapter I of this book.

The important point in designing the SVM classifier was the choice of the kernel function. The simplest linear kernel was inefficient due to the lack of linear separability of the data. The polynomial kernel checked in the introductory experiments was also found useless since a high degree of polynomial was needed and the system had become badly conditioned. The best results have been obtained through the application of the Gaussian kernel:

$$\kappa(\mathbf{x}, \mathbf{x}_i) = \exp\left(-\frac{\|\mathbf{x} - \mathbf{x}_i\|^2}{\sigma^2}\right), \tag{5}$$

and this kernel has been applied in all further experiments. The hyperparameter σ of the Gaussian function has been adjusted by repeating the learning experiments for the set of its predefined values and choosing the best one at the validation data sets.

On the stage of designing the SVM classifier system, the choice of the regularization constant C is also very important (Schölkopf & Smola, 2002). It controls the trade-off between the complexity of the machine and the number of nonseparable data points used in learning. The small value of C results in the acceptance of more not-separated learning points. At a higher value of C, we get a lower number of classification errors in the learning data points, but a more complex network structure. The optimal values of C were determined for each pair of classes independently after additional series of learning experiments through the use of the validation test sets. The processes of optimizing the values of C and σ were done together. Many different values of C and σ combined together in the learning process have been used, and their optimal values are those for which the classification error on the validation data set was the smallest. The SVM networks were trained using the Platt algorithm (Platt, 1998).

To deal with the problem of many classes, we used the one-against-one approach (Hsu & Lin, 2002). In this approach, the SVM networks are trained to recognize between all combinations of two classes of data. For M classes, we have to train M(M-1)/2 individual SVM networks. In the retrieval mode, the vector $\mathbf{x}$ belongs to the class of the highest number of winnings in all combinations of classes.

There are many reasons for choosing the one-against-one instead of the one-against-all method. The most important advantage of using the first choice is having a much more balanced set of learning samples of both classes. In the one-against-all method, one class is opposed to the rest. At approximately the same population of all classes, we get a great imbalance of data (the set of the learning samples of one class against the samples corresponding to the other 16 classes), which has a negative impact on the learning results and decreases the efficiency of the classifier system.

The other reason is that each pair of classes uses an individual set of features selected from the whole set in a way described in the previous section. In such case, more specialized sets of optimal features for the recognition of two classes may be selected. Thanks to such specialization, higher efficiency of the whole classification system is expected.

The Results of Recognition of the Blood Cells

Database of the Blood Cells

The database of the blood cells has been created in cooperation with Hematology Hospital in Warsaw. The bone-marrow smear samples have been collected from more than 40 patients

Table 2. List of classes of blood cells under recognition

Notation of class	class name	Number of samples
1	Proerythroblast	39
2	Basophilic erythroblast	139
3	Polychromatic erythroblast	350
4	Pyknotic erythroblast	227
5	Megaloerythroblast	140
6	Myeloblast/monoblast	115
7	Promyelocyte	94
8	Neutrophilic myelocyte	155
9	Neutrophilic metamyelocyte	128
10	Neutrophilic band	140
11	Neutrophilic segmented	225
12	Eosinophils	127
13	Prolymphocyte	45
14	Lymphocyte	281
15	Proplasmocyte	84
16	Plasmocyte	93
17	Others	206
Total		**2,588**

suffering from myelogenous leukaemia. The images were digitized using an Olympus microscope with magnification of 1000× and a digital camera of resolution 1712×1368 pixels. The picture was saved in RGB format. The smears have been processed by applying the standard method of May-Grunwald-Giemsa (MGG). More than 2,500 blood cells have been acquired in this way.

The results of the experiments will be presented for the 17 types of blood cells, of which 16 belonged to strictly defined classes and the 17th was a heterogeneous class composed of other cells existing in the image of the bone-marrow aspirate (the red blood corpuscles, the so-called shadows of the cells deprived of the nucleus, the new rare cell types, etc.). The overview of all cell types has been presented in the previous section. In further investigations, we will refer to the particular class by its number.

Table 2 presents the list of all considered classes and the number of samples available in each class that have been used in all experiments. The number of samples belonging to different classes changes a lot from class to class. Some of them have been sparsely represented in bone-marrow aspirates of the patients, mainly due to their rare occurrence or short lifetime in the typical process of the development of the illness.

The introductory experiments with the validation data set have enabled us to adjust the best values of hyperparameters (the regularization constant C and the parameter σ of the Gaussian functions). After that, the main experiments started at frozen values of these parameters. The available data set has been split into five exchangeable parts to enable application of the cross-validation procedure. The class representatives have been split equally into all these parts. Four groups have been combined together and used in learning, while the fifth one was used only in testing. The experiments have been repeated five times, exchanging the contents of the four learning subsets and the testing subset. The misclassification ratio in the learning mode has been calculated as the mean of all five runs. The number of the testing error is simply the sum of these errors committed by the system at each cross-correlation run.

To get the objective assessment of the results, we have performed 10 runs of the cross-validation procedure at different compositions of data, forming each group of data. The final results are simply the mean of all runs. The variance of classification errors is also of some value and will be presented, too.

Measures of Performance of the Recognizing System

To assess the quality of the solution, we have to define some performance measure. Two different error definitions have been applied. The most often used is the ordinary relative error defined as the ratio of all misclassifications to the total number of samples:

$$E_1 = \frac{N_{err}}{N}, \tag{6}$$

where N_{err} is the number of misclassifications and N is the total number of samples. This measure is the accurate performance assessment of the classifier for individual classes, but not necessary for all classes taken together. This is due to the unequal number of representatives of each class. With varying numbers of samples belonging to different classes, the highest impact on the final results is on the class containing the largest number of representatives. To get a more objective measure, applicable for many classes of largely changing popula-tions, we have introduced the second error function E_2, defined as the average of the mean relative recognition errors of all classes:

$$E_2 = \frac{1}{N_{cl}} \sum_{k=1}^{N_{cl}} E_{1k}. \tag{7}$$

In this expression, E_{1k} is the error measure E_1 determined for the kth class and N_{cl} is the number of classes under consideration. The second measure, E_2, has the advantage of being independent on the population of each class. This independence follows from the fact that the measure E_2 is just the average of the mean errors for each class, so the population of the class has no direct impact on the final accuracy of the error estimation.

The Numerical Results

The proposed system has been checked for the recognition of the 17 classes of white blood cells. The main task of the experiments was the determination of its accuracy at recogniz-ing all cells appearing in the smear. The first step of the procedure is the creation of the database of the cells on the basis of bone-marrow samples collected in the hematology hospital. We have applied the automatic extraction of cells on the set of images of the bone marrow of 40 patients suffering from myelogenous leukaemia. The next step is to process the individual images of cells in order to generate the textural, statistical, morphological, and geometrical features characterizing each cell. There were 117 features generated in this way. These features form the set of candidates for the components of the vector $\mathbf{x}$, forming the input signals to the SVM classifiers. The application of all features to form the vector $\mathbf{x}$ was not a best solution. The global learning error, defined as the mean of the misclassifica-tion rate of all classes, was equal to $E_1 = 11.2\%$ and $E_2 = 13.8\%$, while the testing error was $E_1 = 22.7\%$ and $E_2 = 24.1\%$, respectively. This is an unacceptable level of errors, indicating the bad generalization ability of the network. To achieve better generalization, we have to reduce some features with little discrimination abilities.

Table 3. The comparison of the overall error rate (E_1) of the recognition of 17 types of blood cells through different selection methods for features in the testing data.

Choice of features	Single-input SVM		Multiple-input SVM		Mean and variance		Correlation with the class	
	E_1	E_2	E_1	E_2	E_1	E_2	E_1	E_2
Set of 30 best features	21.4%.	23.8%	**15.2%**	**18.2%**	22.6%	23.9%	22.7%	24.0%
Set of 30 worst features	32.6%	31.5%	34.4%	36,1%	35.3%	37.9%	35.5%	37.7%
All features	E_1=22.7%, E_2=24.1%							

Table 4. The detailed results of the blood-cell recognition after the application of linear SVM feature ranking (one cross-validation run).

class	Number of learning errors	Percentage of learning errors	Number of testing errors	Percentage of testing errors
1	4	10.2%	9	23.1%
2	29	1.4%	30	21.6%
3	35	10%	41	11.7%
4	22	9.7%	30	13.2%
5	1	0.7%	6	4.4%
6	9	7.8%	16	13.9%
7	20	21.3%	31	33%
8	16	10.3%	31	20%
9	34	26.6%	37	28.9%
10	49	35%	46	32.8%
11	19	8.4%	21	9.3%
12	10	7.9%	18	14.2%
13	7	15.6%	11	24.4%
14	9	3.2%	13	4.6%
15	7	8.3%	19	22.6%
16	16	17.2%	26	28%
17	6	2.9%	9	4.4%
Total	293	E_1=8.89%	394	E_1=15.22%
		E_2=11.56%		E_2=18.23%

We have tried different methods of feature selection. To compare them, we have carried out the experiments of learning the Gaussian kernel SVM-based classifier system using different numbers of features selected in different ways. The most promising results have been obtained by applying only 30 of the best features ranked by the linear multiple-input SVM network of the features working together. To be sure that the selection procedure works well, we have repeated the experiments with the same number of the worst features and compared the results with the case of all features (no reduction). The profits following from the selection of the best features are evident and depicted in Table 3. The best method (the multiple-input linear SVM) has enabled us to reduce the recognition error E_1 from 22.7% to 15.2%.

The application of the worst features has followed the increase of the overall error rate in a significant way compared to the output at the application of all features. These results confirm the correctness of the applied feature-selection procedure. The relative improvement resulting from the application of the multiple-input SVM selection procedure, with respect to all features, is more than 25% both in the E_1 and E_2 measures of errors. This confirms good performance of the proposed selection procedure of the best features. The detailed

Table 5. Sample confusion matrix of the cell recognition for the testing data

class	1	2	3	4	5	6	7	8	9	10	11	12	13	14	15	16	17
1	30	2			2	1	2					1				1	
2	1	109	24									1		1		3	
3		17	309	24													
4			30	197													
5	2	1			134			1								2	
6	1					99	2	5	1		1			5			1
7	1			1	1	6	63	15	3		1				2		1
8						3	12	124	8	3	1			2		1	1
9		1					2	21	91	11	1						1
10						1		4	13	94	27			1			
11		2						1	3	16	204						
12						1	1	5	2	2	1	109					6
13													34	10			1
14			2	1				2					2	268	1		5
15				1	1			2						1	65	14	
16		4	2				2	2						4	12	67	
17				1		1	2					1		4			197

results of the recognition of individual classes of cells after application of this type of feature ranking are presented in Table 4.

Some blood cells have been recognized with large errors (for example, classes 1, 7, 10, 13, and 16). There are two sources of errors. The badly recognized classes are usually those for which a relatively small number of representatives were available in the learning set, and to such cases belong classes 1 and 13. The second reason follows from the similarities among the neighbouring blood cells in their development line (classes 7, 10, and 16). Observe that the white blood cells are categorized by age, which is the continuous variable. The transition from one cell type to the neighbouring one is continuous, and even an expert is in trouble when recognizing the exact moment of transition from one class to the next neighboring one.

Table 6. Summary of the performance of the classifier at the testing data for the recognition of 17 classes, neglecting the errors following from the neighborhood of cells in their development line

class	Number of testing errors	Percentage of testing errors
1	7	17.8%
2	5	3.6%
3	0	0
4	0	0
5	6	4.3%
6	14	12.1%
7	10	10.6%
8	11	7.1%
9	5	3.9%
10	6	4.3%
11	5	2.2%
12	18	14.2%
13	1	2.25%
14	11	3.9%
15	5	5.9%
16	14	15.0%
17	9	4.4%
Total	**120**	E_1=**4.91%**
		E_2=**6.58%**

In our data set there are cells close to each other in their development stage. For example, the cells belonging to classes 1, 2, 3, and 4 represent the succeeding stages of cells within the erythrocyte development line. Similarly, the cells belonging to classes 6, 7, 8, 9, 10, and 11 form the granulocytic line. The cells 13 and 14 are members of the lymphocytes, while 15 and 16 are the plasma line. The recognition between two neighbouring cells in the same development line is dubious since the images of both cells are very alike and thus difficult to recognize. Close analysis of our misclassification cases reveals that most errors have been committed at the recognition of the neighbouring cells in their development lines.

Table 5 presents the details of class recognition related to the optimal set of features following from the linear SVM ranking. It is done in the form of the so-called confusion matrix, represented as the summed results of one cross-validation procedure for the testing data. The diagonal entries represent the numbers of properly recognized classes. Each entry outside the diagonal means an error. The entry in the (i,j)th position of the matrix means a false assignment of ith class to the jth one.

Figure 7. Statistical results of blood-cell recognition

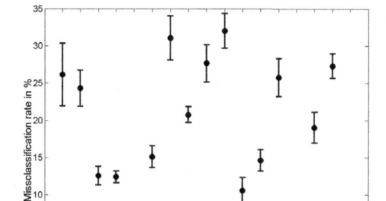

Observe that in our experiments, most misclassifications for classes 1, 2, 3, and 4 are grouped along the diagonal, that is, they are committed for the neighbouring cells in their erythrocyte development line. The same is true for classes 6, 7, 8, 9, 10, and 11 (granulocytic line), classes 13 and 14 (lymphocyte line), and classes 15 and 16 (plasma line). They have been marked by the bold lines in the table. If we neglect such misclassifications, we obtain different (greatly reduced) misclassification rates.

Table 6 presents the summary of the misclassifications when omitting such dubious cases. As we can see, for the worst recognized class 7, the misclassification rate has been radically reduced from 33% to 10.6% (most errors have been committed for the neighbouring classes). The total average misclassification rate in the testing mode has been now reduced to only 6.58% (E_2 measure) or 4.91% (E_1 measure). The highest error for the individual class has dropped to 17.8% for the class 1 (only 39 samples available for experiments) and 15% for the class 16, containing only 93 representatives.

Note, finally, that all misclassification rates mentioned above have been calculated as the ordinary mean of error rates committed for each class. On the basis of this, two total error measures (E_1 and E_2) have been calculated. The E_1 measure is usually more optimistic and E_2 more realistic for the actually uneven number of representatives of each class. With a balanced number of class representatives, both measures approach each other. Moreover, the important observation is that increasing the population of the classes at the stage of learning has a generally positive impact on the accuracy of the automatic classifying system.

It is interesting to compare the statistical variation of the results at many repetitions of cross-validation procedures. Figure 7 presents the results of the 17-class recognition in the form of the mean (the circle) and standard deviation (the vertical lines) of the misclassification errors for 10 independent runs of the cross-validation procedure. In each run, the randomly generated data samples have taken part in different groups of data. The highest variances of misclassification results correspond usually to the classes of smallest population (classes 1, 7, and 13). The results depicted in figure 7 confirm generally that the classifier system is stable and is highly independent on the data-set composition used in the experiments. Hence, there is a good hope to obtain satisfactory performance on the data acquired for new patients.

Verification of Results in the Form of Myelogram

The results of testing, shown in the previous section, have been aimed at the presentation of the potentiality of the presented system. However, in hospital practice, we do not use all potentialities of it. From the medical point of view, the most important is the so-called myelogram, the special protocol containing the numbers and percentage of the blood cells detected in the bone marrow. Such a protocol is normally prepared separately for each patient suffering from leukaemia.

Table 7. Comparison of the Myelogram prepared by the automatic system and the human expert for one patient

Type of cell	Number of cells (human expert)	Rate (human expert)	Number of cells (automatic system)	Rate (automatic system)
ERYTHROPOIESIS	66	58.4%	68	55.7%
Basophilic erythroblast	14	12.4%%	16	13.1%
Polychromatophilic erythroblast	34	30.1%	34	27.8%
Orthochromatic erythroblast	18	15.9%	18	14.8%
GRANULOPOIESIS	38	33.6%	43	35.2%
Promyelocyte	6	5.3%	10	8.2%
Myelocyte	9	8%	10	8.2%
Metamyelocyte	13	11.5%	9	7.4%
Neutrophilic band	7	6.2%	6	4.9%
Neutrophilic segmented	3	2.7%	7	5.7%
Eosinophilic cell	0	0	1	0.8%
LIMPHOCYTE SYSTEM	9	8%	11	9%
Limphocyte	9	8%	11	9%
SHADOWS OF CELLS & BLOOD CORPUSCLE	80		71	
TOTAL NUMBER OF CELLS IN MYELOGRAM	113		122	

Figure 8. Diagram of the cumulative contribution of three main development lines for three patients (E is erythropiesis, G is granulopoiesis, and L is lymphocyte system)

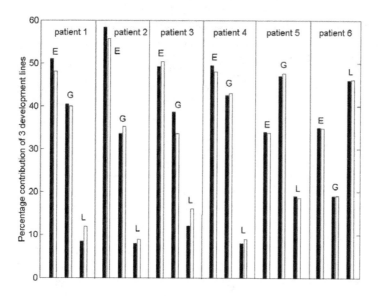

To check the usefulness of the system in the hospital practice, we have tested it on the totally new data sets not taking part in learning. These data have been obtained from new patients entering the hospital. The results of the tests have been compared with the scores obtained independently by the human experts. We have noticed a very good agreement between the results of our system and the human expert. In this experiment, the SVM classifier system has been trained on all samples of the available data, used previously in the cross-validation procedure. After learning, the parameters of the SVM classifier system have been frozen, and the trained system was used for the recognition of the data acquired for these new patients. Table 7 presents the summary of this comparison in the form of a typical myelogram for one chosen patient. As it is seen, the agreement of both results is very good. Small differences among corresponding values are acceptable from the medical point of view.

Note that the total numbers of cells in the myelogram are slightly different in both scores. This follows from the automatic procedure of the extraction of cells. However, it does not influence significantly the relative contribution of each cell type in the myleogram.

Figure 8 presents the diagram of the cumulative percentage contribution of three main development lines—erythropoiesis (E), granulopoiesis (G), and the lymphocyte system (L)—detected in the bone marrow of six patients. The black color denotes the human expert's estimation, while the transparent section represents the results of the automatic system. As it is seen, the differences of scores between the proposed automatic system and of the human expert are negligible.

It would be interesting in the future to compare the performance of our cell-classification system with the online mode in the normal operation of the hospital, as well as on other large data sets containing blood cells from other sources. Unfortunately, at the moment, such a data set in the public domain does not exist.

The last, but not the least, aspect of the solution is the speed of the proposed automatic system since it applies quite complex data processing. The preparation of the myelogram for one patient takes from 10 to 15 minutes for the well-qualified human expert. The same task is done by our system within approximately the same time by using a two-processor computer running at 2GHz with 1M of RAM. The computation time may be greatly reduced in the future after introducing more technologically advanced processors. However, the main advantage of the automatic system is the elimination of the very tedious and prone-to-error human task.

Conclusion

The system for white blood cell recognition in leukaemia patients on the basis of the image of the bone-marrow smear has been presented in this chapter. Our investigations have been aimed at the development of a fully automatic system capable to do the recognition task of the white blood cells with accuracy comparable to the human expert. The following fundamental problems have been addressed and discussed: the extraction of the individual cells from the smear of bone marrow, generation of different features of the cell, selection of the best features, and final recognition using an efficient classifier network based on the Gaussian kernel SVM. The complete system solving all these problems has been presented and discussed.

Good performance of the developed automatic cell-recognition system has been obtained thanks to the efficient solution of all separate stages of the classification task. They include the application of the watershed algorithm for the cell extraction; generation of the well-discriminating features based on texture, geometry, morphology, and the statistical description of the intensity of the image; optimal feature selection using linear SVM; and the final classification by applying a set of Gaussian kernel SVMs working in one-against-one mode.

The results of numerical experiments in the recognition of up to 17 classes of blood cells of myelogenous leukaemia and a few thousand cell samples have shown that the proposed system does quite well, with accuracy comparable to the human expert. Also, the application of the system to the preparation of the myelogram protocol for the data acquired for new patients of the hematology hospital has shown good agreement with the human expert's results. Hence, there is a chance to apply this automatic system of cell recognition in the clinical practice.

References

Beksac, M., Beksac, M. S., Tippi, V. B., Duru, H. A., Karakas, M. U., & Nurcakar, A. (1997). An artificial intelligent diagnostic system on differential recognition of haematopoietic cells from microscopic images. *Cytometry, 30*, 145-150.

Bennett, J. M., Catovsky, D., Daniel, M. T., Flandrin, G., Galton, D. A., Gralnick, H. R., et al. (1976). Proposals for the classification of the acute leukaemias. *Hematology, 33*, 451-458.

Duda, R. O., Hart, P. E., & Stork, P. (2003). *Pattern classification and scene analysis.* New York: Wiley.

Guyon, I., & Elisseeff, A. (2003). An introduction to variable and feature selection. *Journal of Machine Learning Research, 3*, 1158-1182.

Guyon, I., Weston, J., Barnhill, S., & Vapnik, V. (2002). Gene selection for cancer classification using support vector machines. *Machine Learning, 46*, 389-422.

Haykin, S. (1999). *Neural networks, comprehensive foundation.* NJ: Prentice Hall.

Hsu, C. W., & Lin, C. J. (2002). A comparison method for multi class support vector machines. *IEEE Transactions on Neural Networks, 13*, 415-425.

Lewandowski, K., & Hellmann, A. (2001). *Haematology atlas.* Gdansk, Poland: Multimedia Medical Publisher.

Markiewicz, T., Osowski, S., Mariańska, B., & Moszczyński, L. (2005). Automatic recognition of the blood cells of myelogenous leukaemia using SVM. *International Joint Conference on Neural Networks (IJCNN)*, 2496-2501.

Matlab user guide: Image processing toolbox. (1999). Natick, MA: MathWorks.

Osowski, S., Markiewicz, T., Mariańska, B., & Moszczyński, L. (2004). Feature generation for the cell image recognition of myelogenous leukemia. *IEEE International Conference EUSIPCO*, 753-756.

Osowski, S., & Tran Hoai, L. (2003). On-line heart beat recognition using Hermite polynomials and neuro-fuzzy network. *IEEE Transactions on Instrumentation and Measurements, 52*, 1224-1231.

Otsu, N. (1979). A threshold selection method from gray-level histograms. *IEEE Transactions SMC, 9*, 62-66.

Platt, L. (1998). Fast training of SVM using sequential optimization. In B. Schölkopf, B. Burges, & A. Smola (Eds.), *Advances in kernel methods: Support vector learning* (pp. 185-208). Cambridge, MA: MIT Press.

Pratt, W. (1991). *Digital image processing.* New York: Wiley.

Schölkopf, B., & Smola, A. (2002). *Learning with kernels.* Cambridge, MA: MIT Press.

Schurmann, J. (1996). *Pattern classification: A unified view of statistical and neural approaches.* New York: Wiley.

Sohn, S. (1999). *Bone marrow white blood cell classification.* Unpublished master's thesis, University of Missouri, Columbia.

Soille, P. (2003). *Morphological image analysis, principles and applications.* Berlin, Germany: Springer.

Theera-Umpon, N., & Gader, P. (2002). System-level training of neural networks for counting white blood cells. *IEEE Transactions SMC-C, 32*, 48-53.

Vapnik, V. (1998). *Statistical learning theory.* New York: Wiley.

Wagner, T. (1999). Texture analysis. In B. Jahne, H. Haussecker, & P. Geisser (Eds.), *Handbook of computer vision and application* (pp. 275-309). Boston: Academic Press.

Chapter V

Classification of Multiple Interleaved Human Brain Tasks in Functional Magnetic Resonance Imaging

Manel Martínez-Ramón, Universidad Carlos III de Madrid, Spain

Vladimir Koltchinskii, Georgia Institute of Technology, USA

Gregory L. Heileman, University of New Mexico, USA

Stefan Posse, University of New Mexico, USA

Abstract

Pattern recognition in functional magnetic resource imaging (fMRI) is a novel technique that may lead to a quantity of discovery tools in neuroscience. It is intended to automatically identify differences in distributed neural substrates resulting from cognitive tasks. Previous works in fMRI classification revealed that information is organized in coarse areas in the neural tissues rather than in small neural microstructures. This fact opens a field of study of the functional areas of the brain from the multivariate analysis of the rather coarse images provided by fMRI. Nevertheless, reliable pattern classification is challenging due to the high dimensionality of fMRI data, the small number of available data sets, interindividual differences, and dependence on the acquisition methodology. The application of kernel methods and, in particular, SVMs, to pattern recognition of fMRI is a reasonable approach to deal with these difficulties and has given reasonable results in accuracy and generalization ability. Some of the most relevant fMRI classification studies using SVMs are analyzed in this chapter. All of them were applied in individual subjects using ad hoc techniques to isolate small brain areas in order to reduce the dimensionality of the problem. Some of them included blind techniques for feature selection; others used the previous knowledge of the human brain to isolate the areas in which the information is presumed to lie. Nevertheless, these methods do not explicitly address the dimensionality, small data sets, or cross-subject classification issues. We present an approach to improve multiclass classification across groups of subjects, field strengths, and fMRI methods. We use an approach based on the segmentation of the brain in functional areas using a neuroanatomical atlas, and each map is classified separately using local classifiers. A single multiclass output is applied using an Adaboost aggregation of the classifier's outputs. This Adaboost combined the region-specific classifiers to achieve improved classification accuracy with respect to conventional techniques without previous ad hoc area or voxel selection.

Introduction

Brain activation changes in response to even simple sensory input, and motor tasks encompass a widely distributed network of functional brain areas. Information embedded in the spatial shape and extent of these activation patterns, and differences in voxel-to-voxel time courses, are not easily quantified with conventional analysis tools, such as statistical parametric mapping (SPM; Kiebel & Friston, 2004a, 2004b). Pattern classification in functional magnetic resonance imaging (fMRI) is a novel approach that promises to characterize subtle differences in activation patterns between different tasks. Roughly speaking, fMRI uses MRI techniques to detect regional changes in blood flow, volume, or oxygenation in response to task activation. The most popular technique uses blood oxygenation level dependent (BOLD) contrast, which is based on the different magnetic properties of the oxygenated and deoxygenated blood. Oxygenated blood presents diamagnetic properties while deoxygenated blood presents paramagnetic properties. These differences in susceptibility produce small differences in MR image intensity. Rapid image techniques together with statistical tools are used to generate fMRI images from sets of raw time-series data scans. The most general framework to obtain fMRI activation maps is the general linear model (GLM; Friston, Holmes, Worsley, Poline, Frith, & Frackowiak, 1995). The aim of this model is to explain the variation of the time course in terms of a linear combination of explanatory variables and an error term. The GLM can be written as $X=G\beta+e$, where X is a matrix containing the acquired data. It has a column for each voxel (a voxel, or volume pixel, is a three-dimensional pixel, or a quantity of 3-D data), and a row for each scan. G is the so-called design matrix, and it has one row per time point in the original data, and one column for every explanatory variable in the model. In an fMRI experiment, G contains indicators of the level of a certain activity reflecting the experimental design (e.g., zeros and ones for a required activation) or other kinds of information not related to the experiments (covariates of global cerebral blood flow, drift, respiration, etc.). Matrix β is the parameter matrix and **e** is the vector of error terms. In order to obtain β, least squares are applied. Provided that one can split matrices **G** and β into four parts containing indicators and covariates of interesting and confounding effects, a range of statistical analyses can be performed on the GLM. The student t-test (t-map) can be viewed as a particular case of the GLM, and it is one of the most used techniques in fMRI. Student t-tests and other statistical analyses can be viewed as particular cases of the GLM.

The automatic and reliable classification of patterns is challenging due to the high dimensionality of fMRI data, which contain 10,000 to 100,000 voxels per image; the small number of available data sets; interindividual differences in activation patterns; and the dependence on the image-acquisition methodology.

Recent work by Cox and Savoy (2003) demonstrated that linear discriminant analysis (LDA) and support vector machines (SVMs) allow the discrimination of 10-class visual activation patterns evoked by the visual presentation of various categories of objects on a trial-by-trial basis within individual subjects. In Kamitani and Tong (2005), a linear SVM is used to show that even if the orientation information for visual stimuli is held in structures that cannot be seen using fMRI, this information can be retrieved by observing the corresponding brain areas by this technique, thus demonstrating that the information is structured in a coarse way in these areas.

LaConte, Strother, Cherkassky, Anderson, and Hu (2005), and LaConte, Strother, Cherkassky, and Hu (2003) used a linear SVM for the online pattern recognition of left and right motor activation in single subjects. They compared the results using an SVM to those of a canonical variates analysis (CVA). Wang, Hutchinson, and Mitchell (2004) applied an SVM classifier to detect brain cognitive states across multiple subjects. Mitchell, Hutchinson, Niculescu, Pereira, and Wang (2004) compare the classification accuracies of Gaussian naïve Bayes classifiers (GNBC), k-nearest neighbors (KNN), and linear SVM applied to various fMRI classification tasks. Here, the authors show that a feature selection that reduces the dimensionality significantly improves the accuracy of the classifiers.

In these papers, with the exception of Mitchell et al. (2004), the dimensionality problem was not addressed, although better results in generalization ability can be achieved by reducing the dimensionality of the data. Some authors suggest the reduction of the resolution as a way to reduce dimensionality. Nevertheless, reducing the resolution implies a low-pass filtering of the signal, so a possible loss of information can preclude good classification performance. Other techniques look for those dimensions that contain information. Principal component analysis (PCA) is widely used as a preprocessing tool for dimensionality reduction for single-subject and group space-time source separation (e.g., Calhoun, Adali, Pearlson, & Pekar, 2001). But here two additional problems arise. PCA needs to deal with square matrices containing as many columns and rows as dimensions; the resulting computational burden makes the algorithm unsuitable for real-time implementations. On the other hand, this technique is only accurate if the total amount of data is large, but only small data sets are available in t-map classification tasks.

In Martínez-Ramón, Koltchinskii, Heileman, and Posse (2005a, 2005b), a work has been presented that splits the activation maps into areas, applying a local (or base) classifier to each one. In Koltchinskii, Martinez, and Posse (2005), theoretical bounds on the performance of the method for the binary case have been presented, and in Martínez-Ramón,

Koltchinskii, Heileman, and Posse (2006), a more general method and a set of experiments are introduced. When splitting the activation maps in smaller areas, the dimension of each area will be smaller than the dimension of the whole activation map. Local SVMs are then trained in each of the areas. An optimal aggregation of these local classifiers through boosting is able to select those areas in which useful information is present, discarding the others, and improving the classification performance with respect to the performance of the local classifiers. Also, the output of boosting in the form of boosting maps that highlight relevant activated areas can be directly compared with the output from conventional fMRI analysis that are reported as maxima of activation clusters. As local classifiers, multiclass SVMs have been applied (Burges, 1998; Hsu & Lin, 2002, 2002). See also Chapter 1 for an introduction to SVM.

From one point of view, one can think of the present SVM plus the distributed boosting algorithm as a combination of two kernel strategies. Both boosting algorithms and SVMs can be considered as algorithms in which input data is mapped to some representation through a hidden layer (Müller, Mika, Rätsch, Tsuda, & Schölkopf, 2001). An interesting fundamental similarity between boosting and kernel SVM emerges, as both can be described as methods for regularized optimization in high-dimensional predictor space (Rosset, Zhu, & Hastie, 2004).

In next section, the works by Cox and Savoy (2003) and Kamitani and Tong (2005) are summarized. LaConte et al. (2005) were the first authors to present the SVM as a tool that has superior performance for the brain imaging community, and they presented several methods for model interpretation from the analysis of the SVM parameters. This paper is also summarized. Then, we present the work introduced in Martínez-Ramón et al. (2006), in which distributed boosting is introduced as a tool that takes advantage of the fact that the distribution of the information in the brain is sparse. Finally, several results using this approach are provided.

Application of SVM to fMRI Classification

Classification of Object Recognition in Visual Cortex

Cox and Savoy (2003) were among the first authors to apply a classifier to the analysis of fMRI data, and to compare it to the univariate analysis of it. The main claim of the work is that univariate analysis of fMRI data relies exclusively on the information contained in the time course of individual voxels, but multivariate analysis may take advantage of the information contained in activity patterns across space from multiple voxels. Multivariate analysis has the potential to expand the amount of information extracted from fMRI data sets. In their study, an SVM was used to classify patterns of fMRI activation evoked by the visual presentation of various categories of objects. Results were compared to the ones of a linear discriminant.

The classification experiment is made showing an object (among a set of 10 objects) to a participant. The classifier was trained to detect which object was shown from the observation of the fMRI data in the visual cortex of the participant. Ten participants were used, and the total amount of data for training was relatively small; less than 200 data items were available for training, and the user classifiers were a linear and a polynomial kernel SVM.

In the first set of experiments, authors trained the machine with the fMRI data obtained during the observation of the 10 objects. A total of 10 blocks of 20 different observations were taken. The test was done using fMRI data taken during later sessions, but using the same objects.

In a second experiment, different objects of the same 10 classes were used for testing. The resolution of the fMRI images were of 3×3×5 mm per voxel, and the imaging matrix was 64×64×21 voxels. A total of 27,000 voxels were measured in the images, which could preclude a good generalization as only 200 images were available for classification. A method was applied to reduce the dimensionality of the images, consisting of an ANOVA (analysis of variance) test that automatically includes voxels that are out of the visual cortex. This is reasonable due to the visual nature of the experiments. The number of picked voxels was less than or equal to 200.

The authors compared a linear discriminant to a linear and a polynomial SVM for different numbers of voxels and different numbers of training data items. The used SVM implementation was the popular OSU SVM (http://sourceforge.net/projects/svm/), and the multiclass strategy was one against one (see, e.g., Hsu & Lin, 2002), so a total of 45 binary SVMs were used in the experiments.

Accuracies varied from 52 to 97% depending on the participant, and they were better for the linear SVM. Although differences between the linear and polynomial have no statistical significance, in almost all cases, the tendency is favorable for the linear SVM.

The work presented in that paper reveals that neuron activity is organized in a coarse scale and that the information is distributed as it is not possible to make a classification using a single voxel, but it is possible to do it when a number of voxels is used. Even if each voxel contains the averaged activity of thousands or millions of neurons, one can extract the information by looking at a coarse pattern made by a few hundred voxels.

On the other hand, experiments were done using a number of voxels that was similar to the number of available data for training. The rest of the voxels were discarded prior to the experiments. Also, all the experiments were made with a single participant; no interparticipant experiments were reported.

Orientation Detection in Visual Cortex

Kamitani and Tong (2005) went deeper inside the idea that a multivariate analysis is able to retrieve the information being processed by the neurons, even if the fMRI resolution is several million times the dimension of a single neuron because the information is structured in a coarse fashion in the neural tissue. To support this claim, they used the classification results given by a standard SVM. In particular, they focused on the fact that there is neurophysiological evidence of orientation tuning in cortical columns and single neurons in cat and monkey visual areas (Bartfeld & Grinvald, 1992; Blasdel, 1992; Hubel & Wiesel, 1962, 1968). However, there is no possibility of checking this in humans due to the invasive nature of the needed experiments. Practical noninvasive methods have been useless due to the low resolution of the brain image of the available technologies. As a consequence, there is not much knowledge of the neural basis of orientation selectivity in the human visual system or about how these features are represented during perception.

The work is intended to introduce a framework for the readout of the visual orientation in the human cortex using fMRI. As this technique was not able to reach the necessary resolution to look for orientation patterns in individual neurons or microstructures, it looked for macroscopic patterns that are different depending on the orientation of the stimuli presented to the participants. If differences were present in these macroscopic patterns, a multivariate analysis consisting of a classifier applied to a group of voxels located in the visual cortex could be able to classify different orientations.

The chosen base classifier was a linear SVM, and the multiclass strategy was the one-against-all multiclass classifier. The experiment consisted of the presentation of a circle with a grating inside and a fixation cross in its center. The participants observed among a total of eight different orientations between 0 and 157.5 degrees. Each participant views a total of 24 different images, whose corresponding fMRI images are used as training data. The volume introduced in the classifier consisted of 400 voxels located in the early visual area.

During the test phase, participants observed a total of 16 images with different orientations. The fMRI data was fed into the classifier, and the average test error was computed. Only single-participant experiments were reported. Results were statistically significant and suggested that a pattern of orientation exists in the ensemble of used voxels. A similar experiment is presented in Haynes and Rees (2005), which suggests that there is a subconscious *aftereffect* of the orientation visualization in the human cortex.

Online Motor Task Classification

Laconte et al. (2005) recently presented a work in which they applied a classifier to detect different motor tasks using fMRI images. One of the differences between this work and the works summarized above is that the previous ones used statistical parametric maps that represent a statistical test over a series of fMRI images taken during the task period. In Kamitani and Tong, (2005), the used images are a student t-study of the time-series images (see "Introduction"). In Cox and Savoy (2003), averages of raw data images rather than t-maps are used. In LaConte et al. (2005), the authors classify the individual scans of the time series on a TR-by-TR basis. The authors justify the use of raw time-series data rather than t-maps or other statistical parametric mapping by the fact that, from a Bayesian perspective, there is no mathematical advantage for choosing to estimate a spatial summary map from our knowledge of the experiment (e.g. general linear model approaches (Friston et al., 1995)) over trying to estimate these experimental parameters from our input patterns (LaConte et al., 2005, p. 1).

In fact, if the reference vector does not exactly reflect the actual time course in the region of interest, the resulting statistical map may be corrupted.

A strategy like SVM can be useful to construct summary maps from the time series. SVMs construct the classification or regression machines by explicitly computing their parameters as a linear combination of some of the training patterns, the so-called support vectors. These support vectors are among those data that are closer to the classification margin, that is, from those data that are difficult to classify. Authors propose several methods to construct summary maps. Among them, they propose to compute a correlation test for every voxel time series, but instead of using a reference vector of two levels (on and off), they propose to weight this reference with a distance measure from the separation margin. So, a voxel corresponding to an image that is close to the margin will produce a small weight in the reference vector, thus having less importance in the summary map.

Also, an SVM can be constructed using the data of a single experiment as a set of images will be available. However, this possibility does not exist if t-maps are used because the number of images is reduced: Typically, one image per experiment is obtained. This is, of course, true as long as the prior information to construct the design matrix of the GLM (see Friston et al., 1995) is wrong, incomplete, or inaccurate.

The authors use the time series to train and test different SVMs using resampling techniques to select the parameters. fMRI experiments were performed with 16 right-handed participants. The aim was to discriminate between left- and right-hand motor tasks. Tests were done with linear and polynomial SVMs and CVA. The best results were obtained using linear SVMs, which showed good generalization ability. Also, the authors compare their SVM summary maps from those obtained using conventional correlation techniques, showing that much better results can be obtained using SVMs.

Finally, this work opens a framework for real-time fMRI classification as there is no need for batch preprocessing before the training or the test of the classifier. The classifier can be trained or tested as the time-series images are produced.

A Spatially Distributed Classifier for Multiple Interleaved Tasks

The previously summarized works introduced the use of SVMs in fMRI classification due to the properties of the generalization of such machines over other linear approaches like linear Fisher discriminant analysis. Also, they introduced neuroanatomical and neurofunctional knowledge from the results of the presented experiments. Nevertheless, the dimension of the used images is about 10^4 to 10^5, and the total number of images that are available for training purposes is about 100. So, the problem of the dimensionality still remains in these works. The approaches taken in these works include the following:

- Dimensionality reduction by selecting a small area that is presumed to contain the information needed for the classification.
- Classification among binary and relatively simple tasks.

- Classification using linear machines (with low complexity).
- If raw time-series scans are used, a larger amount of data for training purposes.

The approach that is presented in this section has been extracted from 0 and is intended to reduce the problem of the dimensionality of the images without dramatically reducing the total number of used voxels, and using small data sets for training. The approach is based on the fact that the information in the brain is sparse, so only a few areas of it will contain relevant information for the classification tasks.

With this idea in mind, a reasonable segmentation of the activation map in anatomically constrained functional areas (FA) can be performed. Then, each area of the map will contain a smaller number of voxels. A local classifier applied to one FA that contains information relevant to the classification might show an improved generalization performance with respect to a classifier applied to the whole map. However, the classifiers that present poor classification performance must be removed from the classification task. Moreover, a good classifier must average the outputs of all classifiers following their classification performance. A boosting algorithm (Schapire, 1999) can be applied to perform this task.

Boosting algorithms can be viewed as algorithms that perform empirical risk minimization with convex loss over a linear span of a given base class of functions (classifiers) using an iterative gradient functional descent method. This is typically implemented by maintaining a distribution of weights over the training set. At each iteration, the algorithm attempts to minimize the weighted training error over the base class, and then it updates the weights of the training examples in such a way that those samples that are misclassified at the current iteration will have a higher weight at the next iteration. In this way, the learning machine will focus on the examples that are hard to classify at the current iteration. The algorithm also assigns nonnegative coefficients to the base classifiers obtained at each iteration, and, at the end, outputs a convex combination of these classifiers. It can be shown that this strategy indeed implements a version of gradient functional descent. We introduce a modification of the Adaboost algorithm (Freund & Schapire, 1996; Schapire, 1999) to apply it to a set of distributed classifiers. In Chapter 16 by Bruzzone, Gomez-Chova, Marconcini, and Camps-

Figure 1. Structure of the classifier (Martinez et al., 2006, reproduced with permission of Elsevier)

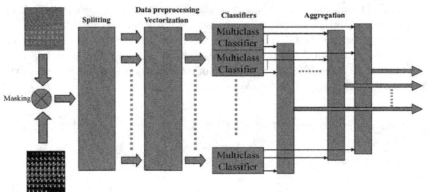

Figure 2. Fourteen masks used to extract the functional areas (Martinez et al., 2006, reproduced with permission of Elsevier)

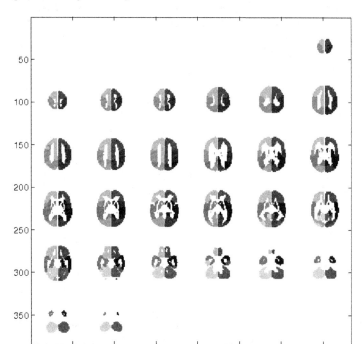

Valls, the authors use a regularized version of the Adaboost algorithm in the context of hyperspectral image classification.

Using this approach, a set of nonlinear SVMs can be applied that outperform the classification performance of their linear counterparts. That way, one can apply kernel functions without jeopardizing the generalization ability due to the dimensionality of the input data. In particular, Gaussian SVMs are applied as local classifiers.

A set of multiclass local classifiers $\mathbf{h}_j$, $1 \leq j \leq N$ are constructed and trained, one for each of the N FAs. All classifiers provide a vector of L outputs, L being the number of classes. The chosen schema for multiclass classification is the direct multiclass SVM classifier as described in Weston and Watkins (1999). This approach produced more accurate results than the classical one-against-one, one-against-all, error-correcting-output-codes (Dietterich & Bakiri, 1995; Hsu & Lin, 2002), or directed-acyclic-graphs (Platt, Cristianini, & Shawe-Taylor, 2000) strategies when used for the present fMRI classification task. Nevertheless, following Rifkin and Klautau (2004), there is no clear evidence of the advantage of using one or another approach. The classifier consists of the modules shown in Figure 1.

The activation maps are segmented into FAs based on the atlas of Talairach and Tournoux (1988) using Analysis of Functional NeuroImages (AFNI) fMRI analysis software (http://afni.nimh.nih.gov/afni/). A total of 14 masks were used to extract the FAs, grouped into left and right brainstem, cerebellum, parietal, temporal, occipital, subcortical, and frontal lobes (see Figure 2). The dimension of the data introduced to each classifier is roughly 10 times lower than the dimension of the whole t-map. Additional masks including brainstem, cerebellum, parietal, temporal, occipital, subcortical areas, and frontal cortex were created using BRAINS2 image analysis software (Magnotta, Harris, Andreasen, Yuh, & Heckel, 2002), which can be obtained by request at http://www.psychiatry.uiowa.edu/.

The outputs of the local classifiers are linearly aggregated as:

$$\mathbf{h} = \sum_{j=1}^{N} \lambda_j \mathbf{h}_j, \tag{1}$$

λ_j being the weighting parameter for the aggregation. The classifiers that yield good performance are boosted by increasing their aggregation parameter. As a result, a parameter λ is assigned to each FA, which measures its importance for the given classification task. Then, a boosting map of the brain can be constructed highlighting those FAs containing relevant information for the classification.

Optimal Aggregation of a Set of Spatially Distributed Classifiers

In our application, the base class for boosting consists of a finite number of local classifiers trained in advance in each of the FAs, and our method can be viewed as a distributed version of boosting, very natural in the classification of images. At each iteration, boosting picks one of the classifiers that minimize the current weighted training error. The output of the algorithm is, in this case, a convex combination of local classifiers, which can be viewed as a method of their optimal aggregation to produce a classifier with the smallest empirical risk. The coefficients of the convex combination show the relative importance of local classifiers and corresponding FAs for a particular classification problem, and they are used to construct a boosting map.

Assume that a set of pairs $\{\mathbf{x}_i, \mathbf{y}_i\}$ is available for classification tasks, where $y_i^{(l)}$ is 1 if the pattern belongs to class l, and -1 otherwise. In our fMRI pattern-classification task, each pattern x_i is a vector constructed by placing all voxels of a t-map in a row. If the classification task involves more than two classes of t-maps, the labels associated with the patterns are vectors. In the classification tasks, there are four classes of patterns, corresponding to visual, motor, cognitive, and auditory. Arbitrarily, one can assign the label $\mathbf{y}_i = \{-1, 1, -1, 1\}$ to the visual patterns, $\mathbf{y}_i = \{-1, 1, -1, 1\}$ to the motor ones, and so on.

The local classifiers will produce a vector output equal to one of the L possible labels. Here, the multiclass Adaboost procedure of Allwein, Schapire, and Singer (2000) is followed. The procedure is the following one.

For each j, l, do the following:

- Initialize an error distribution matrix $D_0(i,j,l) = \frac{1}{n}$ for each data x_i and each class, and initialize a set of aggregation parameters $\lambda_{j,0}^{(l)} = 0$.

- Repeat for $t = 1...T$.

  - For each classifier, compute the classification error $\varepsilon_t(j,l)$:

$$\varepsilon_t(j,l) = \sum_{i=1}^{n} D_t(i,j,l) I\{h_j^{(l)}(\mathbf{x}_i) \neq y_i^{(l)}\}, \qquad (2)$$

  where $I\{h_j^{(l)}(\mathbf{x}_i) \neq y_i^{(l)}\}$ is 1 if $h_j^{(l)}(\mathbf{x}_i) \neq y_i^{(l)}$ and 0 otherwise.

  - Choose the best classifier, or the classifier that produces the lowest error.

  - Compute an update term $\alpha_t^{(l)}$ for the aggregation parameters $\lambda_j^{(l)}$ corresponding to the best classifier:

$$\alpha_t^{(l)} = \frac{1}{2} \ln \left(\frac{1 - \varepsilon_t(\hat{j},l)}{\varepsilon_t(\hat{j},l)} \right). \qquad (3)$$

  - Update the aggregation parameter:

$$\lambda_{\hat{j},t+1}^{(l)} = \lambda_{\hat{j},t}^{(l)} + \alpha_t^{(l)}. \qquad (4)$$

  - Update the error distribution:

$$D_{t+1}(i,j,l) = \frac{D_t(i,j,l)}{2\sqrt{\varepsilon_t(\hat{j},l)(1-\varepsilon_t(\hat{j},l))}} \exp(-\alpha y_i^{(l)} h_j^{(l)}(\mathbf{x}_i)). \qquad (5)$$

- End.

- Normalize the aggregation set so that $\sum_j \lambda_j^{(l)} = 1$.

The strategy produces a set of L-dimensional parameters $\lambda_j = [\lambda_j^{(1)} \cdots \lambda_j^{(L)}]$ that weight the local classifiers as:

$$h^{(l)} = \sum_{j=1}^{N} \lambda_j^{(l)} h_j^{(l)}. \qquad (6)$$

Here, a set of parameters $\lambda_{j,l}$, $1 \leq l \leq L$ have been updated to separately aggregate each of the L binary outputs of the local classifiers. As a result, L separate boosting maps have been obtained, one corresponding to each class.

Since we have to deal with a small number of training examples (less than 100), the following randomization technique was useful. We split the training data at random into two subsets as

Figure 3. Application of a local classifier for each of the 14 brain mask areas (Martinez et al., 2006, reproduced with permission of Elsevier)

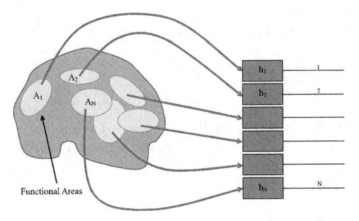

follows: For each class, half of the data is randomly picked and put into one of the subsets, and the remainder is put into the other subset. Thus, both subsets have approximately the same fraction of patterns of each class as the original set.

The first subset is used to train the local classifiers and the second is used for boosting the aggregation of these classifiers. This procedure is repeated independently a number of times.

Figure 4. Combination of classifier outputs to generate boosting maps, reproduced with permission

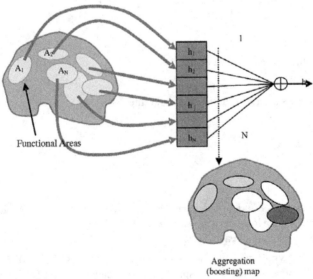

Figure 5. Representative visual stimuli used in interleaved paradigm

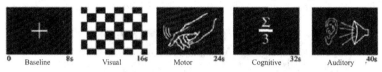

| 0 | Baseline | 8s | Visual | 16s | Motor | 24s | Cognitive | 32s | Auditory | 40s |

The aggregation coefficients are then averaged. At the end, local classifiers are trained again based on the whole training data and an aggregate classifier is created by applying to them the average boosting coefficients.

Functional Magnetic Resonance Imaging Experiment

Participants and Paradigm

Ten healthy participants were studied using a 1.5 Tesla Siemens Sonata scanner, and another 10 using a 4.0 Tesla Brucker MedSpec scanner. Informed consent based on institutionally reviewed guidelines was obtained prior to participation in the study. Stimuli were presented via MR-compatible LCD goggles and headphones (Resonance Technology Inc., Northridge, CA). The paradigm consists of four interleaved tasks: visual (checkerboard stimulation at 8 Hz), motor (right index finger tapping at 2 Hz), auditory (syllable discrimination), and cognitive (mental calculation). These tasks are arranged in a randomized block design (8 seconds per block), with a crosshair serving as baseline for a total of 132 seconds per scan (Figure 5). The total duration for each condition was thus approximately 27 seconds. Visual stimulation consisted of reversing black and white checkerboards at 8 Hz. Finger tapping in the motor task was paced with an auditory tone (1 kHz). Participants were asked to tap with

Table 1. Number of t-maps acquired with different field strengths, spatial resolutions, and read-out bandwidths

Field	# t-maps	Resolution	# t-maps	BW	# t-maps
-1.5T	-101	-32×32	-76	LB	55
				HB	21
		64×64	25	LB	25
-4.0T	-81	-32×32	-52	LB	47
				HB	5
		64×64	29	LB	29

Figure 6. Activation t-maps corresponding to (a) visual, (b) motor, (c) cognitive, and (d) auditory activations (Martinez et al., 2006, reproduced with permission of Elsevier)

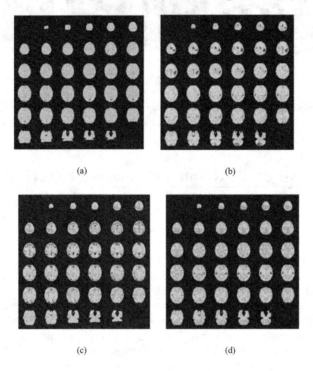

(a)   (b)

(c)   (d)

maximum extension of the finger onto a button-response pad (Cedrus Corp., San Pedro, CA). During the auditory task, participants listened to recorded syllables (i.e., "Ah, Ba, Ha, Ka, Ra") and pressed a button when they heard the target syllable "Ta" (25% of syllables). The cognitive task consisted of mental calculations. Participants were asked to sum three aurally presented numbers and divide the sum by three, responding with a button press when the sum was divisible by three without remainder (50% of trials). Participants were instructed to attend to each task with a constant effort across scans and field strengths.

Data Acquisition

fMRI data were acquired using single-shot echo-planar imaging with repetition time (TR) of 2 seconds, echo time (TE) of 50 msec, flip angle of 90 degrees, matrix size of 64×64 or 32×32 pixels, and field of view (FOV) of 192 mm. Data with the 32v32 matrix were acquired with different bandwidths, either with1200 Hz/pixel (low bandwidth – LBW) or with 2400 Hz/pixel (high bandwidth – HBW), which changes the degree of geometrical distortion and the signal-to-noise ratio. Slices were 6 mm thick, with 25% gap; 66 volumes were collected for a total measurement time of 132 seconds per run.

The available data set consists of 184 t-maps taken from 18 different participants. Details of the data set are provided in Table 1.

Data Analysis

Statistical parametric mapping using SPM2 (Kiebel & Friston, 2004a, 2004b) was performed to generate t-maps that represent brain activation changes. Preprocessing steps included motion correction, slice-time correction, spatial normalization, and spatial smoothing. Statistical analysis using a design matrix with four conditions (motor, visual, auditory, cognitive) was performed with corrected amplitude threshold ($p < 0.05$) and 132-second high-pass filter. Examples of the obtained t-maps in Figure 6 show in part overlapping activation patterns due to auditory stimulus presentation in motor, cognitive, and auditory tasks, and button responses in motor, cognitive, and auditory tasks. T-maps have the same normalization as the masks, shown in Figure 2. Nevertheless, distortion may appear during the normalization of the t-maps, which can make the masking procedure inaccurate. For all used images, activations lied in the corresponding masks. For example, the visual activation of Figure 6a will lie in the occipital masks, where the visual areas are located. Activations of Figure 6b will lie in the frontal masks, and activations of Figure 6d will lie in the parietal mask, corresponding to the auditory areas. Cognitive activations (Figure 6c) will lie in different areas as the information is highly distributed around the brain.

In order to measure the performance of the classifier, the following tests were conducted.

1. **Dynamics of the boosting parameters.** In order to test the time behavior of the Adaboost, we ran the algorithm for all the 1.5 Tesla data and looked at the behavior of the aggregation parameters and error rates.

2. **Misclassification results for cross-modality training.** Different tests were run to measure the cross-modality performance of the classifier.

   - Training with all 1.5 T (4.0 T) t-maps and test with the 4.0 T (1.5 T) t-maps. The number of 1.5 T t-maps is 101, where there are 81 4.0 T t-maps.

   - Training with high- (low-) resolution and test with low- (high-) resolution t-maps. There are 128 low-resolution t-maps and 54 high-resolution t-maps.

   - Training with low- (high-) bandwidth and test with low- (high-) resolution t-maps. There are 156 low-bandwidth t-maps and 26 high-bandwidth t-maps.

3. **Test with all data.** We performed a leave-one-out test using all the available activation maps. This procedure consisted of training the algorithm with 218 maps, leaving one out for testing, which results in 219 different trainings and tests.

4. **Relative contribution of different classes to mixed activation patterns.** The interleaved task design in the present study leads to a partial overlap of activation patterns from different classes, and the classifier assigns multiple labels in accordance with the relative contribution of different activation patterns. It can be said that the activation

Figure 7. Evolution of the test misclassification rate as a function of the number of averaged Adaboost parameters using the Distributed Adaboost and RBF-SVM local classifiers (30 different realizations of the experiment have been averaged to obtain this graph) (Martinez et al., 2006, reproduced with permission of Elsevier)

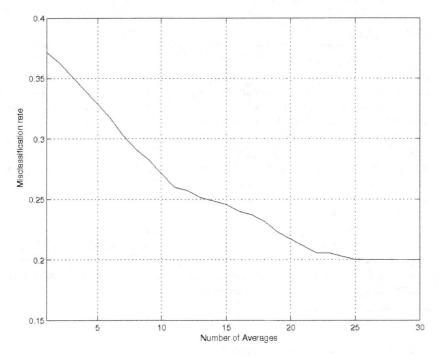

maps used in the experiments are often multilabeled, that is, they belong to more than one class.

Provided that the activations belonging to different tasks have different locations in the brain, the introduced classification method has some ability to detect multilabel patterns because it consists of the aggregation of the outputs of local classifiers that work based on different brain areas.

In order to detect different classes of activations, instead of just aggregating all of the local classifier outputs, one may group the classifiers whose outputs belong to each class and aggregate them separately using the obtained aggregation parameters of Algorithm. One can define the following quantities:

$$o_l = \frac{\sum_{i:h_{i,j}=1} \lambda_{i,l}}{\sum_{l=1}^{L} \sum_{i:h_{i,j}=1} \lambda_{i,l}}, 1 \le l \le L, \tag{7}$$

Figure 8. Evolution of the aggregation parameters λ as a function of the number of randomized boosting iterations using the distributed Adaboost Algorithm and RBF-SVM local classifiers (Martinez et al., 2006, reproduced with permission of Elsevier)

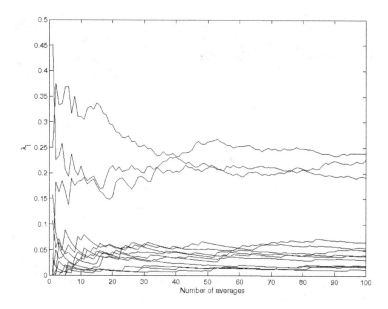

Figure 9. Boosting maps for (a) visual, (b) motor, (c) cognitive, and (d) auditory activation (Martinez et al., 2006, reproduced with permission of Elsevier)

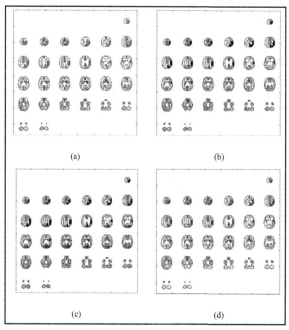

Figure 10. Map of the output of all classifiers and the aggregation of them (Σ) for all test data (four tones represent visual, motor, cognitive, and auditory classifications) (Martinez et al., 2006, reproduced with permission of Elsevier)

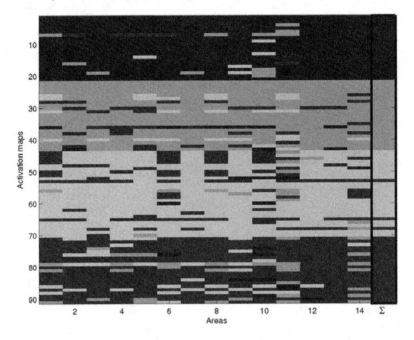

which represent the fraction of detected activation for each class. Here, the aggregation parameters weight the predicted labels of each classifier. This is a weighting of the predicted labels: Those classifiers that have shown poor classification performance during the training of the boosting aggregation will have low-valued aggregation parameters, so their predicted label will be weighted with a low value, and the ones with good performance will be weighted with a higher value. This can be viewed as the "best" classifiers being given a better credibility in the classification. The output will be not only a label, but a vector of L scalars, each one with a weight indicating the fraction of each predicted activation.

Results

Dynamics of the Boosting Parameters

The local classifiers consisted of SVMs with the Gaussian radial basis function (RBF) kernel function. The Adaboost training was repeated up to 100 times, and the resulting sets of aggregation parameters were averaged and normalized to 1, as described previously. Specifically, in each training of Adaboost, 25 t-maps from the training data set were randomly picked and used to train the local classifiers. The other 25 were used to train the parameters.

Figure 7 shows the error rate as a function of the number of averaged Adaboost parameters. To compute the error rate, the local classifiers are trained with the entire training data set and then the aggregation is tested with the averaged Adaboost parameters.

The error rate as a function of time corresponding to the Adaboost algorithm shows the same behavior. We can see in Figure 7 that the performance increases with the number of averages (although, with the current amount of data, there is no statistical significance on the improvement). As the amount of data is small, the resulting aggregation parameters from each Adaboost training are inaccurate, but for this test set, averaging 25 aggregation parameters is enough to obtain stable results.

Figure 8 shows the behavior of the aggregation parameters of the algorithm from the previous experiments. Each graph in the figure is the average over l of all parameters $\lambda_{j, l}$. The parameters are quite stable after 40 iterations, although the results of Figure 7 suggest 20 to 25 iterations may be enough to achieve good generalization performance for this experiment.

Figure 9 shows the four boosting maps produced by the algorithm. The visual map does not show high values exclusively in the occipital areas because all areas contain information that can be used for classification. For example, the right subcortical and temporal areas can be used for the classification due to the fact that there is no activation in them during the visual activity but there is during all other activities. On the other hand, activity in the cerebellum is present during motor tasks, which extends partly into the occipital cortex due to spatial normalization and smoothing. The activation map corresponding to motor activation shows a high value in the right parietal area, where the motor activation is present. For the case of the cognitive and auditory maps, the right temporal area is relevant for the classification, but not the left one; it typically contains more noise or interleaved activation in the images used for training, which precludes its use for classification. Interestingly, the occipital areas are used for classification of the cognitive activity

Figure 10 shows the classification given by all local classifiers for all test activation maps, plus the decision given by the boosting aggregation. The four intensities represent the four possible answers of the classifiers. Each row of the graph corresponds to each of the classifier outputs for an activation map, sorted as left and right brainstem, cerebellum, frontal, occipital, parietal, subcortical, and temporal. Each column shows the output of one classifier for all of

Table 2. Misclassification rates for single classifier and boosting classifier using Gaussian radial basis function kernels

Tr:	4T	1.5T	32×32	64×64	HB	LB
Test:	1.5T	4T	64×64	32×32	LB	HB
Alg. II	7.9%	7.4%	3.7%	8.6%	3.9%	9.6%
Single	14.8%	14.8	21%	23.3%	19%	23.1%

Table 3. Confusion matrices for: (left) Training with 4 T data and testing with 1.5 T data, and (right) training with high read-out bandwidth and test with low read-out bandwidth data. Gaussian RBF kernel were used for local classifiers. Columns: actual class; rows: predicted class. 1: visual; 2: motor; 3: cognitive; 4: auditory.

4T vs 1.5T						HBW vs LBW				
1	2	3	4			1	2	3	4	
1	14 0	0	0			1	36 1	0	0	
2	0	23 0	1			2	0	38 0	0	
3	0	0	23 0			3	3	1	37 4	
4	0	0	5	15		4	0	1	5	30

the activation maps. We sorted the activation maps according to their corresponding label, first the visual, then motor, cognitive, and finally auditory. The last column (into the black frame) shows the aggregated output for all activation maps. It can be seen that the aggregation shows the best performance, with only three misclassified cognitive activations.

Misclassification Results for Cross-Modality Training

The results of the tests are shown in Table 2. We can see that in all cases, distributed Adaboost performs better than the single classifier. This might be related to the fact that the boosting classifier has a special structure. Specifically, it is a convex combination of local classifiers related to specified functional areas of the brain. In the case when there are only few functional areas that contain relevant information for a particular classification problem, the convex combination becomes sparse, which leads to a reduction in the complexity of the classifier and the improvement of its generalization performance. Global SVM classifiers cannot achieve this goal unless they are based on a specially designed kernel that takes the

Table 4. Relative contributions of task mixures in the activation maps shown in Figures 6 and 11

t-map	Visual	Motor	Cognitive	Auditory
Fig. 6a	1	0	0	0
Fig. 11a	0.91	0.06	0.03	0
Fig. 6b	0	1	0	0
Fig. 11b	0	0.67	0.32	0
Fig. 6c	0	0	1	0
Fig. 11c	0	0.14	0.58	0.28
Fig. 6d	0	0	0	1
Fig. 11d	0.01	0.24	0.03	0.72

Figure 11. Examples of activation t-maps corresponding to (a) visual, (b) motor, (c) cognitive, and (d) auditory activations showing mixtures of activation patterns (Martinez et al., 2006, reproduced with permission of Elsevier)

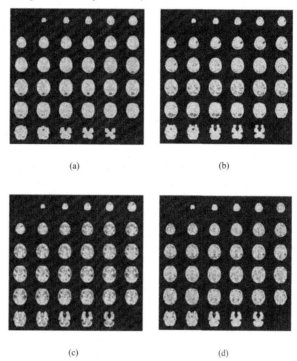

(a)   (b)

(c)   (d)

functional areas into account. Because of this, global SVMs tend to overfit as compared to distributed boosting.

Almost all misclassifications were in the auditory activation classification, where the information is not as sparse as in visual or motor activations, and where other kinds of activations were present, mainly cognitive and motor. As an example, Table 3 shows the confusion matrix for the experiment of 4 T vs. 1.5 T data. Among the 20 auditory activations, only 15 were correctly classified, where 5 of them were classified as cognitive. All visual and cognitive activations were correctly classified and only 1 out of 23 motor activations were misclassified. The table also shows the result of the high bandwidth vs. low bandwidth test, with similar behavior.

The same set of tests was run for linear and second-degree polynomial kernels. In both cases, results were poorer than with Gaussian RBF kernels. Linear classifiers produce poor performance due to the fact that the optimum separation hyperplanes are not linear. For polynomial kernels, we observe high sensitivity of the classification results to small changes in the parameters. For example, slight differences in amplitude scaling or the order of the set of polynomials produce very different results, which make polynomials not well suited for this kind of classification task.

Tests with All Data

Results give a misclassification rate of less than 2% for the boosting scheme, and above 9% for the single classifier, which suggests that the boosting scheme has improved generalization ability.

Relative Contribution of Different Classes to Mixed Activation Patterns

Visual activation maps were very distinct, but most of the other activation maps show mixtures of activation patterns. As an example, the outputs described in equation (7) were computed for the activation maps in Figures 6 and 11. The activation t-maps in Figure 6 do show very distinct activation patterns, and are thus clearly classified as belonging to a single class. The maps in Figure 11 show mixed activation patterns that are classified as belonging to multiple classes. Table 4 contains the fraction of overlapping tasks estimated by the classifier. For example, in the motor activation pattern in Figure 11, there is an estimation of cognitive activity of 32%, which can be explained mainly by the activation in the center of the frontal and temporal areas, which is much less intense in the corresponding motor activation in Figure 6. Also, one can see activation in the parietal area and cerebellum in the auditory map in Figure 11, which suggests motor activation, as detected by the classifier.

Discussion

SVMs have been applied to a variety of fMRI patterns, from which we summarize some of the most recent ones. The first one is related to seen-object classification, and the tested classifiers are linear SVMs and a linear discriminant analysis over sets of averages of fMRI time-series images. The second summarized approach uses linear SVMs to classify among a number of images of grids with 10 different orientations. The used data consisted of sets of fMRI t-maps. The last approach is intended to classify motor activities from each single image of an fMRI time series. This approach can be considered as one of the first real-time fMRI approaches as authors are able to perform an online classification from a single 4-second scan. Linear SVM show better performance than polynomial SVM or CVA. One of the aims of this chapter is to show that multivariate analysis can be useful in the prediction of brain activity from macroscopic brain data as fMRI scans.

All the mentioned approaches suggest that the use of SVM has an advantage over other classical classification algorithms due to the superior generalization ability of SVM. Nevertheless, the linear SVM produced better results than the nonlinear ones, which may be due to the fact that the dimensionality of the addressed problems is very high, thus resulting in overfitting when using nonlinear classifiers.

We introduced a new classification method for application to the multiclass classification of different activations in fMRI t-maps that combines two kernel strategies: a nonlinear SVM classification stage plus a distributed Adaboost stage. The method is based on the segmentation of t-maps into different neuroanatomical areas, and the application of independent local classifiers to each one. The outputs of the classifiers are optimally aggregated using a spatially distributed version of the well-known Adaboost algorithm. The spatially distributed Adaboost chooses the areas with information relevant for the classification, discarding the rest, which makes the classifier sparser and reduces its complexity. The reduction of the complexity makes the method robust across cross-modality training. Also, we observed that the method is robust against variations in the choice of the parameters of the local classifiers. This is interesting for real applications as the user does not need to interact with the algorithm to adjust parameters. In addition, the spatially distributed Adaboost produces a boosting map of the brain. This map is obtained from the amplitudes of the aggregation parameters and helps to highlight those areas of the brain with information relevant for the classification.

We tested the algorithm across different participants, field strengths, resolutions, and bandwidths. We compared the results against those of standard classifiers, showing improved classification accuracy. The most similar results are obtained with tests of different field strengths. This is probably due to the fact that both data sets have a similar number of t-maps. Also, we can observe that the classification accuracy is high compared to others in the same table. Nevertheless, we cannot conclude that this is due to the differences between field strengths. The second and the third experiments have similar results, which is mainly due to the amount of data used for training and testing. When the structure is trained with low-resolution or low-bandwidth data, the number of t-maps for training is high (128 and 156, respectively). The test accuracies are the lowest, and they are similar. This suggests that training with different data does not make any difference, and that accuracy is mainly a matter of the number of training t-maps. For example, if we randomly choose 50 data points of low resolution to train, and then test the network at high resolution, the average misclassification rate is about 10%, similar to the fourth and sixth row of Table 4.

The method has many potential uses in neuroanatomical studies. Rather than using the method to classify previously known activations, which are explicit in the paradigms used to compute the t-maps, we intend to predict hidden variables. These hidden variables may be related to the prediction of diseases, brain computing interfaces, and others. It is well suited for real-time applications as it has a fast classification response and a fast training time. We have recently interfaced the classifier to a real-time fMRI analysis software (*Turbo*Fire, http://mic.health.unm.edu/turbofire; Gao & Posse, 2004; Gembris, Taylor, Schor, Frings, Suter, & Posse, 2000; Posse et al., 2001; Posse et al., 2003).

The limitations of the method are related to the sparsity of the information in the brain. If the information relevant for the classification is distributed in a large area of the brain, the performance of the classifier will degrade. In those cases, it may be better to apply a single classifier to the whole brain t-map. In addition, the method requires a good choice of neuroanatomical areas. A bad choice may result in a decreased performance. Nevertheless, there is no limitation to the number and extent of the applied neuroanatomical areas. They may even overlap, and one can leave the choice of the adequate areas to the distributed Adaboost procedure. Furthermore, one can combine small functional areas with coarse areas and with the whole brain.

It would be good to add a paragraph that compares the new method with previous work mentioned in the introduction and discusses future development. The comparison between the classification of t-maps and raw time series is an important topic.

Acknowledgments

We want to thank H. Jeremy Bockholt and Andrew Mayer (MIND Institute, University of New Mexico, USA) for providing the brain masks and helping us to use them; Kunxiu Gao, Jing Xu, and Ting Li (MIND Institute) for providing all scans made using the software *Turbo*Fire; and Jason Weston and Gökhan Bakir (Max-Plank-Institüt) for sharing their machine-learning library Spider (http://www.kyb.tuebingen.mpg.de/bs/people/spider).

This work has been partially supported by NIH Grant NIBIB 1 RO1 EB002618-01 and NSF Grant DMS-0304861, and the Department of Electrical and Computing Engineering, the Department of Psychiatry, the MIND Institute, and the Department of Mathematics and Statistics of the University of New Mexico.

References

Allwein, E. A., Schapire, R. E., & Singer, Y. (2000). Reducing multiclass to binary: A unifying approach for margin classiffiers. *Journal of Machine Learning Research, 1*, 113-141.

Bartfeld, E., & Grinvald, A. (1992). Relationships between orientation-preference pinwheels, cytochrome oxidate blobs, and oculardominance columns in primate striate cortex. In *Proceedings of the National Academy of Science, 89*, 11905-11909.

Blasdel, G. G. (1992). Orientation selectivity, preference and continuity in monkey striate cortex. *Journal of Neuroscience, 12*, 3139-3161.

Burges, C. (1998). A tutorial on support vector machines for pattern recognition. *Data Mining and Knowledge Discovery, 2*(2), 1-32.

Calhoun, V., Adali, T., Pearlson, G., & Pekar, J. (2001). Group ICA of functional MRI data: Separability, stationarity, and inference. In *Proceedings of ICA2001*, San Diego, CA.

Cox, D. D., & Savoy, R. L. (2003). Functional magnetic resonance imaging (fMRI) "brain reading": Detecting and classifying distributed patterns of fMRI activity in human visual cortex. *Neuroimage, 19*(2), 261-270.

Dietterich, T. G., & Bakiri, G. (1995). Solving multiclass learning problems via error correcting output codes. *Journal of Artificial Intelligence Research, 2*, 263-286.

Freund, Y., & Schapire, R. (1996). A decision theoretic generalization of on-line learning and an application to boosting. In *Proceedings of the Ninth Annual Conference on Computational Learning Theory* (pp. 325-332).

Friston, K. J., Holmes, A. P., Worsley, K. J., Poline, J.-B., Frith, C. D., & Frackowiak, R. S. J. (1995). Statistical parametric maps in functional imaging: A general linear approach. *Human Brain Mapping, 2*, 189-210.

Gao, K., & Posse, S. (2004). TurboFire: Real-time fMRI with automated spatial normalization and Talairach Daemon Database. *Neuroimage, 19*(2), 838.

Gembris, D., Taylor, J. G., Schor, S., Frings, W., Suter, D., & Posse, S. (2000). Functional MR imaging in real-time using a sliding-window correlation technique. *Magnetic Resonance in Medicine, 43*, 259-268.

Haynes, J. D., & Rees, G. (2005). Predicting the orientation of invisible stimuli from activity in human primary visual cortex. *Nature Neuroscience, 8*(5), 686-691.

Hsu, C. W., & Lin, C.-J. (2002). A comparison of methods for support vector machines. *IEEE Transactions on Neural Networks, 13*, 415-425.

Hubel, D. H., & Wiesel, T. N. (1962). Receptive fields, binocular interaction and functional architecture in the cat's visual cortex. *Journal of Physiology, 160*, 106-154.

Hubel, D. H., & Wiesel, T. N. (1968). Receptive fields and functional architecture of monkey's striate cortex. *Journal of Physiology, 195*, 215-243.

Kamitani, Y., & Tong, F. (2005). Decoding the visual and subjective contents of the human brain. *Nature Neuroscience, 8*(5), 679-685.

Kiebel, S. J., & Friston, K. J. (2004a). Statistical parametric mapping: I. Generic considerations. *Neuroimage, 2*, 402-502.

Kiebel, S. J., & Friston, K. J. (2004b). Statistical parametric mapping: II. A hierarchical temporal model. *Neuroimage, 2*, 503-520.

Koltchinskii, V., Martínez-Ramón, M., & Posse, S. (2005). Optimal aggregation of classifiers and boosting maps in functional magnetic resonance imaging. *Advances in Neural Information Processing Systems, 17*, 705-712.

LaConte, S., Strother, S., Cherkassky, V., Anderson, J., & Hu, X. (2005). Support vector machines for temporal classification of block design fMRI data. *Neuroimage, 26*, 317-329.

LaConte, S., Strother, S., Cherkassky, V., & Hu, X. (2003). Predicting motor tasks in fMRI data with support vector machines. In *Proceedings of the ISMRM 11th Scientific Meeting and Exhibition,* Toronto, Ontario, Canada.

Magnotta, V. A., Harris, G., Andreasen, N. C., Yuh, W., & Heckel, D. (2002). Structural MR image processing using the brains2 toolbox. *Computerized Medical Imaging and Graphics, 26*, 251-264.

Martínez-Ramón, M., Koltchinskii, V., Heileman, G., & Posse, S. (2005a). Pattern classification in functional MRI using optimally aggregated adaboost. In *Proceedings of the International Society for Magnetic Resonance in Medicine 13th Scientific Meeting,* Miami, FL.

Martínez-Ramón, M., Koltchinskii, V., Heileman, G., & Posse, S. (2005b). Pattern classification in functional MRI using optimally aggregated ada-boosting. *Organization of Human Brain Mapping, 11th Annual Meeting*, 909.

Martínez-Ramón, M., Koltchinskii, V., Heileman, G., & Posse, S. (2006). fMRI pattern classification using neuroanatomically constrained boosting. *Neuroimage, 31*, 1129-1141.

Mitchell, T. M., Hutchinson, R., Niculescu, R. S., Pereira, F., & Wang, X. (2004). Learning to decode cognitive states from brain images. *Machine Learning, 57*, 145-175.

Müller, K.-R., Mika, S., Rätsch, G., Tsuda, K., & Schölkopf, B. (2001). An introduction to kernel- based learning algorithms. *IEEE Transactions on Neural Networks, 12*(2), 181-202.

Platt, J., Cristianini, N., & Shawe-Taylor, J. (2000). Large margin DAG's for multiclass classification. *Advances in Neural Information Processing Systems, 12*, 547-553.

Posse, S., Binkofski, F., Schneider, F., Gembris, D., Frings, W., Salloum, U. H. J. B., et al. (2001). A new approach to measure single event related brain activity using real-time fMRI: Feasibility of sensory, motor, and higher cognitive tasks. *Human Brain Mapping, 12*(1), 25-41.

Posse, S., Fitzgerald, D., Gao, K., Habel, U., Rosenberg, D., Moore, G. J., et al. (2003). Real-time fMRI of temporo-limbic regions detects amygdala activation during single trial self-induced sadness. *Neuroimage, 18*, 760-768.

Rifkin, R., & Klautau, A. (2004). In defense of one-vs-all classification. *Journal of Machine Learning Research, 5*, 101-141.

Rosset, S., Zhu, J., & Hastie, T. (2004). Boosting as a regularized path to a maximum margin classifier. *Journal of Machine Learning research, 5*, 941-973.

Schapire, R. (1999). A brief introduction to boosting. In *Proceedings of the Sixteenth International Conference on Artificial Intelligence*, 1401-1406.

Talairach, J., & Tournoux, P. (1988). *Co-planar stereotaxic atlas of the human brain.* New York: Thieme.

Wang, X., Hutchinson, R., & Mitchell, T. M. (2004). Training fMRI classifiers to discriminate cognitive states across multiple subjects. *Advances in Neural Information Processing Systems, 16*, 709-716.

Weston, J., & Watkins, C. (1999). Multi-class support vector machines. In *Proceedings of ESANN99*, Brussels, Belgium.

Section II

Signal Processing

Chapter VI

Discrete Time Signal Processing Framework with Support Vector Machines

José Luis Rojo-Álvarez, Universidad Rey Juan Carlos, Spain

Manel Martínez-Ramón, Universidad Carlos III de Madrid, Spain

Gustavo Camps-Valls, Universitat de València, Spain

Carlos E. Martínez-Cruz, Universidad Carlos III de Madrid, Spain

Carlos Figuera, Universidad Rey Juan Carlos, Spain

Abstract

Digital signal processing (DSP) of time series using SVM has been addressed in the litera-ture with a straightforward application of the SVM kernel regression, but the assumption of independently distributed samples in regression models is not fulfilled by a time-series prob-lem. Therefore, a new branch of SVM algorithms has to be developed for the advantageous application of SVM concepts when we process data with underlying time-series structure. In this chapter, we summarize our past, present, and future proposal for the SVM-DSP frame-work, which consists of several principles for creating linear and nonlinear SVM algorithms devoted to DSP problems. First, the statement of linear signal models in the primal problem (primal signal models) allows us to obtain robust estimators of the model coefficients in classical DSP problems. Next, nonlinear SVM-DSP algorithms can be addressed from two different approaches: (a) reproducing kernel Hilbert spaces (RKHS) signal models, which state the signal model equation in the feature space, and (b) dual signal models, which are based on the nonlinear regression of the time instants with appropriate Mercer's kernels. This way, concepts like filtering, time interpolation, and convolution are considered and analyzed, and they open the field for future development on signal processing algorithms following this SVM-DSP framework.

Introduction

Support vector machines (SVMs) were originally conceived as efficient methods for pattern recognition and classification (Vapnik, 1995), and support vector regression (SVR) was subsequently proposed as the SVM implementation for regression and function approximation (e.g., Smola & Schölkopf, 2004). Many other digital signal processing (DSP) supervised and unsupervised schemes have also been stated from SVM principles, such as discriminant analysis (Baudat & Anouar, 2000), clustering (Ben-Hur, Hom, Siegelmann, & Vapnik, 2001), principal and independent component analysis (Bach & Jordan, 2002; Schölkopf, 1997), or mutual information extraction (Gretton, Herbrich, & Smola, 2003). Also, an interesting perspective for signal processing using SVM can be found in Mattera (2005), which relies on a different point of view of signal processing.

The use of time series with supervised SVM algorithms has mainly focused on two DSP problems: (a) nonlinear system identification of the underlying relationship between two simultaneously recorded discrete-time processes, and (b) time-series prediction (Drezet & Harrison 1998; Gretton, Doucet, Herbrich, Rayner, & Schölkopf, 2001; Suykens, 2001). In both of them, the conventional SVR considers lagged and buffered samples of the available signals as its input vectors. Although good results in terms of signal-prediction accuracy are achieved with this approach, several concerns can be raised from a conceptual point of view. First, the basic assumption for the regression problem is that observations are independent and identically distributed; however, the requirement of independence among samples is not fulfilled at all by time-series data. Moreover, if we do not take into account the temporal dependence, we could be neglecting highly relevant structures, such as correlation or cross-correlation information. Second, most of the preceding DSP approaches use Vapnik's ε-insensitive cost function, which is a linear cost (that includes an insensitivity region). Nevertheless, when Gaussian noise is present in the data, a quadratic cost function should also be considered. Third, the previously mentioned methods take advantage of the well-known "kernel trick" (Aizerman, Braverman, & Rozoner, 1964) to develop nonlinear algorithms from a well-established linear signal processing technique. However, the SVM methodology has many other advantages, additional to the flexible use of Mercer's kernels, which are still of great interest for many DSP problems that consider linear signal models. Finally, if we consider only SVR-based schemes, the analysis of an observed discrete-time sequence becomes limited because a wide variety of time-series structures are being ignored. Therefore, our purpose is to establish an appropriate framework for creating SVM algorithms in DSP problems involving time-series analysis. This framework is born from

Figure 1. Scheme of the proposal for a SVM-DSP framework described in this chapter. Our aim is to develop and create a variety of algorithms for time series processing that can benefit from the excellent properties of the SVM in a variety of different signal models.

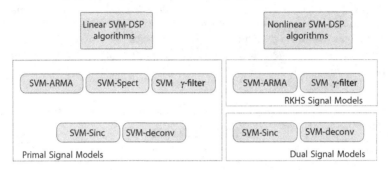

the consideration that discrete-time data should be treated in a conceptually different way from the SVR way in order to develop more advantageous applications of SVM concepts and performance to data with underlying time-series structure. In this chapter, we summarize our past, present, and future proposal for the SVM-DSP framework, which consists of creating SVM algorithms devoted to specific problems of DSP.

A brief scheme of our proposal is presented in Figure 1. On the one hand, the statement of linear signal models in the primal problem, which will be called *SVM primal signal models*, will allow us to obtain robust estimators of the model coefficients (Rojo-Álvarez et al., 2005) in classical DSP problems, such as auto-regressive and moving-averaged (ARMA) modeling, the γ-filter, and the spectral analysis (Camps-Valls, Martínez-Ramón, Rojo-Álvarez, & Soria-Olivas, 2004; Rojo-Álvarez, Martínez-Ramón, Figueiras-Vidal, dePrado Cumplido, & Artés-Rodríguez, 2004; Rojo-Álvarez, Martínez-Ramón, Figueiras-Vidal, García-Armada, & Artés-Rodríguez, 2003). On the other hand, the consideration of nonlinear SVM-DSP algorithms can be addressed from two different approaches: (a) *RKHS signal models*, which state the signal model equation in the feature space (Martínez-Ramón, Rojo-Álvarez, Camps-Valls, Muñoz-Marí, Navia-Vázquez, Soria-Olivas, & Figueiras-Vidal, in press), and (b) *dual signal models*, which are based on the nonlinear regression of each single time instant with appropriate Mercer's kernels (Rojo-Álvarez et al., 2006). While RKHS signal models allow us to scrutinize the statistical properties in the feature space, dual signal models yield an interesting and simple interpretation of the SVM algorithm under study in connection with the classical theory of linear systems.

The rest of the chapter is organized as follows. In the next section, the ε-Huber cost function (Mattera & Haykin, 1999; Rojo-Álvarez et al., 2003) is described, and the algorithm based on a generic primal signal model is introduced. SVM linear algorithms are then created for well-known time-series structures (spectral analysis, ARMA system identification, and the γ-filter). An example of an algorithm statement from an RKHS signal model, the nonlinear ARMA system identification, is then presented. After that, SVM algorithms for time-series sinc interpolation and for nonblind deconvolution are obtained from dual signal models. A separate section presents simple application examples. Finally, some conclusions and several proposals for future work are considered.

Primal Signal Models: SVM for Linear DSP

A first class of SVM-DSP algorithms are those obtained from primal signal models. Rather than the accurate prediction of the observed signal, the main estimation target of the SVM linear framework is a set of model coefficients or parameters that contain relevant information about the time-series data.

In this setting, the use of the ε-Huber cost function of the residuals allows us to deal with Gaussian noise in all the SVM-DSP algorithms, while still yielding robust estimations of the model coefficients. Taking into account that many derivation steps are similar when proposing different SVM algorithms, a general model is next included that highlights the common and the problem-specific steps of several preceding proposed algorithms (Rojo-Álvarez et al., 2005). Examples of the use of this general signal model for stating new SVM-DSP linear algorithms are given by creating an SVM algorithm version for the spectral analysis, the ARMA system identification, and the γ-filter structure.

The ε-Huber Cost

As previously mentioned, the DSP of time series using SVM methodology has mainly focused on two supervised problems (nonlinear time-series prediction and nonlinear system identification; Drezet & Harrison 1998; Gretton et al., 2001; Suykens, 2001), and both have been addressed from the straight application of the SVR algorithm. We start by noting that the conventional SVR minimizes the regularized Vapnik ε-insensitive cost, which is in essence a linear cost. Hence, this is not the most suitable loss function in the presence of Gaussian noise, which will be a usual situation in time-series analysis. This fact was previously taken into account in the formulation of LS-SVM (Suykens, 2001), where a regularized quadratic cost is used for a variety of signal problems, but in this case, nonsparse solutions are obtained.

Figure 2. (a) In the ε-Huber cost function, three different regions allow to adapt to different kinds of noise. (b) The nonlinear relationship between the residuals and the Lagrange multipliers provides with robust estimates of model coefficients.

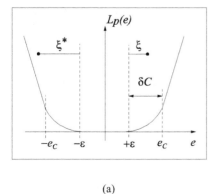
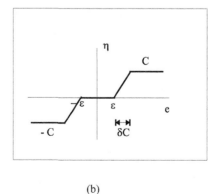

(a)   (b)

An alternative cost function of the residuals, the ε-Huber cost, has been proposed (Mattera & Haykin, 1999; Rojo-Álvarez et al., 2003), which just combines both the quadratic and the ε-insensitive cost functions. It has been shown to be a more appropriate residual cost, not only for time-series problems, but also for SVR in general (Camps-Valls, Bruzzone, Rojo-Álvarez, & Melgani, 2006). The ε-Huber cost is represented in Figure 2a, and is given by:

$$
L^{\varepsilon H}(e_n) = \begin{cases} 0, & |e_n| \le \varepsilon \\ \dfrac{1}{2\delta}(|e_n| - \varepsilon)^2, & \varepsilon \le |e_n| \le e_C \\ C(|e_n| - \varepsilon) - \dfrac{1}{2}\delta C^2, & |e_n| \ge e_C \end{cases} \tag{1}
$$

where e_n is the residual that corresponds to the nth observation for a given model, $e_c = \varepsilon + \delta C$; ε is the insensitive parameter, and δ and C control the trade-off between the regularization and the losses. The three different regions allow us to deal with different kinds of noise: the ε-insensitive zone ignores absolute residuals lower than ε; the quadratic cost zone uses the L_2-norm of errors, which is appropriate for Gaussian noise; and the linear cost zone is an efficient limit for the impact of the outliers in the solution model coefficients. Note that equation (1) represents the Vapnik ε-insensitive cost function when δ is small enough, the least squares (LS) cost function for $\delta C \to \infty$ and $\varepsilon = 0$, and the Huber cost function when $\varepsilon = 0$.

The Primal Signal Model

Let $\{y_n\}$ be a discrete-time series from which a set of N consecutive samples are measured and grouped into a vector of observations:

$$
\mathbf{y}_n = [y_1, y_2, ..., y_N]', \tag{2}
$$

and let the set of vectors $\{\mathbf{z}^p\}$ be a set of basis vectors spanning a P-dimensional subspace E^P of the N-dimensional Hilbert signal space E^N. These vectors are described by:

$$
\mathbf{z}^p = [z_1^p, z_2^p, ..., z_N^p]', \qquad p = 1, ..., P. \tag{3}
$$

Each observed signal vector y can be represented as a linear combination of elements of this basis set, plus an error vector $\mathbf{e} = [e_1, ..., e_N]'$ modeling the measurement errors:

$$
\mathbf{y} = \sum_{p=1}^{P} w^p \mathbf{z}^p + \mathbf{e}. \tag{4}
$$

For a given time instant n, a linear time-series model can be written as:

$$y_n = \sum_{p=1}^{P} w^p z_n^p + e_n = \mathbf{w}'\mathbf{v}_n + \mathbf{e}_n, \tag{5}$$

where $\mathbf{w} = [w^1, ..., w^P]'$ is the model weight vector to be estimated, and $\mathbf{v}_n = [z_n^1, ..., z_n^P]'$ represents the input space E^I at time instant n. Equation (5) will be called the *general primal signal model*, and it defines the time-series structure of the observations. This equation represents the functional relationship between the observations, the data (signals generating the projected signal subspace), and the model residuals. In practice, the general primal signal model equation is fulfilled by the n available observations.

Note that input space E^I is closely related to Hilbert signal subspace E^P because the input vector at time instant n is given by the nth element of each of the basis space vectors of E^P. For instance, in the case of a nonparametric spectral estimation, the basis of E^P are the sinusoidal harmonics, whereas in the case of ARMA system identification, the basis of E^P are the input signal and the delayed versions of input and output signals.

The problem of estimating the coefficients can be stated as the minimization of:

$$\frac{1}{2}\|\mathbf{w}\|^2 + \sum_{n=1}^{N} L^{\varepsilon H}(e_n). \tag{6}$$

Equivalently, by plugging equation (1) into equation (6), we have the following functional:

$$\frac{1}{2}\|\mathbf{w}\|^2 + \frac{1}{2\delta}\sum_{n\in I_1}(\xi_n^2 + \xi_n^{*2}) + C\sum_{n\in I_2}(\xi_n + \xi_n^*) - \sum_{n\in I_2}\frac{\delta C^2}{2} \tag{7}$$

to be minimized with respect to $\mathbf{w}$ and $\{\xi_n^{(*)}\}$, and constrained to

$$y_n - \mathbf{w}'\mathbf{v}_n \le \varepsilon + \xi_n \tag{8}$$

$$-y_n + \mathbf{w}'\mathbf{v}_n \le \varepsilon + \xi_n^* \tag{9}$$

$$\xi_n, \xi_n^* \ge 0 \tag{10}$$

for $n = 1, ..., N$, where I_1 and I_2 are the observation indices whose residuals are in the quadratic and in the linear cost zone, respectively. The following expression for the coefficients is then obtained:

$$w^p = \sum_{n=1}^{N} \eta_n z_n^p \tag{11}$$

where $\eta_n = \alpha_n - \alpha_n^*$.
Several properties of the method can be observed from these expressions.

1.   Coefficient vector $\mathbf{w}$ can be expressed as a (possibly sparse) linear combination of input space vectors.

2.   A straightforward relationship between the residuals and the Lagrange multipliers can be derived (e.g., Rojo-Álvarez et al., 2004) from the Karush-Khun-Tucker conditions:

$$\eta_n = \begin{cases} sign(e_n)C, & |e_n| \geq e_C \\ sign(e_n)\dfrac{1}{\delta}(|e_n| - \varepsilon), & \varepsilon \leq |e_n| \leq e_C \\ 0, & |e_n| < \varepsilon \end{cases} \tag{12}$$

which is depicted in Figure 2b. It can be conveniently controlled through the cost function parameters, hence yielding robust estimators of the model coefficients in the presence of impulse noise.

3.   Equation (11) reveals that the pth coefficient is obtained as the dot product between the (nonlinearly transformed) residuals and the pth element of the base of the projection signal space.

By stating the primal-dual Lagrangian functional and making zero its gradient, we identify the cross-correlation matrix of input space vectors, denoted as:

$$\mathbf{R}_v(s, t) = \mathbf{v}_s' \mathbf{v}_t, \tag{13}$$

and then, the dual problem is obtained and expressed, in matrix form, as the maximization of:

$$-\frac{1}{2}(\boldsymbol{\alpha} - \boldsymbol{\alpha}^*)'[\mathbf{R}_v + \delta \mathbf{I}](\boldsymbol{\alpha} - \boldsymbol{\alpha}^*) + (\boldsymbol{\alpha} - \boldsymbol{\alpha}^*)' \mathbf{y} - \varepsilon \mathbf{1}'(\boldsymbol{\alpha} - \boldsymbol{\alpha}^*) \tag{14}$$

constrained to $0 \leq \boldsymbol{\alpha}, \boldsymbol{\alpha}^* \leq C$. After obtaining Lagrange multipliers $\boldsymbol{\alpha}^*$, the time-series model for a new sample at time instant m can be readily expressed as:

$$\hat{y}_m = \sum_{n=1}^{N} \eta_n \mathbf{v}_n' \mathbf{v}_m. \tag{15}$$

Therefore, by taking into account the primal signal model in equation (5) that is used for a given DSP problem, we can determine signals z_n^p that generate the Hilbert subspace where the observations are projected, and then the remaining elements and steps of the SVM methodology (such as the input space, the input space correlation matrix, the dual quadratic programming problem, and the solution) can be easily and immediately obtained.

To illustrate this procedure, we next use this approach to propose three different linear SVM-DSP algorithms.

SVM Spectral Analysis

The SVM algorithm for spectral analysis (SVM-Spect; Rojo-Álvarez et al., 2003) can be stated as follows. Let $\{y_{t_n}\}$ be a time series obtained by possibly nonuniformly sampling at the corresponding time instants $\{t_1, \cdots, t_N\}$ of a continuous-time function $y(t)$. A signal model using sinusoidal functions can be stated as:

$$y_{t_n} = \sum_{i=1}^{N_\omega} A_i \cos(\omega_i t_n + \phi_i) + e_n = \sum_{i=1}^{N_\omega} c_i \cos(\omega_i t_n) + d_i \sin(\omega_i t_n) + e_n, \tag{16}$$

where the unknown parameters are amplitudes A_i, phases ϕ_i, and angular frequencies ω_i for a number N_ω of sinusoidal components. The signals generating Hilbert subspace E^p are the discretized sinusoidal functions (phase and quadrature components), and hence, the model coefficients are obtained as:

$$c_l = \sum_{k=1}^{N_\omega} \eta_k \cos(\omega_l t_k); \qquad d_l = \sum_{k=1}^{N_\omega} \eta_k \sin(\omega_l t_k). \tag{17}$$

The input space matrix correlation is given by the sum of two terms:

$$\mathbf{R}_{\cos}(m,k) = \sum_{i=1}^{N_\omega} \cos(\omega_i t_m) \cos(\omega_i t_k) \tag{18}$$

and

$$\mathbf{R}_{\sin}(m,k) = \sum_{i=1}^{N_\omega} \sin(\omega_i t_m) \sin(\omega_i t_k), \tag{19}$$

and the dual functional to be maximized is:

$$-\frac{1}{2}(\boldsymbol{\alpha}-\boldsymbol{\alpha}^*)'[\mathbf{R}_{cos}+\mathbf{R}_{sin}+\delta](\boldsymbol{\alpha}-\boldsymbol{\alpha}^*)+(\boldsymbol{\alpha}-\boldsymbol{\alpha}^*)'\mathbf{y}-\varepsilon\mathbf{1}'(\boldsymbol{\alpha}+\boldsymbol{\alpha}^*),\tag{20}$$

constrained to $0\le\boldsymbol{\alpha},\boldsymbol{\alpha}^*\le C$.

SVM-ARMA System Identification

The SVM algorithm for system identification basing on an explicit linear ARMA model[1] was proposed in Rojo-Álvarez et al. (2004). Assuming that $\{x_n\}$ and $\{y_n\}$ are the input and the output, respectively, of a rational linear, time-invariant system, the corresponding difference equation is:

$$y_n=\sum_{i=1}^{M}a_iy_{n-i}+\sum_{j=1}^{Q}b_jx_{n-j+1}+e_n,\tag{21}$$

where $\{a_i\}$ and $\{b_j\}$ are the M autoregressive and Q moving-averaged coefficients of the system, respectively. Here, the output signal in the present time lag is built as a weighted sum of the M-lag delayed versions of the same output signal, the input signal, and the Q-lag delayed versions of the input signal, and hence, these signals generate E^P. The model coefficients are:

$$a_i=\sum_{n=1}^{N}\eta_n y_{n-i}\qquad b_j=\sum_{n=1}^{N}\eta_n x_{n-j+1},\tag{22}$$

and the input space correlation matrix is again the sum of two terms:

$$\mathbf{R}_y^{M}(m,k)=\sum_{i=1}^{M}y_{m-i}y_{k-i}\tag{23}$$

and

$$\mathbf{R}_x^{Q}(m,k)=\sum_{j=1}^{Q}x_{m-j+1}y_{k-i+1}.\tag{24}$$

These equations represent the time-local Mth and Qth order sample estimators of the values of the (non-Toeplitz) autocorrelation functions of the input and the output discrete-time processes, respectively. The dual problem consists of maximizing:

$$-\frac{1}{2}(\boldsymbol{\alpha}-\boldsymbol{\alpha}^*)'[\mathbf{R}_x^{Q}+\mathbf{R}_y^{M}+\varphi](\boldsymbol{\alpha}-\boldsymbol{\alpha}^*)+(\boldsymbol{\alpha}-\boldsymbol{\alpha}^*)'\mathbf{y}-\varepsilon\mathbf{1}'(\boldsymbol{\alpha}+\boldsymbol{\alpha}^*),\tag{25}$$

constrained to $0\le\boldsymbol{\alpha},\boldsymbol{\alpha}^*\le C$.

SVM γ-Filter

The use of the primal signal model approach for stating an SVM version of the γ-filter (Camps-Valls et al., 2004) is presented next. An important issue in time-series parametric modeling is how to ensure that the obtained model is causal and stable, which can be a requirement for AR time-series prediction and for ARMA system identification. A remarkable compromise between the stability and simplicity of adaptation can be provided by the γ-filter, which was first proposed in Principe, deVries, and de Oliveira (1993). The γ-filter can be regarded as a particular case of the generalized feed-forward filter, an infinite impulse response (IIR) digital filter with restricted feedback architecture. The γ-structure, when used as a linear adaptive filter, results in a more parsimonious filter, and it has been used for echo cancellation (Palkar & Principe, 1994), time-series prediction (Kuo, Celebi, & Principe, 1994), system identification (Principe et al., 1999), and noise reduction (Kuo & Principe, 1994). Previous work on γ-filters claims two main advantages: (a) It provides stable models, and (b) it permits the study of the memory depth of a model, that is, how much past information the model can retain.

The γ-filter is defined by using the difference equations of the linear ARMA model of a discrete-time series $\{y_n\}$ as a function of a given input sequence $\{x_n\}$, as follows:

$$y_n = \sum_{p=1}^{P} w^p x_n^p + e_n \qquad (26)$$

$$x_n^p = \begin{cases} x_n, & p = 1 \\ (1-\mu)x_{n-1}^p + \mu\, x_{n-1}^{p-1}, & p = 2,\dots,P \end{cases} \qquad (27)$$

where μ is a free parameter of the model. For $\mu=1$, the structure reduces to Widrow's adaline, whereas for $\mu \neq 1$, it has an IIR transfer function due to the recursion in equation (27). The stability is trivially obtained with $0 < \mu < 1$ for a low-pass transfer function, and with

Figure 3. The gamma structure; the gamma filter can be seen as the cascade of IIR filters where loops are kept local and loop gain is constant

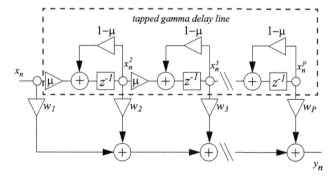

$1 < \mu < 2$ for a high-pass transfer function. Figure 3 shows the γ-filter structure corresponding to these equations. In comparison to general IIR filters, the feedback structure in the γ-filter presents two complementary conditions: *locality*, since the loops are kept local with respect to the taps, and *globality*, since all the loops have the same loop gain $1-\mu$. A proposed measurement of the memory depth of a model, which allows us to quantify the past information retained, is given by $M = \frac{P}{\mu}$, and it has units of time samples (Principe et al., 1993).

For creating a linear SVM algorithmic version of the γ-filter, we must identify the base of Hilbert signal subspace E^P, which is just:

$$\mathbf{z}^p = [x_1^p, x_2^p, \ldots, x_N^p]', \qquad p = 1, \ldots P \qquad (28)$$

that is, the signals generating E^P are the output signals after each γ unit loop. Note that, for a previously fixed value of μ, the generating signal vectors of the Hilbert projection space are straightforwardly determined. By denoting, as before, $\mathbf{v}_n = \left[z_n^1, \ldots, z_n^P \right]'$, the generic primal signal model in equation (5) can be used, the input space correlation matrix being given by equation (13), the dual problem by equation (14), and the output prediction model by equation (15). More details on the SVM γ-filter can be found in Camps-Valls et al. (2004) and Rojo-Álvarez et al. (2005).

RKHS Signal Models: Nonlinear SVM-ARMA

Nonlinear SVM-DSP algorithms can be developed from two different general approaches, which are presented in this section and in the next one. Another class of SVM-DSP algorithms consists of stating the signal model of the time-series structure in the RKHS, and hence they will be called RKHS signal model based algorithms. The major interest of this approach is the combination of flexibility (provided by the nonlinearity to the algorithm) together with the possibility of scrutinizing the time-series structure of the model and the solution, despite the nonlinearity.

In this section, the SVR algorithm for nonlinear system identification is briefly examined in order to check that, though efficient, this approach does not correspond explicitly to an ARMA model. Then, a nonlinear version of the linear SVM-ARMA algorithm is provided by using an explicit ARMA model on the RKHS. Nonlinear SVM-ARMA modeling is an example of the possibilities of the RKHS signal model approach for creating SVM-DSP algorithms, and the approach could be used with other DSP problems, for example, the γ-filter, which is not discussed here (Camps-Valls, Requena-Carrión, Rojo-Álvarez, & Martínez-Ramón, 2006).

SVR System Identification

The SVR system identification algorithm (Gretton et al., 2001) can be described as follows. Let $\{x_n\}$ and $\{y_n\}$ be two discrete-time signals, which are the input and the output, respectively, of a nonlinear system. Let $\mathbf{y}_{n-1} = [y_{n-1}, y_{n-2}, \ldots, y_{n-M}]'$ and $\mathbf{x}_n = [x_n, x_{n-1}, \ldots, x_{n-Q+1}]'$ denote the states of input and output at discrete-time instant n. Assuming a nonlinear transformation $\phi([\mathbf{y}_{n-1}; \mathbf{x}_n])$ for the concatenation of the input and output discrete-time processes to a B-dimensional feature space, $\phi : R^{M+Q} \to F$, a linear regression model, can be built in F, and its equation is:

$$y_n = \mathbf{g}'\phi([\mathbf{y}_{n-1}; \mathbf{x}_n]) + e_n, \tag{29}$$

where $\mathbf{g} = [g_1, \ldots, g_B]'$ is a vector of coefficients in the RKHS, and $\{e_n\}$ are the residuals. By following the usual SVM methodology, the solution vector is:

$$\mathbf{g} = \sum_{n=1}^{N} \eta_n \phi([\mathbf{y}_{n-1}; \mathbf{x}_n]) \tag{30}$$

and the following Gram matrix containing the dot products can be identified:

$$\mathbf{G}(m,k) = \phi([\mathbf{y}_{m-1}, \mathbf{x}_m])' \phi([\mathbf{y}_{k-1}, \mathbf{x}_k]) = \kappa([\mathbf{y}_{m-1}; \mathbf{x}_m], [\mathbf{y}_{k-1}; \mathbf{x}_k]), \tag{31}$$

where the nonlinear mappings do not need to be explicitly calculated, but instead the dot product in RKHS can be replaced by Mercer's kernels. The problem consists of maximizing the constrained functional:

$$\frac{1}{2}(\boldsymbol{\alpha} - \boldsymbol{\alpha}^*)'[\mathbf{G} + \delta\mathbf{I}](\boldsymbol{\alpha} - \boldsymbol{\alpha}^*) + (\boldsymbol{\alpha} - \boldsymbol{\alpha}^*)'\mathbf{y} - \varepsilon\mathbf{1}'(\boldsymbol{\alpha} + \boldsymbol{\alpha}^*). \tag{32}$$

The predicted output for newly observed $[\mathbf{y}_{m-1}; \mathbf{x}_m]$ is given by:

$$\hat{y}_m = \sum_{n=1}^{N} \eta_n \kappa([\mathbf{y}_{n-1}, \mathbf{x}_n], [\mathbf{y}_{m-1}, \mathbf{x}_m]). \tag{33}$$

Note that equation (29) is the expression for a general nonlinear system identification model in the RKHS rather than an explicit ARMA structure. Moreover, though the reported performance of the algorithm is high when compared with other approaches, this formulation does not allow us to scrutinize the statistical properties of the time series that are being modeled in terms of autocorrelation and/or cross-correlation between the input and the output signals.

SVM-ARMA in RKHS

An explicit SVM-ARMA filter model can be stated in the RKHS by taking advantage of Mercer's kernels' properties. Assume that the state vectors of both the input and the output discrete-time signals can be separately mapped to two (possibly different) RKHSs by using a nonlinear mapping $\phi_x(\mathbf{x}_n) : \mathbb{R}^Q \to F_x$ and $\phi_y(\mathbf{y}_{n-1}) : \mathbb{R}^M \to F_y$. If a linear ARMA model is built in each of those RKHSs for the AR and for the MA model components, the corresponding difference equation is given by:

$$y_n = \mathbf{a}'\phi_y(\mathbf{y}_{n-1}) + \mathbf{b}'\phi_x(\mathbf{x}_n) + \mathbf{e}_n, \tag{34}$$

where $\mathbf{a} = [a_1, ..., a_{B_y}]'$ and $\mathbf{b} = [b_1, ..., b_{B_x}]'$ are vectors determining the AR and the MA coefficients of the system, respectively, in the RKHSs, and B_y and B_x are the space dimensions.

By writing down the primal problem, and then the primal-dual Lagrangian functional, the vector coefficients can be shown to be:

$$\mathbf{a} = \sum_{n=1}^{N} \eta_n \phi_y(\mathbf{y}_{n-1}); \qquad \mathbf{b} = \sum_{n=1}^{N} \eta_n \phi_x(\mathbf{x}_n). \tag{35}$$

We can identify two different kernel matrices: one for the input and another for the output vector, denoted and calculated as:

$$R_{y;m(m,k)} = \phi_y(\mathbf{y}_{m-1})'\phi_y(\mathbf{y}_{k-1}) = \kappa_y(\mathbf{y}_{m-1}, \mathbf{y}_{k-1}) \tag{36}$$

and

$$R_{x;m(m,k)} = \phi_x(\mathbf{x}_m)'\phi_x(\mathbf{x}_k) = \kappa_x(\mathbf{x}_m, \mathbf{x}_k). \tag{37}$$

These equations account for the sample estimators of input and output time-series autocorrelation functions (Papoulis, 1991), respectively, in the RKHS space. Specifically, they are proportional to the non-Toeplitz estimator of each time-series autocorrelation matrix.

The dual problem consists of maximizing, with the usual constraints, the functional:

$$-\frac{1}{2}(\boldsymbol{\alpha} - \boldsymbol{\alpha}^*)'[\mathbf{R}_x + \mathbf{R}_y + \delta\mathbf{I}](\boldsymbol{\alpha} - \boldsymbol{\alpha}^*) + (\boldsymbol{\alpha} - \boldsymbol{\alpha}^*)'\mathbf{y} - \varepsilon\mathbf{1}'(\boldsymbol{\alpha} + \boldsymbol{\alpha}^*). \tag{38}$$

The output for a new observation vector is obtained through:

$$\hat{y}_m = \sum_{n=1}^{N} \eta_n(\kappa_y(\mathbf{y}_{n-1}, \mathbf{y}_{m-1}) + \kappa_x(\mathbf{x}_n + \mathbf{x}_m)). \tag{39}$$

Note that this prediction model is different from equation (33), and for different real-data problems, we will be able to choose from one or another of the presented proposals.

Dual Signal Models:
Sinc Interpolation and Deconvolution

An additional class of nonlinear SVM-DSP algorithms can be obtained by considering the nonlinear regression of the time lags or instants of the observed signals and using appropriate Mercer's kernels. This class is known as the *dual signal* model based SVM algorithms. Here, we present this approach and pay attention to the interesting and simple interpretation of these SVM algorithms in connection with theory of linear systems. Although in dual signal models we use nonlinear kernels for their formulation, the resulting signal models are still linear (in the parameters) if we consider the final prediction equation.

In this section, the statement of the sinc interpolation SVM algorithm is addressed following both a primal signal model and a dual signal model (Rojo-Álvarez et al., 2006). Given that the resulting dual signal model can be seen as the convolution of a sparse sequence (Lagrange multipliers) with the impulse response of a noncausal, linear, time-invariant system, given by the sinc kernel, the sinc model suggests the introduction of the SVM non-blind deconvolution algorithm, thus yielding a comparison between the resulting schemes for the primal and the dual signal models (Martínez-Cruz, Rojo-Álvarez, Camps-Valls, & Martínez-Ramón, 2006).

SVM Sinc Interpolation

A classical DSP problem is the discrete time series interpolation with a noncausal sinc filter, which, in the absence of noise, gives the perfect reconstruction of uniformly sampled signals (Oppenheim & Schafer, 1989). However, the sinc reconstruction of a possibly nonuniformly sampled time series in the presence of noise is a hard problem to solve, and it has received special attention in the literature (Choi & Munson, 1995, 1998; Yen, 1956).

The general problem can be stated as follows. Let $x(t)$ be a band-limited, possibly Gaussian-noise-corrupted signal, and let $\{x_i = x(t_i), i = 1, ..., N\}$ be a set of N nonuniformly sampled observations. The sinc interpolation problem consists of finding an approximating function $\hat{y}(t)$ fitting the data, given by:

$$y(t) = \hat{y}(t) + e(t) = \sum_{i=1}^{N} a_i \operatorname{sinc}(\sigma_0(t - t_i)) + e(t), \tag{40}$$

where $\operatorname{sinc}(t) = \frac{\sin(t)}{t}$, $\sigma_0 = \frac{\pi}{T_0}$ is the bandwidth of the interpolating sinc units, and $e(t)$ represents the noise. The previous continuous-time model, after nonuniform sampling, is expressed as the following discrete-time model:

$$y_j = \hat{y}(t_j) + e(t_j) = \sum_{i=1}^{N} a_i \operatorname{sinc}(\sigma_0(t_j - t_i)) + e(t_j). \tag{41}$$

An optimal band-limited interpolation algorithm, in the LS sense, was first proposed by Yen (1956). Given that we have as many free parameters as observations, this can become an ill-posed problem. In fact, in the presence of (even a low level of) noise, the coefficient estimations can often grow dramatically, leading to huge interpolation errors far away from the observed samples. To overcome this limitation, the regularization of the quadratic loss has also been proposed.

The good properties of generalization and regularization of the SVM make it attractive to explore the possibility of creating SVM algorithms for sinc interpolation. From a primal signal model formulation, the signal model is equation (41), and the functions generating the projection signal subspace E^P are the sinc functions centred at each sampling time instant, $\{z_n^p\} = \{\mathrm{sinc}(\sigma_0(t_n - t_p))\}$, for $p = 1, ..., N$. Therefore, the input space product matrix is:

$$\mathbf{T}(k, m) = \sum_{n=1}^{N} \mathrm{sinc}(\sigma_0(t_n - t_k))\mathrm{sinc}(\sigma_0(t_n - t_m)), \tag{42}$$

And the primal coefficients $\{a_j\}$ are given by:

$$a_j = \sum_{i=1}^{N} \eta_i \mathrm{sinc}(\sigma_0(t_i - t_j)). \tag{43}$$

The dual Lagrangian problem can now be stated as usual.

A different SVM algorithm for sinc interpolation can be obtained by using the conventional SVR as follows. Given observations $\{y_n\}$ at time instants $\{t_n\}$, we map the *time instants* to a feature space F by using nonlinear transformation ϕ, that is, $\phi : \mathbb{R} \rightarrow F$ maps $t \in \mathbb{R} \rightarrow \phi(t) \in F$. In the RKHS, a linear approximation to the transformed time instant can properly fit the observations:

$$\hat{y}_n = \mathbf{w}'\phi(t_n) \tag{44}$$

for $n = 1, ..., N$, the weight vector in F is given by

$$w = \sum_{j=1}^{N} \eta_j \phi(t_j). \tag{45}$$

The following Gram matrix is identified:

$$\mathbf{G}(k, m) = \phi(t_k)'\phi(t_m) = \kappa(t_k, t_m), \tag{46}$$

where $\kappa(t_k, t_m)$ is a Mercer's kernel, and, as usual, it allows one to obviate the explicit knowledge of nonlinear mapping $\phi(\cdot)$. The dual problem consists now of maximizing:

$$-\frac{1}{2}(\boldsymbol{\alpha} - \boldsymbol{\alpha}^*)'[\mathbf{G} + \delta \mathbf{I}](\boldsymbol{\alpha} - \boldsymbol{\alpha}^*) + (\boldsymbol{\alpha} - \boldsymbol{\alpha}^*)'\mathbf{x} - \varepsilon \mathbf{1}'(\boldsymbol{\alpha} + \boldsymbol{\alpha}^*), \tag{47}$$

constrained to $0 \le \boldsymbol{\alpha}^{(*)} \le C$. The final solution is expressed as:

$$\hat{y}_m = \sum_{n=1}^{N} \eta_n \kappa(t_n, t_m). \tag{48}$$

Moreover, we can define here $\kappa(t_k, t_n) = \mathrm{sinc}(\sigma(t_k - t_n))$ as it is possible to show that it is a valid Mercer's kernel (Zhang, Weida, & Jiao, 2004), called *sinc Mercer's kernel*. Therefore, when using the sinc Mercer's kernel, equation (48) can be seen as the nonuniform interpolation model given in equation (41). Note that other Mercer's kernels could be easily used; for instance, if we define:

$$\kappa(t_k, t_n) = \exp\left(-\frac{|t_k - t_n|^2}{2\sigma_0^2}\right),$$

we obtain the Gaussian interpolator.

Finally, we can observe that, for uniform sampling, equation (48) can be interpreted as the reconstruction of the observations given by a linear filter, where the impulse response of the filter is the sinc function, and the input signal is given by the sequence of the Lagrange multipliers corresponding to each time instant. That is, if we assume that $\{\eta_n\}$ are observations from discrete-time process $\eta[n]$, and that $\{\kappa(t_n)\}$ are the samples of the discrete-time version of the sinc kernel, given by $\kappa[n]$, then solution $\hat{y}[n]$ can be written as a convolutional model given by:

$$\hat{y}[n] = \eta[n] * \kappa[n], \tag{49}$$

where $*$ denotes the discrete-time convolution operator.

Note that this expression is valid as far as we use an even Mercer's kernel because in this case, the impulse response is symmetric. By allowing ε to be nonzero, only a subset of the Lagrange multipliers will be nonzero, thus providing a sparse solution that is a highly desirable property in the sinc interpolation problem.

SVM Nonblind Deconvolution

Another DSP problem that can be stated from an SVM approach is nonblind deconvolution. Given the observations of two discrete-time sequences $\{y_n\}$ and $\{h_n\}$, we need to find the discrete-time sequence $\{x_n\}$ fulfilling:

$$y_n = x_n * h_n + e_n. \tag{50}$$

Similar to the SVM sinc interpolation case, we have two different approaches to this problem. The first one is a dual signal model approach, similar to the case of the SVM sinc interpolation. The solution of the nonlinear regression of the time instants is:

$$\hat{y}_n = \sum_{i=1}^{N} \eta_i \kappa(t_i, t_n), \tag{51}$$

and hence $y[n] = \eta[n]*\kappa[n]+e$ $[n]$ is the convolutional model if we identify the Mercer's kernel with the impulse response and the Lagrange multipliers with the input sequence to be estimated. This approach requires an impulse response being compatible with a Mercer's kernel, for instance, being an autocorrelation sequence. However, in this case, one can obtain sparse solutions with an appropriate tuning of the free parameters.

Another approach is the statement of the primal signal model, which is:

$$y_n = \sum_{j=1}^{N} \hat{x}_j h_{n-j+1} + e_n . \tag{52}$$

The signals generating the projection subspace are lagged versions of the impulse response:

$$\{z_n^p\} = \{h[n-p]\} = \{h_{n-p+1}\}. \tag{53}$$

The dual problem is the standard one, with the following correlation matrix:

$$\mathbf{T}(k,m) = \sum_{n=1}^{N} h_{n-k+1} h_{n-m+1}. \tag{54}$$

The main characteristics of the algorithm from the primal signal model are that the solution is, in general, nonsparse, and that any impulse response can be used (and not only Mercer's kernels).

Additionally, by noting that the solution can be expressed as:

$$\hat{x}_n = \sum_{i=1}^{N} \eta_i h_{i-n+1}, \tag{55}$$

an implicit signal model can be seen, which is:

$$\hat{x}_k = \sum_{i=Q}^{N} \eta_i h_{i-k+1} = \eta_k * h_{-k+Q} = \eta_k * h_{-k} * \delta_{k+Q} , \tag{56}$$

where δ_{k+Q} denotes the samples of a Kronecker delta function that has been delayed Q samples, that is, the samples of discrete-time function $\delta[k+Q]$. Hence, the estimated signal is built

Figure 4. Algorithms for nonblind deconvolution. Schemes of the primal signal model (left) and for the dual signal model (right).

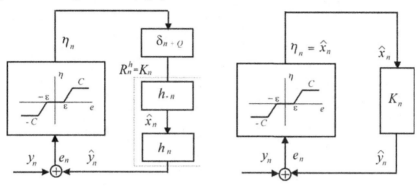

as the convolution of the Lagrange multipliers with the time-reversed impulse response and with a Q-lag time-offset delta function.

Figure 4 shows the schemes of both SVM algorithms. The residuals between the observations and the model output are used to control the Lagrange multipliers. In the dual signal model based SVM algorithm, the Lagrange multipliers are the input to a linear, time-invariant, noncausal system whose impulse response is the Mercer's kernel. Interestingly, in the primal signal model based SVM algorithm, the Lagrange multipliers can be seen as the input to a single linear, time-invariant system whose global input response is $h_{eq}[n]$ = $h[n]* h[-n]*\delta [n+Q]$. It is easy to show that $h_{eq}[n]$ is the expression that corresponds (except for the delay) to a valid Mercer's kernel, which emerges naturally from the primal dual model SVM formulation.

This last point of view provides a new direction to explore the properties of the primal signal model SVM algorithms in connection with classical linear system theory, which is currently being studied. In particular, an intermediate method for providing sparse solutions while allowing us to use causal impulse responses in the model could benefit from the advantages of both kinds of approaches (Martínez-Cruz et al., 2006).

Some Application Examples

In this section, several examples are used to highlight the usefulness and capabilities of the SVM-DSP framework. An example of the SVM-Spect algorithm (Rojo-Álvarez et al., 2003) is used to show the insensitivity to impulse noise, using considerations that are also valid for the other schemes described in this chapter. Then, the properties of memory depth and regularization are studied for the SVM γ-filter structure (Camps-Valls et al., 2004; Rojo-Álvarez et al., 2005). The application of SVR and the described SVM-ARMA algorithms in a nonlinear system estimation is included, as presented in Martínez-Ramón et al. (in press). Finally, an example using SVM sinc in nonuniform interpolation is summarized (Rojo-Álvarez et al., 2005).

Figure 5. Insensitivity of SVM-Spect to impulse noise. (a) Sinusoid whithin impulsive noise (up) and its Welch periodogram (down). (b) Histogram of the residuals (scaled to δ= 10) and control of the outlier impact onto the solution with C. (c) SVM-Spect spectral estimators for different values of insensitivity, which is controlled by the product δC.

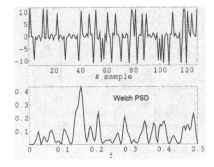
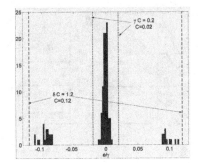

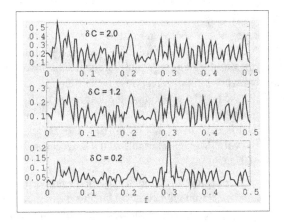

SVM-Spect and Insensitivity to Outliers

A simple synthetic data example is first presented to show the capacity of SVM-Spect to deal with outliers. A discrete-time process is given by:

$$y_n = \sin(2\pi\, fn) + v_n + j_n, \tag{57}$$

where $f = 0.3$; v_n is a white, Gaussian-noise sequence with zero mean and variance $\sigma^2 = 0.1$; and j_n is an impulsive noise process, generated as a sparse sequence for which 30% of the samples, randomly placed, are high-amplitude values given by $\pm10 + U(-0.5, 0.5)$, where $U()$ denotes the uniform distribution in the given interval, and the remaining are null samples. The number of observed samples is $N=128$, and we set $N_\omega = N/2 = 64$ (Figure 5a). A previous simulation showed that $\varepsilon = 0$ was a proper choice. A low value of δ leads to a major emphasis on minimizing the losses so that overfitting to the observations occurs in this case. We select a moderately high value of $\delta = 10$.

The appropriate *a priori* choice of free parameter C can be addressed by considering that, according to equation (22) the solution coefficients are a function of the multipliers and the data. Also, equations (12) and (13) reveal that a high amplitude residual, corresponding to an outlier, will produce a high amplitude multiplier, which will distort the solution. However, if the maximum value that the multiplier can take is properly limited by C, the impact of the outlier on the solution is lessened. Figure 5b shows that C should be low enough to exclude the residual amplitudes greater than the base level. This level can be obtained from previous methods of estimation of the prediction error, from *a priori* knowledge of the problem, or from training data. Figure 5c shows the results for $\delta C = 2, 1.2$, and 0.2, the last one allowing us to recover the spectral peak. Other experiments, not included here, show that similar solutions are obtained for a range of values of δC being low enough.

Figure 6. Performance criterion for the identification of an elliptic filter by the LS γ-filter (thin) and the SVM γ-filter (thick) for different orders (P between 1 and 4). The optimal μ parameter is also indicated for all the methods.

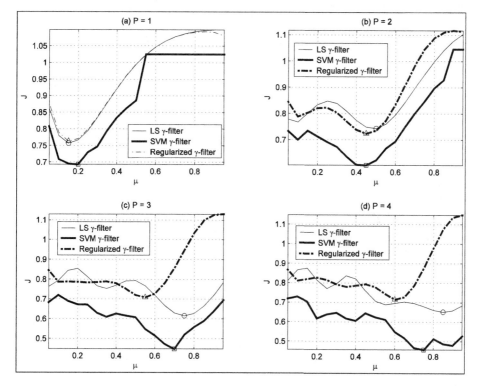

Example with SVM γ-Filter

The performance of the SVM γ-filter is examined next in terms of memory depth and regularization. In this experiment, we focused on the main advantages of both the γ-filter structure (stability and memory depth) and the SVM (regularization). We compared the memory parameter μ in the LS, the SVM, and the regularized γ-filters. The last one used the leaky LS algorithm described in Harris, Juan, and Principe (1999), which was introduced to alleviate the stalling of the filter coefficients in a real-time hardware implementation. We identified the following third-order elliptic low-pass filter:

$$H(z) = \frac{0.0563 - 0.0009z^{-1} + 0.0009z^{-2} + 0.0563z^{-3}}{1 - 2.129z^{-1} + 1.7834z^{-2} + 0.5435z^{-3}}, \tag{58}$$

which was previously analyzed in Principe et al. (1993) because of its long impulse response. A 100-sample input discrete process $\{x_n\}$ is a white, Gaussian-noise sequence with zero mean and unit variance. The corresponding output signal $\{y_n\}$ was corrupted by additive, small-variance ($\sigma_e^2 = 0.1$), random processes, modeling the measurement errors. An independent set of 100 samples was used for testing, and the experiment was repeated 100 times.

Figure 6 shows the chosen performance criterion $J_{min} = var(e_n)/var(y_n)$ (Principe et al., 1993) as a function of μ and P in the test set. It is noteworthy that, in all cases, the adaline structure (μ =1) performs worse than the γ structures. In addition, the SVM γ-filter clearly improves the results of the LS and the regularized versions in terms of J_{min}. The memory depth M for a fixed P increases with lower values of μ. This trend (observed for the three methods) is especially significant for the regularized γ-filter, but it occurs at the expense of poor performance of the criterion. Nevertheless, the SVM γ-filter still presents a good trade-off between memory depth and performance.

Figure 7. Nonlinear system used for SVR and SVM-ARMA system identification example

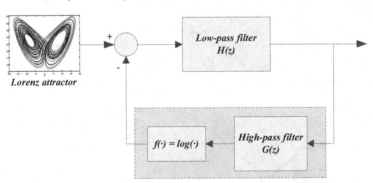

Table 1. Mean error (ME), mean-squared error (MSE), mean absolute error (ABSE), correlation (r), and normalized MSE (with respect of variance), for the models at the test set.

	Eq.	ME	MSE	ABSE	r	nMSE
SVR	(33)	0.28	3.07	1.08	0.99	-0.82
SVM-ARMA	(39)	0.14	2.08	0.88	0.99	-0.92

SVR and SVM-ARMA Non-Linear System Identification

We will now compare the performance in nonlinear system identification of SVR to the SVM-ARMA formulation provided in the chapter. We used the RBF kernel, which gives universal nonlinear mapping capabilities, and because only one kernel free parameter has to be tuned.

For illustration purposes, we run an example with explicit input-output relationships. The system that generated the data is illustrated in detail in Figure 7. The input discrete-time signal to the system is generated using a Lorenz system, which is described by the solution of the following three simultaneous differential equations:

$$dx / dt = -\rho x + \rho y \tag{59}$$

$$dy / dt = -xz + rx - y \tag{60}$$

$$dz / dt = xy - bz \tag{61}$$

with $\rho = 10$, $r = 28$, and $b = 8/3$. The chaotic nature of the time series is made explicit by plotting a projection of the trajectory in the x–z plane. Only the x component was used as an input signal to the system, and thus the model must perform the more difficult task of state estimation. This signal was then passed through an eighth-order low-pass finite impulse response (FIR) filter, $H(z)$, with cutoff frequency $\omega_n = 0.5$ and normalized gain of -6dB at ω_n. The output signal was then passed through a feedback loop consisting of a high-pass minimum-phase channel:

$$G(z) = \frac{1}{1.00 + 2.01z^{-1} + 1.46z^{-2} + 0.39z^{-3}}, \tag{62}$$

and further distorted with the nonlinearity $f(\cdot) = log(\cdot)$. The resulting system performs an extremely complex operation, in which the relationship between the input and output signals has an important effect in the time-series dynamics.

The described system was used to generate 1,000 input and output samples, which were split into two sets: a cross-validation data set to select the optimal free parameter consisting of 50 samples, and a test set to assess model performance, containing the following 500 samples. In all experiments, we selected the model order, σ, C, ε, and δ by following the usual cross-

Figure 8. SVM sinc interpolation from primal and dual signal models.(a) Training, test, and reconstructed signals in the time domain. (b) Training, test, and reconstructed signals in the spectral domain. (c) Spectral representation of the test signal and of the optimum kernel after validation.

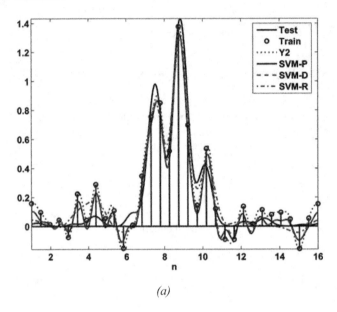

(a)

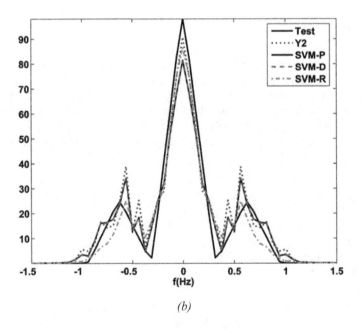

(b)

Figure 8. Continued

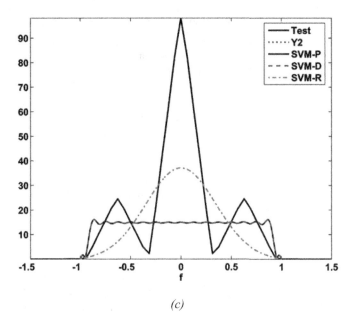

(c)

validation method. The experiment was repeated 100 times with randomly selected starting points in the time series. Averaged results are shown in Table 1, where it can be seen a general reduction in several merit figures for SVM-ARMA system identification.

SVM Sinc Interpolation

In order to see the basic features of the primal and dual signal model SVM algorithms for sinc interpolation, the recovery of a signal with relatively lower power energy on high frequency was addressed. This signal was chosen to explore the potential effect that regularization could have on the high-frequency components. The observed signals consisted of the sum of two squared sincs, one of them being a lower level, amplitude-modulated version of the baseband component, thus producing the following band-limited signal:

$$y(t) = \operatorname{sinc}^2(\frac{\pi}{T_0}t)(1 + \frac{1}{2}\sin(2\pi\,ft)) + e(t), \tag{63}$$

where $f = 0.4$ Hz. A set of $L = 32$ samples was used with averaged sampling interval $T = 0.5s$. Sampling intervals falling outside $[0, LT]$ were wrapped inside. The sampling instants were uniform. The signal-to-noise ratio was 10dB. The performance of the interpolators was measured by building a test set consisting of a noise-free, uniformly sampled version of the output signal with sampling interval $T/16$ as an approximation of the continuous-time signal, and by comparing it with the predicted interpolator outputs at the same time instants.

Figure 8 represents the resulting training and test signals, in the temporal (a) and in the spectral (b) domains, together with the results of the interpolation of the primal and dual signal model with the sinc kernel (SVM-P and SVM-D, respectively), the dual signal model with the RBF kernel (SVM-R), and the regularized Yen algorithm (Y2). Figure 8c shows that the spectral bandwidth of the optimum kernels after validation matched closely to the test signal bandwidth. As can be seen in Figure 9b, the spectral shape of the Lagrange multipliers always clearly provides the spectral shape of the test signal, either very similar to the sinc kernel, or compensating for the fading spectral shape of the RBF kernel. The time representation of the Lagrange multipliers (Figure 9a) shows that the coefficients and the Lagrange multipliers in the primal dual model and the Lagrange multipliers in the dual signal model are very similar (though not exactly the same), but the sparseness obtained by the RBF kernel is higher than that obtained by the sinc kernel.

Figure 9. SVM sinc interpolation. (a) Temporal representation of the Lagrange multipliers. (b) Spectral representation of the Lagrange multipliers. Primal: Lagrange multipliers for SVM-P; primal coefs: coefficients for SVM-P; dual: Lagrange multipliers for SVM-D; RBF: Lagrange multipliers for SVM-R.

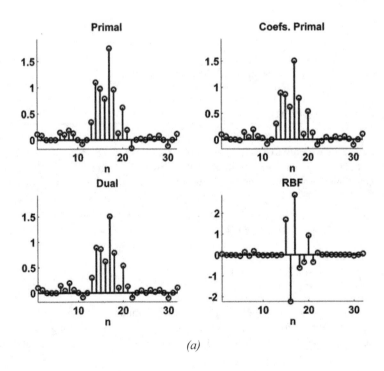

(a)

Figure 9. Continued

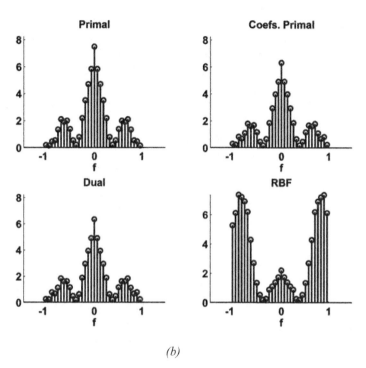

(b)

Future Directions

This chapter has summarized the SVM-DSP framework, which pursuits to exploit the SVM properties in signal processing problems by taking into account the temporal structure of the data to be modeled. To our understanding, this approach opens several research directions, and our aim here has been just to summarize the wide variety of methods that emerge when simple properties, such as the model equation, are considered. A more formalized statement of these concepts should be elaborated. An interesting research direction for the SVM-DSP framework is the use of complex arithmetic, which opens the fields of both digital communications and array processing to the possibilities of SVM methodology. These topics are analyzed in Chapters VII and VIII.

There are many other topics that will deserve special attention, some of them being the following:

- **Free-parameter selection:** The choice of the free parameters of both the ε-Huber cost and the used kernel is not always a trivial task, and a theoretical and practical analysis of the resampling techniques used to date (e.g., k-fold and bootstrap resampling) should be addressed. Additionally, the Bayesian point of view using the regularized expectation-maximization (EM) algorithm could be explored. The temporal structure of the DSP problems should be taken into account in this setting.

- **Computational burden:** Due to the use of quadratic programming and to the need for free-parameter selection, the computational burden required by these algorithms can preclude its use to online signal processing applications and to adaptive versions.

- **The choice of an appropriate kernel:** For nonlinear models, the SVM in general requires the choice of an appropriate Mercer's kernel among a variety of available known ones. A systematic procedure for determining which kernel is appropriate for a given real problem would be desirable.

- **Detailed comparison for each algorithm:** Our presentation does not address the detailed comparison of SVM-DSP algorithms to advanced methods, but this is a topic to consider in each new SVM algorithm.

Acknowledgments

Portions reprinted, with permission, from Rojo-Álvarez et al. (2004) and Rojo-Álvarez et al. (2003; © 2006 IEEE). Portions reprinted, with permission, from Rojo-Álvarez et al. (2005; © 2006 Elsevier). C. E. Martínez-Cruz is partially supported by Alban (EU Programme of High Level Scholarships for Latin America) scholarship No. E04M037994SV.

References

Aizerman, A., Braverman, E. M., & Rozoner, L. I. (1964). Theoretical foundations of the potential function method in pattern recognition learning. *Automation and Remote Control, 25*, 821-837.

Bach, F. R., & Jordan, M. I. (2002). Kernel independent component analysis. *Journal of Machine Learning Research, 3*, 1-48.

Baudat, G., & Anouar, F. (2000). Generalized discriminant analysis using a kernel approach. *Neural Computation, 12*(2), 2385-2404.

Ben-Hur, A., Horn, D., Siegelmann, H., & Vapnik, V. (2001). Support vector clustering. *Journal of Machine Learning Research, 2*, 125-137.

Camps-Valls, G., Bruzzone, L., Rojo-Álvarez, J. L., & Melgani, F. (2006). Robust support vector regression for biophysical parameter estimation from remotely sensed images. *IEEE Geoscience and Remote Sensing Letters, 3*(3), 339-343.

Camps-Valls, G., Martínez-Ramón, M., Rojo-Álvarez, J. L., & Soria-Olivas, E. (2004). Robust gamma-filter using support vector machines. *Neurocomputing, 62*, 493-499.

Camps-Valls, G., Requena-Carrión, J., Rojo-Álvarez, J. L., & Martínez-Ramón, M. (2006). *Nonlinear gamma-filter using support vector machines* (Tech. Rep. No. TR-DIE-TSC-22/07/2006). Spain: University of Valencia & University Carlos III of Madrid.

Choi, H., & Munson, D. C., Jr. (1995). Analysis and design of minimax-optimal interpolators. In *Proceedings of IEEE International Conference on Acoustics, Speech, and Signal Processing (ICASSP'95)* (Vol. 2, pp. 885-888).

Choi, H., & Munson, D. C., Jr. (1998). Analysis and design of minimax-optimal interpolators. *IEEE Transactions on Signal Processing, 46*(6), 1571-1579.

Drezet, P., & Harrison, R. (1998). Support vector machines for system identification. *UKACC International Conference on Control'98* (Vol. 1, pp. 688-692).

Gretton, A., Doucet, A., Herbrich, R., Rayner, P., & Schölkopf, B. (2001). Support vector regression for black-box system identification. *11ᵗʰ IEEE Workshop on Statistical Signal Processing* (pp. 341-344).

Gretton, A., Herbrich, R., & Smola, A. (2003). The kernel mutual information. In *Proceedings of the IEEE International Conference on Acoustics, Speech, and Signal Processing (ICASSP'03)* (Vol. 4, pp. 880-883).

Harris, J. G., Juan, J.-K., & Principe, J. C. (1999). Analog hardware implementation of continuous-time adaptive filter structures. *Journal of Analog Integrated Circuits and Signal Processing, 18*(2), 209-227.

Kuo, J. M., Celebi, S., & Principe, J. (1994). Adaptation of memory depth in the gamma filter. In *Proceedings of IEEE International Conference on Acoustics, Speech, and Signal Processing (ICASSP94)* (Vol. 5, pp. 373-376).

Kuo, J. M., & Principe, J. (1994). Noise reduction in state space using the focused gamma model. In *Proceedings of IEEE International Conference on Acoustics, Speech, and Signal Processing (ICASSP94)* (Vol. 2, pp. 533-536).

Martínez-Cruz, C. E., Rojo-Álvarez, J. L., Martínez-Ramón, M., Camps-Valls, G., Muñoz-Marí, J., & Figueiras-Vidal, A. R. (2006). *Sparse deconvolution using support vector machines* (Tech. Rep. No. TR-DIE-TSC-10/09/2006). Spain: University Carlos III of Madrid & University of Valencia.

Martínez-Ramón, M., Rojo-Álvarez, J., Camps-Valls, G., Muñoz-Marí, J., Navia-Vázquez, A., Soria-Olivas, E., & Figueiras-Vidal, A.R. (in press). Support vector machines for non-linear kernel arma system identification. *IEEE Transactions on Neural Networks*.

Mattera, D. (2005). Support vector machines for signal processing. In L. Wang (Ed.), *Support vector machines: Theory and applications* (pp. 321-342). Springer.

Mattera, D., & Haykin, S. (1999). Support vector machines for dynamic reconstruction of chaotic systems. In B. Schölkopf, C. Burges, & A. Smola (Eds.), *Advances in kernel methods* (pp. 211-242). MIT Press.

Oppenheim, A., & Schafer, R. (1989). *Discrete-time signal processing*. Englewood Cliffs, NJ: Prentice Hall.

Palkar, M., & Principe, J. (1994). Echo cancellation with the gamma filter. In *Proceedings of IEEE International Conference on Acoustics, Speech and Signal Processing (ICASSP94)* (Vol. 3, pp. 369-372).

Papoulis, A. (1991). *Probability random variables and stochastic processes* (3rd ed.). New York: McGraw-Hill.

Principe, J. C., deVries, B., & de Oliveira, P. G. (1993). The gamma filter: A new class of adaptive IIR filters with restricted feedback. *IEEE Transactions on Signal Processing, 41*(2), 649-656.

Reed, M., & Simon, B. (1980). *Functional analysis.* London: Academic Press.

Rojo-Álvarez, J. L., Camps-Valls, G., Martínez-Ramón, M., Soria-Olivas, E., Navia Vázquez, A., & Figueiras-Vidal, A. R. (2005). Support vector machines framework for linear signal processing. *Signal Processing, 85*(12), 2316-2326.

Rojo-Álvarez, J.L., Figuera, C., Martínez-Cruz, C., Camps-Valls, G., & Martínez-Ramón, M. (2006). *Sinc kernel nonuniform interpolation of time series with support vector machines* (Tech. Rep. No. TR-DIE-TSC-01/07/2006). Spain: University Carlos III of Madrid & University of Valencia.

Rojo-Álvarez, J.L., Martínez-Ramón, M., Figueiras-Vidal, A. R., dePrado Cumplido, M., & Artés-Rodríguez, A. (2004). Support vector method for ARMA system identification. *IEEE Transactions on Signal Processing, 52*(1), 155-164.

Rojo-Álvarez, J. L., Martínez-Ramón, M., Figueiras-Vidal, A. R., García-Armada, A., & Artés-Rodríguez, A. (2003). A robust support vector algorithm for non-parametric spectral analysis. *IEEE Signal Processing Letters, 10*(11), 320-323.

Schölkopf, B. (1997). *Support vector learning.* Munich, Germany: R. Oldenbourg Verlag.

Smola, A. J., & Schölkopf, B. (2004). A tutorial on support vector regression. *Statistics and Computing, 14*(3), 199-222.

Suykens, J. (2001). Support vector machines: A nonlinear modelling and control perspective. *European Journal of Control, 7*(2-3), 311-327.

Vapnik, V. (1995). *The nature of statistical learning theory.* New York: Springer.

Yen, J. L. (1956). On nonuniform sampling of bandwidth-limited signals. *IRE Transactions on Circuit Theory, CT-3*, 251-257.

Zhang, L., Weida, Z., & Jiao, L. (2004). Wavelet support vector machine. *IEEE Transactions on System, Man and Cybernetics B, 34*(1), 34-39.

Endnote

[1]   The notation of ARMA is used according to the consideration of an ARMA filter structure, however, from a system identification point of view, the model is an ARX (exogenous).

Chapter VII

A Complex Support Vector Machine Approach to OFDM Coherent Demodulation

M. Julia Fernández-Getino García, Universidad Carlos III de Madrid, Spain

José Luis Rojo-Álvarez, Universidad Rey Juan Carlos, Spain

Víctor P. Gil-Jiménez, Universidad Carlos III de Madrid, Spain

Felipe Alonso-Atienza, Universidad Carlos III de Madrid, Spain

Ana García-Armada, Universidad Carlos III de Madrid, Spain

Abstract

Most of the approaches to digital communication applications using support vector machines (SVMs) rely on the conventional classification and regression SVM algorithms. However, the introduction of complex algebra in the SVM formulation can provide us with a more flexible and natural framework when dealing with complex constellations and symbols. In this chapter, an SVM algorithm for coherent robust demodulation in orthogonal frequency division multiplexing (OFDM) systems is studied. We present a complex regression SVM formulation specifically adapted to a pilot-based OFDM signal, which provides us with a simpler scheme than an SVM multiclassification method. The feasibility of this approach is substantiated by computer simulation results obtained for Institute of Electrical and Electronic Engineers (IEEE) 802.16 broadband fixed wireless channel models. These experiments allow us to scrutinize the performance of the OFDM-SVM system and the suitability of the ε-Huber cost function in the presence of non-Gaussian impulse noise interfering with OFDM pilot symbols.

Introduction

Orthogonal frequency division multiplexing (*OFDM*) is a very attractive technique for high bit rate transmission in wireless environments (Sampath, Talwar, Tellado, Erceg, & Paulraj, 2002). Data symbols are frequency multiplexed with orthogonal subcarriers to minimize the effects of multipath delay spread. Thus, a frequency-selective channel is transformed into a set of parallel flat-fading Gaussian subchannels, which makes equalization a simpler task. Moreover, this transmission technique can be efficiently implemented via (inverse) Discrete Fourier Transform (IDFT/DFT) operations. *Channel estimation* is usually carried out based on *pilot symbols* with an estimation algorithm such as the least squares (LS) criterion (Edfors, Sandell, van de Beek, Wilson, & Börjesson, 1996). However, in a practical environment where **impulse noise** can be present, this channel-estimation method may not be effective for this non-Gaussian noise.

The use of *support vector machines* (SVMs) has already been proposed to solve a variety of digital communications problems. The decision feedback equalizer (Chen, Gunn, & Harris, 2000; Sebald & Buclew, 2000) and the adaptive multiuser detector for direct-sequence code division multiple access (CDMA) signals in multipath channels (Chen, Samingan, & Hanzo, 2001) have been addressed by means of binary SVM nonlinear classifiers. In Rahman, Saito, Okada, and Yamamoto (2004), signal equalization and detection for a multicarrier (MC) CDMA system is based on an SVM linear classification algorithm. Nonlinear channel estimation based on SVM multiregression for multiple-input, multiple-output (MIMO) systems has also been scrutinized (Sánchez-Fernández, de Prado-Cumplido, Arenas-García, & Pérez-Cruz, 2004). In all these applications, SVM techniques outperform classical methods.

This chapter, which is an extended version of the proposal presented in Fernández-Getino García, Rojo-Álvarez, Alonso-Atienza, and Martínez-Ramón (2006), analyzes an SVM-based robust algorithm for channel estimation that is specifically adapted to a typical OFDM data structure. There are two main features in this approach. First, a *complex* regression SVM formulation is developed, which provides us with a simpler scheme than describing OFDM signals with either multilevel or nested binary SVM classification algorithms. Second, the adequacy of free parameters in the ε-Huber *robust cost function* (Mattera & Haykin, 1999; Rojo-Álvarez, Camps-Valls, Martínez-Ramón, Soria-Olivas, Navia Vázquez, & Figueiras-Vidal, 2005) is investigated since the properties of this cost function are suitable for impulse noise scenarios. A detailed description of the ε-Huber robust cost function can be found in Chapter VI. Although the robustness of some digital communication receivers against impulse noise had been examined by using *M*-estimates (Bai, He, Jiang, & Li, 2003; Ghosh, 1996), there were no previous works about the performance of SVM algorithms in digital communications under this condition. For the sake of simplicity, a linear dispersive channel with non-Gaussian noise is analyzed here. The extension of the proposed linear OFDM-SVM scheme to nonlinear scenarios can be easily introduced by using Mercer's kernels in a similar way as proposed for other communication schemes (Sebald & Buclew, 2000). It should also be noted that two of the most common robust cost functions (regularized LS and Huber cost) are particular cases of this SVM approach.

This chapter is organized as follows. In the next section, the algorithm for SVM complex regression is derived in detail. Then, the OFDM system and impulse noise model are described. The coherent demodulation of OFDM signals with SVM is addressed next, and some simulation results are presented. Finally, some conclusions and future directions are drawn.

Complex SVM Formulation

Most SVM-based solutions to complex-valued problems have been addressed in practice by reformulating complex single-dimensional vector spaces into real, two-dimensional vector spaces. However, not only the explicit complex-valued SVM formulation is possible, but also complex-variable algebra in SVM regression yields a constrained optimization problem that is formally analogous to the real-variable problem statement. The complex-algebra representation can be appropriate in problems such as digital communication systems and array processing (see Chapter VIII), where complex numbers are often used for calculations. A short version of the algorithm for complex support vector regression (SVR) can be found in Rojo-Álvarez et al. (2005). In this section, we present (for the first time) a detailed derivation of the general complex SVR algorithm, which will be also used in Chapter VIII.

Primal Functional

Let us consider a set of N pairs of observations $\{\mathbf{x}_n \in \mathbb{C}^Q, y_n \in \mathbb{C}\}$ with $n = 1,...,N$ that are related by a linear, complex-coefficients regression model defined by:

$$y_n = \sum_{m=1}^{Q} w^m x_n^m + e_n = \mathbf{w}^H \mathbf{x}_n + e_n \tag{1}$$

where $\mathbf{w} = [w^1,...,w^Q]^T$ is a Q-complex regression vector; $\mathbf{x}_n = [x_n^1,...,x_n^Q]^T$ and y_n are the nth complex input and output data, respectively; and e_n is the complex error or residual noise. Note that superscripts $*$, T, and H denote the conjugated, transposed, and hermitic (transposed and conjugated) matrix or vector, respectively. This notation is adopted in this chapter for convenience, though it slightly deviates from the notation in the other chapters.

The risk of an estimator consists of two terms: an empirical risk term, which is measured directly on the residuals by using an appropriate cost function, and a structural risk term, which comprises a bound on the complexity of the resulting model. If the empirical risk can be reduced to zero, then minimizing the structural risk term corresponds to maximizing the estimator generalization capabilities, as shown in Vapnik (1998). Besides this, for a linear machine such as equation (1), the procedure reduces to finding maximal margin solutions by minimizing the norm of the model coefficients **w**. Therefore, we have to minimize:

$$\frac{1}{2}\| \mathbf{w} \|^2,\tag{2}$$

constrained to

$$\Re\left(y_n - \mathbf{w}^H \mathbf{x}_n\right) \le \varepsilon$$
$$\Re\left(-y_n + \mathbf{w}^H \mathbf{x}_n\right) \le \varepsilon$$
$$\Im\left(y_n - \mathbf{w}^H \mathbf{x}_n\right) \le \varepsilon$$
$$\Im\left(-y_n + \mathbf{w}^H \mathbf{x}_n\right) \le \varepsilon\tag{3}$$

where ε is an error-tolerance parameter, and $\Re$ and $\Im$ denote the real and the imaginary part of a complex number, respectively. Given a data set of noisy observations, not all of the samples will satisfy the conditions in equation (3); instead, some of them will produce errors above ε. In this case, empirical error terms have to be included by using an appropriate cost function of the model residuals. In the real-valued SVR (Burges, 1998), empirical errors are introduced by using the ε-insensitive cost function, which is given by:

$$L^{\varepsilon}(e,\varepsilon) = \begin{cases} |e| - \varepsilon, |e| \ge \varepsilon \\ 0, |e| \le \varepsilon. \end{cases}\tag{4}$$

A more general cost function (Mattera & Haykin, 1999; Rojo-Álvarez et al., 2005), which additionally considers a quadratic cost zone (see Chapter VI), is the ε-Huber cost, given by:

$$L^{\varepsilon H}(e,\varepsilon,\delta,C) = \begin{cases} 0, |e| \le \varepsilon \\ \frac{1}{2\delta}(|e| - \varepsilon)^2, \ \varepsilon \le |e| \le \delta C + \varepsilon \\ C(|e| - \varepsilon) - \frac{1}{2}\delta C^2, |e| \ge \delta C + \varepsilon \end{cases}\tag{5}$$

where δ and C are free parameters that control the shape of the cost function. This residual cost function can be useful in communications environments, where additive, white, Gaussian noise is not the only kind of noise that can be present in the input signal. In the presence of sub-Gaussian noise (such as impulse or multiuser noise), whose density function can be approximated by a two-sided exponential, the joint density function is the convolution of both densities. Then, equation (5) can be viewed as an approximation to the maximum likelihood (ML) cost function for such a noise. Provided that Gaussian noise is thermal, and hence it is known by the receiver, the parameters in equation (5) can be estimated. At a low noise level, Gaussian noise will predominate, and then the L_2 or quadratic part of the function will be the optimal one so that a reasonable choice for $\delta C + \varepsilon$ is to be equal to Gaussian-noise variance σ_N. A theoretical optimal value for δ has not been given in the literature yet, but a proper

Figure 1. Complex-valued observation y$_{n}$, its corresponding ε-insensitivity zone, and relationship between errors (e$_{n}$) and losses.

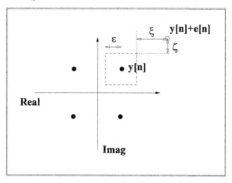

heuristic choice is to set it small, with typical values ranging from 10^{-3} to 10^{-9}. Beyond the low noise level, Gaussian-noise contribution will be negligible, and other noise sources will predominate so that a linear cost function will perform better.

Therefore, when losses are considered (see Figure 1), the problem is to minimize:

$$L = \frac{1}{2}\|\mathbf{w}\|^2 + \sum_{n=1}^{N}(L^{\varepsilon H}(\Re(e_n),\varepsilon,\delta,C) + L^{\varepsilon H}(\Im(e_n),\varepsilon,\delta,C)). \tag{6}$$

Equivalently, we have to minimize:

$$L = \frac{1}{2}\|\mathbf{w}\|^2 + C\sum_{n\in I_1}(\xi_n + \xi_n^+) + C\sum_{n\in I_3}(\zeta_n + \zeta_n^+)$$
$$+ \frac{1}{2\delta}\sum_{n\in I_2}(\xi_n^2 + \xi_n^{+2}) + \frac{1}{2\delta}\sum_{n\in I_4}(\zeta_n^2 + \zeta_n^{+2}) - \sum_{n\in I_1,I_3}(\delta C^2) \tag{7}$$

constrained to

$$\Re\left(y_n - \mathbf{w}^H\mathbf{x}_n\right) \le \varepsilon + \xi_n$$
$$\Re\left(-y_n + \mathbf{w}^H\mathbf{x}_n\right) \le \varepsilon + \xi_n^+$$
$$\Im\left(y_n - \mathbf{w}^H\mathbf{x}_n\right) \le \varepsilon + \zeta_n$$
$$\Im\left(-y_n + \mathbf{w}^H\mathbf{x}_n\right) \le \varepsilon + \zeta_n^+$$
$$\xi_n,\xi_n^+,\zeta_n,\zeta_n^+ \ge 0 \tag{8}$$

where data have been split according to the following sets of indices:

$$I_1 = \{n : \xi_n, \xi_n^+ \geq \delta C\}$$

$$I_2 = \{n : 0 \leq \xi_n, \xi_n^+ \leq \delta C\}$$

$$I_3 = \{n : \zeta_n, \zeta_n^+ \geq \delta C\}$$

$$I_4 = \{n : 0 \leq \zeta_n, \zeta_n^+ \leq \delta C\}, \tag{9}$$

and where $\xi_n(\xi_n^+)$ are called *slack* variables or losses, and they stand for positive (negative) errors in the real part of the output, and analogously for $\zeta_n(\zeta_n^+)$ in the imaginary part of the output. Note that errors are either negative or positive and, therefore, at most one of the losses takes a nonzero value; that is, either ξ_n or ξ_n^+ (either ζ_n or ζ_n^+) is null (or both are null if we are in the insensitivity zone). This constraint can be written as $\xi_n \xi_n^+ = 0$ ($\zeta_n \zeta_n^+ = 0$). Finally, as in other SVM formulations, parameter C can be seen as a trade-off factor between the empirical risk and the structural risk.

Primal-Dual Functional

As usual, in the SVM methodology it is possible to transform the minimization of the primal functional in equation (7), subject to constraints in equation (8), into the optimization of a dual functional. First, we introduce the constraints into the primal functional by means of Lagrange multipliers, obtaining the following primal-dual functional:

$$
\begin{aligned}
L_{pd} = & \frac{1}{2} \| \mathbf{w} \|^2 + C \sum_{n \in I_1}^{N} (\xi_n + \xi_n^+) + C \sum_{n \in I_3}^{N} (\zeta_n + \zeta_n^+) \\
& + \frac{1}{2\delta} \sum_{n \in I_2}^{N} (\xi_n^2 + \xi_n^{+2}) + \frac{1}{2\delta} \sum_{n \in I_4}^{N} (\zeta_n^2 + \zeta_n^{+2}) - \sum_{n \in I_1, I_3} (\delta C^2) \\
& - \sum_{n=1}^{N} (\lambda_n \xi_n + \lambda_n^+ \xi_n^+) - \sum_{n=1}^{N} (\eta_n \zeta_n + \eta_n^+ \zeta_n^+) \\
& + \sum_{n=1}^{N} \alpha_n [\Re(y_n - \mathbf{w}^H \mathbf{x}_n) - \varepsilon - \xi_n] \\
& + \sum_{n=1}^{N} \alpha_n^+ [\Re(-y_n + \mathbf{w}^H \mathbf{x}_n) - \varepsilon - \xi_n^+] \\
& + \sum_{n=1}^{N} \beta_n [\Im(y_n - \mathbf{w}^H \mathbf{x}_n) - \varepsilon - \zeta_n] \\
& + \sum_{n=1}^{N} \beta_n^+ [\Im(-y_n + \mathbf{w}^H \mathbf{x}_n) - \varepsilon - \zeta_n^+]
\end{aligned}
\tag{10}
$$

where it can be seen that a Lagrange multiplier (or dual variable) has been introduced for each constraint of the primal problem. Lagrange multipliers are constrained to be $\alpha_n^{(+)}, \beta_n^{(+)}, \lambda_n^{(+)}, \eta_n^{(+)} \geq 0$, and so also are $\xi_n^{(+)}, \zeta_n^{(+)} \geq 0$. The following additional constraints must also be fulfilled:

$$\alpha_n \alpha_n^+ = 0$$

$$\beta_n \beta_n^+ = 0. \tag{11}$$

Besides this, the Karush-Kuhn-Tucker (KKT) conditions (Vapnik, 1998) yield $\lambda_n \xi_n = 0$, $\lambda_n^+ \xi_n^+ = 0$, and $\eta_n \zeta_n = 0$, $\eta_n^+ \zeta_n^+ = 0$. Functional in equation (10) has to be minimized with respect to the primal variables and maximized with respect to the dual variables. By maximizing L_{pd} with respect to each w^m, we obtain:

$$\mathbf{w} = \sum_{n=1}^{N} \psi_n \mathbf{x}_n, \tag{12}$$

where $\psi_n = .5[(\alpha_n - \alpha_n^+) - j(\beta_n - \beta_n^+)]$. Note that the solution of equation (12) is a linear combination (by means of complex coefficients) of the input samples, and, as usual, observations with a nonzero coefficient will be called the support vectors. It can be observed that a value of ε different from 0 in equation (5) leads to a sparse solution. Nevertheless, whenever small sample sets are used for training, setting $\varepsilon = 0$ can be more convenient because the algorithm will use the maximum knowledge available from data.

If the gradient of L_{pd} with respect to $\xi_n^{(+)}$ and $\zeta_n^{(+)}$ is set to zero, it yields constraints:

$$0 \leq \lambda_n + \alpha_n \leq C$$

$$0 \leq \eta_n + \beta_n \leq C$$

$$0 \leq \lambda_n^+ + \alpha_n^+ \leq C$$

$$0 \leq \eta_n^+ + \beta_n^+ \leq C \tag{13}$$

for samples in I_1 and I_3, and constrains

$$0 \leq \lambda_n + \alpha_n \leq \frac{1}{\delta} \xi_n$$

$$0 \leq \eta_n + \beta_n \leq \frac{1}{\delta} \zeta_n$$

$$0 \leq \eta_n^+ + \alpha_n^+ \leq \frac{1}{\delta} \xi_n^+$$

$$0 \leq \eta_n^+ + \beta_n^+ \leq \frac{1}{\delta} \zeta_n^+ \tag{14}$$

for samples in I_2 and I_4. From equations (13) and (14), and by applying the KKT conditions:

$$\lambda_n \xi_n = 0$$
$$\eta_n \zeta_n = 0$$
$$\lambda_n^+ \xi_n^+ = 0$$
$$\eta_n^+ \zeta_n^+ = 0, \tag{15}$$

it is straightforward to show that an analytical relationship exists between the residuals and the Lagrange multipliers, given by:

$$(\alpha_n - \alpha_n^+) = \begin{cases} -C, \Re(e_n) \le e_C \\ \frac{1}{\delta}(\Re(e_n) + \varepsilon), -e_C \le \Re(e_n) \le \varepsilon \\ 0, -\varepsilon \le \Re(e_n) \le \varepsilon \\ \frac{1}{\delta}(\Re(e_n) - \varepsilon), -\varepsilon \le \Re(e_n) \le e_C \\ C, e_C \le \Re(e_n) \end{cases} \tag{16}$$

and

$$(\beta_n - \beta_n^+) = \begin{cases} -C, -\Im(e_n) \le e_C \\ \frac{1}{\delta}(-\Im(e_n) + \varepsilon), -e_C \le -\Im(e_n) \le \varepsilon \\ 0, -\varepsilon \le -\Im(e_n) \le \varepsilon \\ \frac{1}{\delta}(-\Im(e_n) - \varepsilon), -\varepsilon \le -\Im(e_n) \le e_C \\ C, e_C \le -\Im(e_n) \end{cases} \tag{17}$$

where $e_C = \varepsilon + \delta C$.

Next, we continue towards the dual formulation of the problem using Quadratic Programming (QP) as it is usually done in the literature. Nevertheless, note that alternative optimization methods, such as those relying on iterative reweighted least squares (IRWLS), have been introduced in Navia-Vázquez, Pérez-Cruz, Artés-Rodríguez, and Figueiras-Vidal (2001), with clear advantages in terms of computational cost and flexibility of operation (Parrado-Hernández, Mora-Jiménez, Arenas-García, Figueiras-Vidal, & Navia-Vázquez, 2003).

Dual Problem

The norm of the complex coefficients can be written as:

$$\| \mathbf{w} \|^2 = \mathbf{w}^H \mathbf{w} = \sum_{n,m=1}^{N} \psi_n^* \psi_m \mathbf{x}_n^H \mathbf{x}_m = \sum_{k=1}^{Q} \sum_{n,m=1}^{N} \psi_n^* \psi_m x_n^{k*} x_m^k. \tag{18}$$

At this point, if we denote the Gram matrix of dot products in equation (18) as:

$$\mathbf{G}(n,m) = \mathbf{x}_n^H \mathbf{x}_m = \sum_{k=1}^{Q} x_n^{k*} x_m^k, \tag{19}$$

then the norm of the coefficients can be written as

$$\| \mathbf{w} \|^2 = \boldsymbol{\psi}^H \mathbf{G} \boldsymbol{\psi}, \tag{20}$$

where $\boldsymbol{\psi} = [\psi_1, ..., \psi_N]^T$. By substituting equation (20) into equation (10), the dual functional to be maximized is as follows:

$$\begin{aligned}
W = &\frac{1}{2} \boldsymbol{\psi}^H \mathbf{G} \boldsymbol{\psi} - \Re[\boldsymbol{\psi}^H \mathbf{G}(\boldsymbol{\alpha} - \boldsymbol{\alpha}^+)] + \\
&+ \Im[\boldsymbol{\psi}^H \mathbf{G}(\boldsymbol{\beta} - \boldsymbol{\beta}^+)] + \\
&+ \Re[(\boldsymbol{\alpha} - \boldsymbol{\alpha}^+)^T \mathbf{y}] - \Im[(\boldsymbol{\beta} - \boldsymbol{\beta}^+)^T \mathbf{y}] - \\
&- (\boldsymbol{\alpha} + \boldsymbol{\alpha}^+)^T \mathbf{1}\boldsymbol{\varepsilon} - (\boldsymbol{\beta} + \boldsymbol{\beta}^+)^T \mathbf{1}\boldsymbol{\varepsilon} + L_C \quad ,
\end{aligned} \tag{21}$$

where L_c is a function of $\boldsymbol{\psi}$, and the vector notation has been introduced for $\boldsymbol{\alpha}^{(+)}, \boldsymbol{\beta}^{(+)}$. In order to describe L_c in equation (21), note that if we have $\xi_n^{(+)}, \zeta_n^{(+)} \neq 0$ in both sets (I_1 and I_2), then KKT conditions yield $\lambda_n^{(+)}, \eta_n^{(+)} = 0$. Different sets must be separately studied, as follows.

- Taking equation (13) into account, we have $\alpha_n^{(+)} = \beta_n^{(+)} = C$ for I_1 and I_3. Then, the last term of the functional for I_1 and I_3 is:

$$L_{C;1,3} = \frac{\delta}{2} \boldsymbol{\psi}_{1,3}^H \mathbf{I} \boldsymbol{\psi}_{1,3} \tag{22}$$

  where $\mathbf{I}$ is the corresponding identity matrix.

- Regarding I_2 and I_4, equation (14) holds so that $\alpha_n^{(+)} = \frac{1}{\delta} \xi_n^{(+)}$ and $\beta_n^{(+)} = \frac{1}{\delta} \zeta_n^{(+)}$. The last term for these intervals is:

$$L_{C;2,4} = \frac{\delta}{2} \boldsymbol{\psi}_{2,4}^H \mathbf{I} \boldsymbol{\psi}_{2,4} \tag{23}$$

  where $\boldsymbol{\psi}_{2,4}$ contains the elements corresponding to intervals I_2 and I_4.

Both terms can be grouped as:

$$L_C = L_{C;1,3} + L_{C;2,4} = \frac{\delta}{2}\psi^H \mathbf{I}\psi. \tag{24}$$

By regrouping terms, equation (21) can be written into a compact form:

$$W = -\frac{1}{2}\psi^H(\mathbf{G}+\delta\mathbf{I})\psi + \Re(\psi^H\mathbf{y}) - (\alpha + \alpha^+ + \beta + \beta^+)\mathbf{1}\varepsilon, \tag{25}$$

where $\mathbf{1}$ is the all-ones column vector. This expression is similar to the real-valued expression of the SVM regression functional, but it takes into account the cross-information contained in the complex-valued data. This represents a more convenient representation for complex-valued problems as it will be shown in the following sections, where an SVM scheme for OFDM coherent demodulation is proposed, and in Chapter VIII for antenna array processing.

OFDM Description

In the following subsections, the basic OFDM concepts will be presented in order to provide a better understanding of the OFDM coherent demodulation problem. Besides this, a brief summary of channel-estimation techniques suitable for OFDM is included.

Figure 2. Channel partitioning concept

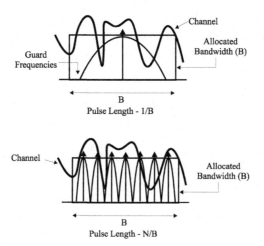

Basic Concepts of OFDM

OFDM is a type of multicarrier modulation. In general, multicarrier systems are based on the *channel-partitioning* concept that divides the bandwidth in N equal subchannels theoretically independent of each other (Cioffi, 2001) as it can be seen in Figure 2. If the subchannel bandwidth is much smaller than the coherence bandwidth, the transmitted signal in each of them will experience a flat fading in the frequency domain and, therefore, the equalization can be easily performed.

Since the allocated bandwidth B is divided into N subcarriers, the frequency spacing will be $T = 1/\Delta f = N/B$ (see Figure 2). Each subcarrier conveys one complex symbol, and all of them are simultaneously transmitted. For this reason, OFDM is usually considered a parallel transmission system. The OFDM-symbol duration will be $T = 1/\Delta f = N/B$. Subcarrier frequencies (related to the carrier frequency) are given by:

$$f_k = f_0 + \frac{k}{T} = f_0 + \frac{kB}{N}, k = 0,...,(N-1) \tag{26}$$

where f_0 is the lower frequency. The signal is obtained by using the following basis of orthogonal waveforms:

$$\phi_k^\ell(t) = g_k(t - \ell T) \tag{27}$$

where the index ℓ represents a symbol index due to the continuous nature of the transmission, the index k corresponds to the transmitted data at the kth subcarrier, and $g_k(t)$ can be written as:

Figure 3. OFDM analog modulator

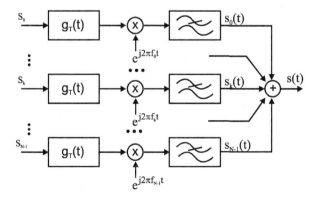

$$g_k(t) = \begin{cases} g_T(t)e^{j2\pi f_k t} & \text{if } t \in [0,T] \\ 0 & \text{otherwise} \end{cases} \tag{28}$$

where $g_T(t)$ denotes the transmission filter with an impulse response duration of T seconds. For the sake of simplicity, it is usually chosen to be rectangular; that is, in this situation, the transmission filter can be omitted. The scheme for an analog OFDM modulator is depicted in Figure 3.

Therefore, by adding all the contributions from different subcarriers, the baseband signal for the ℓth OFDM symbol can be written as:

$$s^\ell(t) = \sum_{k=0}^{N-1} S_k^\ell \phi_k^\ell(t) = \sum_{k=0}^{N-1} S_k^\ell e^{j2\pi \frac{B}{N} k(t - \ell T)}, \tag{29}$$

where S_k^ℓ is a complex symbol belonging to a certain set of signal constellation points (e.g., QPSK), carried at the kth subcarrier in symbol ℓ^{th}.

From this continuous-time model, the discrete one can be derived, where the modulation process is replaced by an IDFT. Similarly, at the receiver side, it can be shown that the corresponding operation is the DFT. When sampling at N samples per OFDM symbol, the discrete-time model can be written as in equation (30), widely used in the literature. It should be noted that this expression corresponds to the IDFT for a given frequency-domain sequence $\mathbf{S}^\ell = [S_0^\ell\ S_1^\ell\ ...S_k^\ell\ ...S_{N-1}^\ell]$:

$$s_n^\ell = \sum_{k=0}^{N-1} S_k^\ell \phi_{k,n}^\ell = \sum_{k=0}^{N-1} S_k^\ell e^{j\frac{2\pi}{N} k(n - \ell N)}, \tag{30}$$

where n denotes the time index. For the sake of simplicity, the symbol index (ℓ) is usually removed, and therefore equation (30) is rewritten as:

$$s_n = \sum_{k=0}^{N-1} S_k e^{j\frac{2\pi}{N} kn}, \tag{31}$$

which is the well-known expression for an OFDM symbol. In Figure 4, the scheme for OFDM transmission is shown, where IDFT and DFT operations are used for the modulation and $\mathbf{r} = [r_0, ..., r_{N-1}]^T$ is the time-domain received sequence after the channel effects and noise addition.

By using OFDM, the signal is transmitted over N orthogonal subcarriers in an efficient way. However, when the signal experiences a time-dispersive channel, as usual in many scenarios, the orthogonality is lost, and Inter-Carrier Interference (ICI) and Inter-Symbol Interference (ISI) appear. In order to avoid these effects while maintaining the orthogonality among subcarriers, the OFDM symbol is extended cyclically (Peled & Ruiz, 1980). This cyclic prefix (CP) is the copy of the last N_{CP} samples of the OFDM symbol at its beginning, configuring a guard period, as shown in Figure 5.

Figure 4. Discrete-time OFDM transmitter/receiver with IDFT/DFT

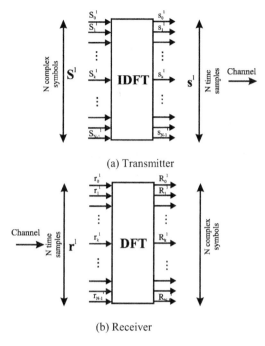

(a) Transmitter

(b) Receiver

The CP is removed at the receiver side, and if its length is longer than the channel duration, then the ISI is avoided because samples affected by ISI are within the guard period and are removed with the CP. However, since samples of the CP are not used at the receiver, the CP introduces a loss in bandwidth efficiency. The loss in signal-to-noise ratio (SNR) can be expressed (Edfors, Sandell, van de Beek, Landström, Sjöberg, 1996) as:

$$SNR_{loss} = -10\log_{10}\left(1 - \frac{T_{CP}}{T + T_{CP}}\right) \tag{32}$$

As mentioned above, the use of the CP maintains the orthogonality among subcarriers and the received signal where T_{CP} is the duration of the cyclic prefix. The length of the CP is

Figure 5. Cyclic prefix in OFDM

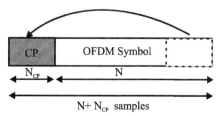

Figure 6. Complex multiplicative model

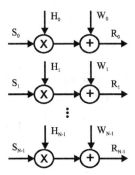

usually small when compared to the symbol length (typically, smaller than $N/5$ samples), thus yielding a loss of less than 1 dB (Nee & Prasad, 2000).

The received signal on each subcarrier is independent from others. Furthermore, provided that N is chosen so that each subchannel is frequency flat, it is only affected by the channel's response at its frequency, as depicted in Figure 6. Therefore, an OFDM system can be modeled as a set of parallel Gaussian subchannels, known as the complex multiplicative model, and then the received signal can be written as follows:

$$R_k = S_k H_k + W_k; \qquad 0 \le k \le N-1, \tag{33}$$

where H_k represents the complex channel coefficient at the kth subcarrier, and R_k and W_k are the DFT of received samples and white Gaussian noise at the kth subchannel, respectively.

Figure 7. Time-frequency grid in OFDM systems

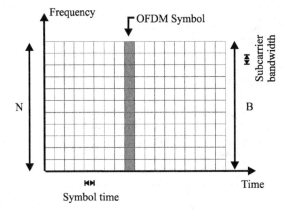

Figure 8. Pilot patterns in time-frequency grid for OFDM, where v_1 and v_2 are two linearly independent vectors to describe each geometry

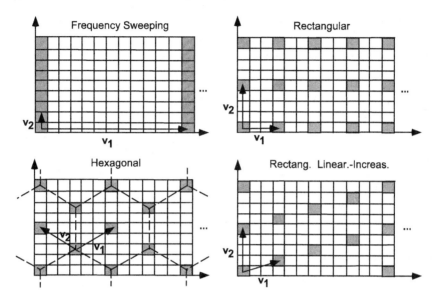

Another classical and useful way of representing an OFDM system is as a lattice in the time-frequency plane, as shown in Figure 7. Each cell of the lattice represents a subcarrier in the frequency domain and a symbol over the time domain.

Insertion of Pilot Symbols

It should be noted that each cell in the time-frequency grid (see Figure 7) is allowed to carry either information or control data independently. Usually, OFDM systems reserve some of the subcarriers for signaling. These data are called *pilots* because they are known at both sides of the transmission link.

Pilots can be used for several purposes, for example, channel estimation, synchronization, signal tracking, automatic gain control, or signal detection. They may also be arranged in the time-frequency grid following different patterns. In Figure 8, the most frequent pilot patterns are depicted. The first one, known as *frequency sweeping*, corresponds to the use of preambles. With this scheme, synchronization and channel estimation are accurate, but on the other hand, the loss in efficiency can be large, and in fast time-varying channels, estimated values are quickly outdated. The *rectangular* pattern allows the tracking of the time variations, and its loss in efficiency is lower than for the frequency-sweeping distribution; however, data must be estimated over the nonpilot subcarriers. This pattern allows us to extract precise information from the same subcarriers, but at different times. In order to improve results by scanning all the subcarriers, two additional patterns are proposed. With *linear increasing*, the pilot's positions are linearly shifted each sampling time, and with the *hexagonal* pattern, the same number of pilots are scattered in a more efficient distribution, thus improving the performance for channel estimation and synchronization methods (Fernández-Getino García, Páez-Borrallo, & Zazo, 1999).

Recalling the transmitted signal from equation (31), the received OFDM symbol after the channel effects and the addition of noise can be expressed as:

$$r_n = \sum_{k=0}^{N-1} S_k H_k e^{j\frac{2\pi}{N}kn} + w_n = \sum_{k \in \{K_p\}} P_k H_k e^{j\frac{2\pi}{N}kn} + \sum_{k \notin \{K_p\}} X_k H_k e^{j\frac{2\pi}{N}kn} + w_n \qquad (34)$$

where r_n, $n = 0, ..., N-1$, are time-domain samples before DFT transformation; P_k and X_k are the complex pilot and data values transmitted at the kth subcarrier, respectively; w_n is the complex, white, Gaussian-noise process in time-domain $N(0, \sigma_w^2)$; and $\{K_p\}$ is the set of indices corresponding to pilots subcarriers.

Therefore, the channel's frequency response can be first estimated over a subset $\{K_p\}$ of subcarriers, with cardinality $N_p = \#\{K_p\}$, and then interpolated over the remaining subcarriers $(N-N_p)$ by using, for example, DFT techniques with zero padding in the time domain (Edfors, Sandell, van de Beek, Wilson, Börjesson, 1996; van de Beek, Edfors, Sandell, Wilson, & Börjesson, 1995).

Channel Estimation for OFDM

When facing the wireless fading channel in OFDM communications, two types of modulation are usually employed, namely, differential or coherent (Proakis, 2000). When using differential modulation, the information is encoded in the difference between two consecutive symbols so that there is no need for channel estimation and complexity is reduced. However, there is a penalty of about 3 dB (Proakis, 2000), and the use of efficient multiamplitude constellations is not allowed. Differential modulation has been adopted in some OFDM-based systems, such as the European DAB (*Digital Audio Broadcasting*, 2001) standard.

On the other hand, coherent schemes allow multiamplitude constellations, and for this reason, when considering high data rates, coherent modulation must be used as in DVB (*Digital Video Broadcasting*, 2004). However, channel estimates are needed in order to apply coherent demodulation, and this estimation is performed at the receiver side. By taking again the complex multiplicative model in equation (33), the equalization process in OFDM only lies in estimating channel coefficients H_k, and then inverting them.

In general, channel-estimation methods can be grouped into two sets, namely, *data aided* (DA) and *decision directed* (DD). DA schemes make use of training OFDM symbols or sequences, pilot tones, or pilot symbols (Cimini, 1985; Classen, Speth, & Meyr, 1995), whereas DD methods are blind but suffer from error propagation and thus are not very common in practical applications.

Regarding DA methods, the channel estimation can be performed in one (1-D) or two (2-D) dimensions. Estimations in 1-D can be achieved by the LS criterion, also known as the zero forcing (ZF) method:

$$\hat{\mathbf{H}}_{LS} = \mathbf{P}^{-1}\mathbf{r},$$ (35)

where $\mathbf{P} = \text{diag}[P_0 \ldots P_{Np-1}]$ is a diagonal matrix whose elements are the pilot tones. The estimation can also be reached by using the optimal method, the linear minimum mean square error (LMMSE) criterion, where only frequency correlations are used for the estimate:

$$\hat{\mathbf{H}}_{LMMSE} = \mathbf{C}_{hh}\left(\mathbf{C}_{hh} + \sigma_w^2\left(\mathbf{P}\mathbf{P}^H\right)^{-1}\right)^{-1}\hat{\mathbf{H}}_{LS},$$ (36)

where $\mathbf{C}_{hh} = E\{\mathbf{H}\mathbf{H}^H\}$ is the channel autocorrelation matrix, $\mathbf{H}$ is an $N{\times}N$ diagonal matrix with the channel coefficients in its main diagonal, and σ_w^2 is the variance of the complex zero-mean, additive, Gaussian noise. Besides these, there is a number of other simpler methods, such as the DFT algorithm (Edfors, Sandell, van de Beek, Wilson, Börjesson, 1996; van de Beek et al., 1995). It is well known that if the channel impulse response has a maximum of L_t resolvable paths (and hence, of degrees of freedom), then N_p must be at least equal to L_t (Fernández-Getino García, Páez-Borrallo, & Zazo, 2001).

For the 2-D estimators, the 2-D Wiener filter is the optimal one (Edfors, Sandell, van de Beek, Wilson, & Börjesson, 1998), but there exist other simpler methods.

Impulse Noise

The use of SVM can provide a more robust channel-estimation algorithm in the presence of impulse noise. By adding this new source of noise to the original equation (34), the complex baseband received signal can be expressed as:

$$r_n = \sum_{k \in \{K_p\}} P_k H_k e^{j\frac{2\pi}{N}kn} + \sum_{k \notin \{K_p\}} X_k H_k e^{j\frac{2\pi}{N}kn} + w_n + b_n g_n.$$ (37)

The impulse noise is modeled as a Bernoulli-Gaussian process, that is, the product of a real Bernoulli process b_n with $Pr(b_n = 1) = p$, and a complex Gaussian process $g_n \sim N(0, \sigma_i^2)$ (Ghosh, 1996). Then, the total noise at the receiver side is given by the sum of both terms $z_n = w_n + b_n g_n$. The scheme of the system is shown in Figure 9.

Figure 9. Scheme of the system

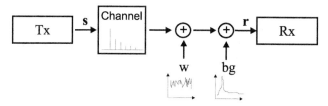

OFDM-SVM Algorithm

The proposed signal model for OFDM-SVM channel estimation is as follows:

$$r_n = \sum_{k \in \{K_p\}} P_k H_k e^{j\frac{2\pi}{N}kn} + e_n, \tag{38}$$

where $e_n = \sum_{k \notin \{K_p\}} X_k H_k e^{j\frac{2\pi}{N}kn} + z_n$ contains the residual noise plus the term due to data symbols. Here, these unknown symbols that carry information will be considered as noise during the estimation process. Channel estimation via the LS cost function is no longer the ML criterion when dealing with this sort of noise (Papoulis, 1991). In order to improve the performance of the estimation algorithm, the ε-Huber robust cost described before is introduced.

The primal problem can then be stated as minimizing:

$$\frac{1}{2} \sum_{k \in \{K_p\}} \left\| H_k \right\|^2 + C \sum_{n \in I_1} (\xi_n + \xi_n^+) + C \sum_{n \in I_3} (\zeta_n + \zeta_n^+)$$

$$+ \frac{1}{2\delta} \sum_{n \in I_2} (\xi_n^2 + \xi_n^{+2}) + \frac{1}{2\delta} \sum_{n \in I_4} (\zeta_n^2 + \zeta_n^{+2}) - \sum_{n \in I_1, I_3} \delta C^2 \tag{39}$$

constrained to

$$\Re(r_n) - \sum_{k \in \{K_p\}} \Re(P_k H_k e^{j\frac{2\pi}{N}kn}) \le \varepsilon + \xi_n, \tag{40}$$

$$\Im(r_n) - \sum_{k \in \{K_p\}} \Im(P_k H_k e^{j\frac{2\pi}{N}kn}) \le \varepsilon + \zeta_n, \tag{41}$$

$$-\Re(r_n) + \sum_{k \in \{K_p\}} \Re(P_k H_k e^{j\frac{2\pi}{N}kn}) \le \varepsilon + \xi_n^+, \tag{42}$$

$$-\Im(r_n) + \sum_{k \in \{K_p\}} \Im(P_k H_k e^{j\frac{2\pi}{N}kn}) \le \varepsilon + \zeta_n^+, \tag{43}$$

$$\xi_n^{(+)}, \zeta_n^{(+)} \ge 0 \tag{44}$$

for $n = 0, \dots, N-1$, where pairs of slack variables are introduced for both real ($\xi_n^{(+)}$) and imaginary ($\zeta_n^{(+)}$) residuals; superscript + and no superscript stand for positive and negative components of residuals, respectively; and $I_1 - I_2$ ($I_3 - I_4$) are the set of samples for which real (imaginary) parts of the residuals are in the quadratic-linear cost zone.

The derivation of the dual problem can be found at the beginning of this chapter, and only the new steps that are specific to our proposal are pointed out next. In brief, the primal-dual functional is obtained by introducing the constraints into the primal functional by means of Lagrange multipliers $\{\alpha_n\},\{\alpha_n^+\},\{\beta_n\},\{\beta_n^+\}$ for the real ($\alpha_n^{(+)}$) and imaginary ($\beta_n^{(+)}$) parts of the residuals. If we set to zero the primal-dual gradient with respect to H_k, we have the following expression for channel- estimated values at pilot positions:

$$\hat{H}_k = \sum_{n=0}^{N-1}\psi_n P_k, \quad k \in \{K_p\}, \tag{45}$$

where again we denote $\psi_n = .5[(\alpha_n - \alpha_n^+) - j(\beta_n - \beta_n^+)]$. For ease of notation, we define the following column vector:

$$\mathbf{v}_n(k) = [P_k e^{j\frac{2\pi}{N}kn}], \quad k \in \{K_p\}, \tag{46}$$

and the following Gram matrix, $\mathbf{R}(n,m) = \mathbf{v}_n^H \mathbf{v}_m$. Now, by placing the optimal solution of equation (45) into the primal-dual functional and grouping terms, a compact form of the functional problem can be stated in vector form that consists of maximizing:

$$-\frac{1}{2}\psi^H(\mathbf{R}+\delta\mathbf{I})\psi + \Re(\psi^H\mathbf{r}) - (\alpha + \alpha^+ + \beta + \beta^+)^T \mathbf{1}\varepsilon, \tag{47}$$

constrained to $0\leq \{\alpha_n\},\{\alpha_n^+\},\{\beta_n\},\{\beta_n^+\} \leq C$, where $\psi = [\psi_0, ..., \psi_{N-1}]^T$. Note that equation (47) is a quadratic form, and thus real valued, and it represents a natural extension of the dual functional in SVM real regression for complex-valued problems. The channel estimated values at pilot positions in equation (45) can be obtained by optimizing equation (47) with respect to $\{\alpha_n\},\{\alpha_n^+\},\{\beta_n\},\{\beta_n^+\}$, and then substituting ψ_n into equation (45).

A Simulation Example

In order to test the performance of the OFDM-SVM scheme, a scenario for the IEEE 802.16 fixed broadband wireless access standard has been considered. For this type of applications below 11 GHz, Non-Line-Of-Sight (NLOS) conditions are present. To simulate this environment, the modified Stanford University Interim SUI-3 channel model for omnidirectional antennas has been employed, with $L_t = 3$ taps, a maximum delay spread of $\tau_{max}=1\mu s$, and maximum Doppler frequency $f_m = 0.4$ Hz (Erceg et al., 2003). The main parameters of this channel are summarized in Table 1. The channel exhibits an Root Mean Square (RMS) delay spread of $\tau_{rms}=0.305$ μs Values for the $K-$ factor shown in Table 1 mean that 90% of the cell locations have K-factors greater than or equal to the K-factor specified; power values are expressed in dB relative to the main tap. Finally, the specified Doppler is the maximum frequency parameter f_m of the round-shaped spectrum (Erceg et al., 2003). Additionally, the

Table 1. SUI-3 channel model parameters for multipath fading

	Tap 1	Tap 2	Tap 3	Units
Delay	0	0.5	1	μs
Power	0	-5	-10	dB
K-factor (90%)	1	0	0	linear
Doppler	0.4	0.4	0.4	Hz

SUI-3 channel model specifies a normalization factor equal to -1.5113 dB, which must be added to each tap power to get the total mean power normalized to unity. Subsequent distortion as impulse noise was modeled with a Bernoulli-Gaussian process (p = 0.05).

This OFDM system consisted of N=64 subcarriers conveying Quaternary Phase Shift Keying (QPSK) symbols. We consider a packet-based transmission, where each packet consists of a header at the beginning of the packet with a known training sequence or preamble to perform channel estimation, followed by 20 OFDM data symbols. At the preamble, we insert two OFDM symbols with N_P =16 pilot subcarriers carrying complex symbols. Note that, due to the short length in samples of the preamble in our OFDM system, there is a low probability of a spike, due to impulse noise, falling into it. For transmission, a channel bandwidth B of

Figure 10. Performance of SVM-OFDM with free parameters, compared to LS in terms of $\Delta log(BER)$: (a) SIR vs C; (b) SIR vs δC; (c) SIR vs ε; and (d) BER as a function of SIR

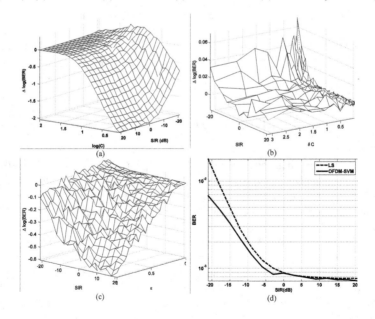

Figure 11. Performance of OFDM-SVM vs LS. MSE as a function of SIR

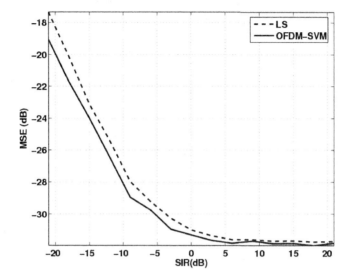

2 MHz has been chosen. Since we sample at Nyquist rate, this yields a sampling interval $T_s = 1/f_s = 0.5\mu s$; this means a minimum length for the cyclic prefix of two samples. After the channel-estimation procedure, we perform ZF equalization.

Channel estimation for the coherent demodulation of this OFDM system was performed with the SVM algorithm. For comparison purposes, LS channel estimates were simultaneously obtained in all cases. The Signal-to-Impulse Ratio (SIR) was defined as $SIR = \frac{E(r_n - z_n)}{E(g_n)}$, and it ranged from - 21 to 21 dB. The free parameters of SVM were explored, according to $C \in (1, 10^2), \delta C \in (10^{-4}, 0.5), \varepsilon \in (0,1)$, at 40 points per interval. Each exploration consisted of 500 realizations.

The comparison between SVM and LS techniques in terms of mean squared error (MSE) and bit error rate (BER) is represented in Figures 10 and 11, respectively. Figures 10d and 11 show that, for high SIR values, a similar performance to LS can be obtained, whereas for low SIR values, SVM outperforms the LS method when we properly choose C, δC, and ε. The expression $\Delta log(BER) = log(BER_{SVM}) - log(BER_{LS})$ has been defined in order to easily detect working zones where SVM works better ($\Delta log(BER) > 0$), similar to ($\Delta log(BER) = 0$), or worse than ($\Delta log(BER) > 0$) LS. Figure 10b shows that the performance of the SVM algorithm is not highly affected by the choice of δC, but low values of this product give rise to better BER performance. This is due to the fact that thermal noise is mainly a zero-mean, low-amplitude contribution, while noise impulses are high-amplitude spikes. Thus, δC must be adjusted to produce a quadratic cost around zero, and linear otherwise. Nevertheless, the choice of these parameters is not critical, showing almost equal performance within a range from $10^{0.5}$ to 10^3. Also, Figure 10c shows that, for almost all noise values, ε must be small and linearly growing with the thermal noise. This result is coherent with Kwok and Tsang (2003) and Cherkassky and Ma (2004), in which two similar rules for the choice of this parameter suggest that a near-optimal value of ε in SVM regressors must be proportional to the power of thermal noise.

Therefore, these figures show that the choice of the parameters is not a critical issue. In order to adjust ε, we only have to roughly know the power of thermal noise, which is usually estimated for other purposes as channel decoding. The choice of δC depends on the power of non-Gaussian noise.

Conclusion and Directions

An SVM algorithm for OFDM coherent demodulation has been presented in this chapter. Instead of a classification-based approach, this formulation is based on a complex regression expression that has been specifically developed for pilot-based OFDM systems. Simulations have confirmed the capabilities of OFDM-SVM in the presence of impulse noise interfering with the pilot symbols. This approach allows a simple implementation and a straightforward choice of free parameters, and its cost function is robust against many different noise scenarios. This scheme turns out to be a framework for the development of new applications of the SVM technique in OFDM systems. The use of the well-known Mercer's theorem will yield a natural extension of this algorithm to nonlinear versions by using Mercer kernels, such as the popular radial basis function. Such an extension may provide a significant benefit for OFDM communications in those scenarios in which nonlinear distortion is present.

References

Bai, W., He, C., Jiang, L. G., & Li, X. X. (2003). Robust channel estimation in MIMO-OFDM systems. *IEEE Electronics Letters, 39*(2), 242-244.

Burges, C. (1998). A tutorial on support vector machines for pattern recognition. *Data Mining and Knowledge Discovery, 2*(2), 1-32.

Chen, S., Gunn, S., & Harris, C. (2000). Decision feedback equaliser design using support vector machines. *IEEE Proceedings of Vision, Image and Signal Processing, 147*(3), 213-219.

Chen, S., Samingan, A. K., & Hanzo, L. (2001). Support vector machine multiuser receiver for DS-CDMA signals in multipath channels. *IEEE Transactions on Neural Networks, 12*(3), 604-611.

Cherkassky, V., & Ma, Y. (2004). Practical selection of SVM parameters and noise estimation for SVM regression. *Neural Networks, 17*(1), 113-126.

Cimini, L. J. (1985). Analysis and simulation of a digital mobile channel using orthogonal frequency-division multiplexing. *IEEE Transactions on Communications, 33*(7), 665-675.

Cioffi, J. (2001). Multichannel modulation. In *Class notes for EE379C: Advanced digital communications* (chap. 4). Stanford, CA: Stanford University.

Classen, F., Speth, M., & Meyr, H. (1995). Channel estimation units for an OFDM system suitable for mobile communications. In *Proceedings of Mobile Kommunikation: ITG-Fachbericht, München, ITG'95, 135*(1), 457-466.

Digital audio broadcasting (DAB): Guidelines and rules for implementation and operation. Part I, II and III (Tech. Rep. No. ETSI TR 101 496-1,2,3 V 1.1.1). (2001).

Digital video broadcasting (DVB): Implementation guidelines for DVB terrestrial services. Transmission aspects (Tech. Rep. No. ETSI TR 101 190 V.1.2.1). (2004).

Edfors, O., Sandell, M., van de Beek, J. J., Landström, D., & Sjöberg, F. (1996). *An introduction to orthogonal frequency division multiplexing* (Research report TULEA). Luleå, Sweden: Luleå University of Technology, Division of Signal Processing.

Edfors, O., Sandell, M., van de Beek, J., Wilson, S., & Börjesson, P. O. (1996). *Analysis of DFT-based channel estimators for OFDM* (Research report TULEA). Sweden: Luleå University of Technology, Division of Signal Processing.

Edfors, O., Sandell, M., van de Beek, J.-J., Wilson, S., & Börjesson, P. O. (1998). OFDM channel estimation by singular value decomposition. *IEEE Transactions on Communications, 46*(7), 931-939.

Erceg, V., Hari, K.V.S., Smith, M.S., Baum, D.S., Soma, P., Greenstein, L.J., et al. (2003). *Channel models for fixed wireless applications* (Tech. Rep. No. IEEE802.16a-03/01). IEEE 802.16 Broadband Wireless Working Group.

Fernández-Getino García, M. J., Páez-Borrallo, J., & Zazo, S. (1999). Novel pilot patterns for channel estimation in OFDM mobile systems over frequency selective fading channels. In *Proceedings of IEEE Personal Indoor Mobile Radio Communications (PIMRC'99)* (Vol. 2, pp. 363-367).

Fernández-Getino García, M. J., Páez-Borrallo, J. M., & Zazo, S. (2001). DFT-based channel estimation in 2D-pilot-symbol-aided OFDM wireless systems. In *Proceedings of IEEE Vehicular Technology Conference* (Vol. 2, pp. 815-819).

Fernández-Getino García, M. J., Rojo-Álvarez, J. L., Alonso-Atienza, F., & Martínez-Ramón, M. (2006). Support vector machines for robust channel estimation in OFDM. *IEEE Signal Processing Letters, 13*(7), 397-400.

Ghosh, M. (1996). Analysis of the effect of impulse noise on multicarrier and single carrier QAM systems. *IEEE Transactions on Communications, 44*(2), 145-147.

Kwok, J. T., & Tsang, I. W. (2003). Linear dependency between ε and the input noise in ε-support vector regression. *IEEE Transactions on Neural Networks, 14*(3), 544 -553.

Mattera, D., & Haykin, S. (1999). Support vector machines for dynamic reconstruction of chaotic systems. In Schölkopf, Burges, & Smola (Eds.), *Advances in kernel methods.* MIT Press.

Navia-Vázquez, A., Pérez-Cruz, F., Artés-Rodríguez, A., & Figueiras-Vidal, A. R. (2001). Weighted least squares training of support vector classifiers leading to compact and adaptive schemes. *IEEE Transactions on Neural Networks, 12*(5), 1047-1059.

Nee, R. V., & Prasad, R. (2000). *OFDM for wireless multimedia communications* (1st ed.). Artech House.

Papoulis, A. (1991). *Probability random variables and stochastic processes* (3rd ed.). New York: McGraw-Hill.

Parrado-Hernández, E., Mora-Jiménez, I., Arenas-García, J., Figueiras-Vidal, A., & Navia-Vázquez, A. (2003). Growing support vector classifiers with controlled complexity. *IEEE Transactions* on *Pattern Recognition, 36*(7), 1479-1488.

Peled, A., & Ruiz, A. (1980). Frequency domain data transmission using reduced computational complexity algorithms. In *Proceedings of IEEE International Conference on Acoustic, Speech and Signal Processing (ICASSP'80), 1*, 964-967.

Proakis, J. (2000). *Digital communications* (4th ed.). McGraw Hill.

Rahman, S., Saito, M., Okada, M., & Yamamoto, H. (2004). An MC-CDMA signal equalization and detection scheme based on support vector machines. In *Proceedings of 1st International Symposium on Wireless Communication Systems* (Vol. 1, pp. 11-15).

Rojo-Álvarez, J. L., Camps-Valls, G., Martínez-Ramón, M., Soria-Olivas, E., Navia Vázquez, A., & Figueiras-Vidal, A. R. (2005). Support vector machines framework for linear signal processing. *Signal Processing, 85*(12), 2316-2326.

Sampath, H., Talwar, S., Tellado, J., Erceg, V., & Paulraj, A. (2002). A fourth-generation MIMO-OFDM broadband wireless system: Design, performance and field trial results. *IEEE Communications Magazine, 40*(9), 143-149.

Sánchez-Fernández, M. P., de Prado-Cumplido, M., Arenas-García, J., & Pérez-Cruz, F. (2004). SVM multiregression for nonlinear channel estimation in multiple-input multiple-output systems. *IEEE Transactions on Signal Processing, 52*(8), 2298-2307.

Sebald, D., & Buclew, A. (2000). Support vector machine techniques for nonlinear equalization. *IEEE Transactions on Signal Processing, 48*(11), 3217-3226.

Van de Beek, J.-J., Edfors, O., Sandell, M., Wilson, S., & Börjesson, P. O. (1995). On channel estimation in OFDM systems. In *Proceedings of IEEE Vehicular Technology Conference (VTC'95)* (Vol. 2, pp. 815-819).

Vapnik, V. (1998). *Statistical learning theory.* John Wiley & Sons.

Chapter VIII

Comparison of Kernel Methods Applied to Smart Antenna Array Processing

Christos Christodoulou, University of New Mexico, USA

Manel Martínez-Ramón, Universidad Carlos III de Madrid, Spain

Abstract

Support vector machines (SVMs) are a good candidate for the solution of antenna array processing problems such as beamforming, detection of the angle of arrival, or sidelobe suppression, due to the fact that these algorithms exhibit superior performance in generalization ability and reduction of computational burden. Here, we introduce three new approaches for antenna array beamforming based on SVMs. The first one relies on the use of a linear support vector regressor to construct a linear beamformer. This algorithm outperforms the minimum variance distortionless method (MVDM) when the sample set used for training is small. It is also an advantageous approach when there is non-Gaussian noise present in the data. The second algorithm uses a nonlinear multiregressor to find the parameters of a linear beamformer. A multiregressor is trained off line to find the optimal parameters using a set of array snapshots. During the beamforming operation, the regressor works in the test mode, thus finding a set of parameters by interpolating among the solutions provided in the training phase. The motivation of this second algorithm is that the number of floating point operations needed is smaller than the number of operations needed by the MVDM since there is no need for matrix inversions. Only a vector-matrix product is needed to find the solution. Also, knowledge of the direction of arrival of the desired signal is not required during the beamforming operation, which leads to simpler and more flexible beamforming realizations. The third one is an implementation of a nonlinear beamformer using a non-linear SVM regressor. The operation of such a regressor is a generalization of the linear SVM one, and it yields better performance in terms of bit error rate (BER) than its linear counterparts. Simulations and comparisons with conventional beamforming strategies are provided, demonstrating the advantages of the SVM approach over the least-squares-based approach.

Introduction

Since the 1990s, there has been significant activity in the theoretical development and applications of support vector machines (SVMs). The first applications of machine learning have been related to data mining, text categorization, and pattern and facial recognition, but very little in the field of electromagnetics. Recently, however, popular binary machine learning algorithms, including SVM, have been applied to wireless communication problems, notably in spread-spectrum receiver design and channel equalization.

A main motivation of the use of SVM is the fact that in communications applications, small data sets are available for training purposes. Also, non-Gaussian noise may appear in wireless and multiuser scenarios. The benefits of the use of SVM in problems in which these situations appear are shown in Martínez-Ramón, Xu, and Christodoulou (2005), Rojo-Álvarez, Martínez-Ramón, De Prado-Cumplido, Artés-Rodríguez, and Figueiras-Vidal (2004), and Rojo-Álvarez, Martínez-Ramón, Figueiras-Vidal, García-Armada, and Artés-Rodríguez (2003). The first one appears as a consequence of a trade-off between the information provided by transmitters in order to train the receivers and the efficiency in the use of the available bandwidth. Many communication channels have small coherence times, so a data burst must be embedded into small time slots; its length is shorter than the time in which one can consider that the received data has stationary properties. In many of the applications, monitoring of the time slot is required in order to account for random delays due to different channel lengths, thus decreasing the actual burst time even more. In these bursts, the receiver must be trained, and then it has to detect and recover the transmitted information. During these time-limited bursts, the transmitter has to place training and data symbols. Each burst is actually transmitted through a different channel due to its variations or because the system arbitrarily switches to another channel, as is the case of mobile communications. So, the receiver has to be trained again, and the previous training data becomes useless. That means that only small data sets will be available for training. There is vast amount of literature on standard communications, from which we highlight Haykin (2001) for adaptive filtering; Benedetto and Biglieri (1999), Haykin (1988), Proakis and Manolakis (1995), and Proakis and Salehi (2001) for digital communications; and Van Trees (2002) for antenna array processing.

In these cases, least squares approaches can result in overfitting, while SVMs offer an approach that controls the generalization ability through a Tikhonov regularization (Tikhonov & Arsenen, 1977; see the introductory chapter).

Also, these channels are often corrupted by multiuser interference, as is sometimes the case in mobile communications, and electromagnetic noise, as, for example, when the system is used in an urban or industrial environment. Least squares approaches use the maximum likelihood (ML) cost function when the noise is Gaussian. This kind of noise always appears in communications since thermal noise is always present in transducers and electronic devices. This, however, may cause a weakness in the algorithm when non-Gaussian outliers appear. If, for example, an impulse noise is present, it may produce a huge cost due to the quadratic nature of the cost function, thus biasing the result. A better approach to deal with impulse noise is to apply a linear cost function. The generated cost will be constant, thus reducing the potential bias. This is the approach that is applied by the SVM.

The high-speed capabilities and learning abilities of support vectors can also be applied to solving complex optimization problems in electromagnetics in the areas of radar, remote sensing, microwaves, and antennas.

Here we introduce the antenna beamforming problem, and then we tackle the problem using linear and nonlinear SVM, but by adapting the algorithms to the particular characteristics of the beamforming problem. First of all, signal processing applications in general and antenna array processing in particular need to deal with complex-valued data. Unlike previously published work on SVM algorithms in signal processing, in which the adopted approaches use real-valued versions of the algorithms to deal with complex-valued data, here we use a direct complex notation to solve the SVM optimization problem. This approach leads to functionals that are a natural and straightforward extension of the standard SVM dual optimization problems. Second, as we pointed out before, both Gaussian and non-Gaussian noise sources are present in communications environments. We use a cost function that is an approximation to the ML cost function for the mixture of thermal noise and interferences. This approach is a combination of the Huber (1972) cost function and the ε-insensitive or Vapnik (1995) cost function. We adapt the cost function in order to make them close to the optimum given the class of noise present in antenna array applications.

In general, there are five main situations that make SVM good candidates for use in electromagnetics. The first of them is the situation in which no close solutions exist, and the only approaches are trial-and-error methods. In these cases, SVM or any other machine-based algorithm can be employed to solve the problem. The second situation is when the application requires operating in real time, but the computation time is limited. In these cases, an SVM algorithm can be trained off line and used in test mode in real time. The algorithm can be embedded in any hardware device such as application-specific integrated circuits (ASICs) or field-programmable gate arrays (FPGAs). Another important case appears when faster convergence rates and smaller errors are required. SVMs have shown that they possess superior performance in generalization ability in many problems. Also, the block optimization and the uniqueness of solutions make the SVM faster than many other methods. Finally, SVMs are good candidates when enough measured data exist to train an SVM for prediction purposes, especially when no analytical tools exist. In this case, one can actually use SVM to solve part of the problem where no analytical solution exists and combine the solution with other existing analytical and closed form solutions.

The organization of this chapter is as follows. The next section addresses the problem of antenna beamforming and how to maximize the received signal-to-noise ratio (SNR) using the standard minimum variance distortionless method (MVDM). In this section, it is shown how to generate training and testing data that are used to optimize the bit error performance and provide an estimator. Then, we present the formulation and use of a linear support vector beamformer. The section after that is related to the design of a nonlinear SVM multiregressor that estimates the beamformer vector using a set of input snapshots. This approach is interesting since there is no need for a priori knowledge of the direction of arrival (DOA) during the beamforming operation. Also, the computation burden is significantly lower than the one needed when using an MVDM or linear SVM beamformer approach. Next the chapter introduces a nonlinear SVM beamformer using Gaussian kernels. This approach has the drawback of a higher computational burden but the benefit of improved performance compared to the linear approaches. These sections include comparisons with standard algorithms. The final section is devoted to the summary and conclusions of the chapter.

Linear Beamforming

Practical beamforming problems face the difficulty of dealing with small data sets available for training purposes, which often jeopardize the generalization ability of the resulting machine. Due to its improved generalization ability, SVM is chosen here to solve this problem.

Array signal processing involves complex signals for which a complex-valued formulation of the SVM is needed. We introduce this formulation by introducing the real and imaginary parts of the error in the primal optimization, and then we proceed to solve a complex-valued constrained optimization problem. The resulting algorithm is a natural counterpart of the real-valued support vector regressor, which can be immediately applied to array signal processing.

In the first section, we use the SVM linear framework to solve linear beamforming problems, whereas in the second section, we apply nonlinear SVM regressors to implement the fast estimation of linear beamformer parameters. The solution presented in the first subsection is robust against interferences and non-Gaussian noise, and it is an alternative to solving problems in which low sample sets are available for training. The second section presents the solution of estimating the beamformer parameters very fast without intense floating point operations due to the fact that the algorithm operates in the test phase rather than in the training phase. The last subsection gives examples of nonlinear beamformers, showing that it is possible to obtain better performance with a nonlinear approach without compromising the generalization ability.

Formulation of the Problem

We first state the beamforming problem as it is usually treated. A beamformer consists of a set of equally spaced sensors or antenna elements that receive a set of electromagnetic signals coming from different DOAs. A signal coming from a DOA reaches each sensor from the same channel, so the only difference between the outputs of a sensor corresponding to a signal is the different phase shift. This assumption is true if the distance between sensors or array spacing and the total dimension of the array is small enough. Usually, the spacing is a fraction of a wavelength. Here we assume that all sensors are identical. Algorithms able to deal with nonequal elements are beyond the purposes of this chapter, but they are an open research topic in which nonlinear SVM may provide good solutions.

Assume that an array of M elements receives a signal coming from the direction of arrival θ_i. The distances traveled by the signal in order to reach two consecutive elements of the array will differ by a quantity of $d \sin(\theta_i)$, where d is the array spacing. Usual radio signals have very high frequencies compared to the bandwidth of the signal, so for practical array design, we assume that the signals are pure tones. In that case, one can also assume that the outputs of the elements contain identical signals, which only differ on their phases. If the wavelength of the signal is λ, then the phase shift will be $k_i = \frac{d}{\lambda} \sin(\theta_i)$.

If we denote the signal by its complex phasor as:

$$S_i[n] = s_i[n] e^{(j 2\pi f t + j\phi_k)}, \tag{1}$$

where f is the frequency of the wave, the expression of the output of the elements can be written as

$$\begin{aligned}
\mathbf{x_i}[n] &= s_i[n][e^{j(2\pi f t + \phi_k)}, e^{j(2\pi f t + \phi_k + k_i)}, \cdots, e^{j(2\pi f t + \phi_k + (M-1)k_i)}]' \\
&= s_i[n] e^{j(2\pi f t + \phi_k)}[1, e^{jk_i}, \cdots, e^{j(M-1)k_i}]'
\end{aligned} \tag{2}$$

The common phase can be introduced in the amplitude $s_i[n]$, so a change of notation gives the expression:

$$\mathbf{x_i}[n] = s_i[n][1, e^{jk_i}, \cdots, e^{j(M-1)k_i}]'. \tag{3}$$

The output of the array given k signals coming from different DOAs can be written in matrix notation as:

$$\mathbf{x}[\mathbf{n}] = \mathbf{A}\mathbf{s}[n] + \mathbf{g}[n], \tag{4}$$

where

$$\begin{aligned}
\mathbf{A} &= [\mathbf{a}(\theta_1) \cdots \mathbf{a}(\theta_k)] \\
\mathbf{a}(\theta_i) &= [1 e^{-jk_i} \cdots e^{-j(M-1)k_i}]' \\
\mathbf{s}[n] &= [s_1[n] \cdots s_k[n]]' \\
\mathbf{g}[n] &= [g_1[n] \cdots g_M[n]]'
\end{aligned} \tag{5}$$

are respectively the $M \times K$ steering matrix and vectors, the received signals, and the thermal noise present at the output of each array element.

Figure 1. Angles of arrival

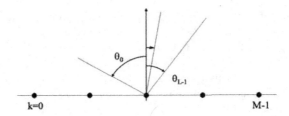

The beamformer computes a linear combination of the outputs $\mathbf{x}[n]$:

$$y[n] = \mathbf{w}^H \mathbf{x}[n]. \tag{6}$$

The optimal beamformer is the one that minimizes the total output power of $y[n]$ while keeping constant the amplitude produced by the steering vector $\mathbf{a}(\theta_d)$ of the desired DOA. Then, the beamformer minimizes the power of the interference signals by placing zeros of reception in their directions of arrival.

In other words, the optimal beamformer needs to satisfy:

$$\min\{\mathbf{w}^H \mathbf{R} \mathbf{w}\}, \tag{7}$$

subject to the constraint

$$\mathbf{w}^H \mathbf{a}(\theta_d) = r, \tag{8}$$

where $\mathbf{R}$ is the spatial correlation matrix of the received signals,

$$\begin{aligned}
\mathbf{R} &= \frac{1}{N} \mathbf{X} \mathbf{X}^H \\
&= E[(\mathbf{A}\mathbf{s}[n] + \mathbf{g}[n])(\mathbf{A}\mathbf{s}[n] + \mathbf{g}[n])^H] \\
&= \mathbf{A} \mathbf{P} \mathbf{A}^H + \sigma_g^2 I
\end{aligned} \tag{9}$$

provided that the signal and noise are independent, where $\mathbf{P}$ is the autocorrelation of $\mathbf{s}[n]$, and σ_g^2 is the noise power.

The solution of equation (7) minimizes the output power subject to the condition that the desired signal $\mathbf{s}_d[n]$ produces a given output $y[n]$. Applying Lagrange multipliers, the constrained optimization problem leads to the solution:

$$\mathbf{w}_{opt} = \mathbf{R}^{-1} \mathbf{a}(\theta_d) [\mathbf{a}^H(\theta_d) \mathbf{R}^{-1} \mathbf{a}(\theta_d)]^{-1} r, \tag{10}$$

where r is the amplitude of the response of the beamformer to an input equal to the steering vector of the desired signal. This method is the MVDM cited above.

Linear SVM Beamformer

Formulation

The beamformer is intended to minimize the error between the output and a reference or desired signal $d[n]$. Introducing the estimation error $\varepsilon[n]$, the expression for the output of the array processor is:

$$y[n] = \mathbf{w}^T \mathbf{x}[n] = d[n] + \varepsilon[n], \tag{11}$$

where $\mathbf{w} = [w_1 \cdots w_M]$.

For a set of N observed samples of $\{x[n]\}$, and when nonzero empirical errors are expected, the functional to be minimized is:

$$\frac{1}{2}\|\mathbf{w}\|^2 + \sum_{n=1}^{N} L(e[n]), \tag{12}$$

where L is a cost function. If we apply the ε-Huber to the real and imaginary parts of the error, this leads to the minimization of (Rojo-Álvarez et al., 2003; see also Chapter VI of this book):

$$\frac{1}{2}\|\mathbf{w}\|^2 + \sum L_{HR}\left(\xi_n + \xi_n^+\right) + \sum L_{HR}\left(\zeta_n + \zeta_n^+\right), \tag{13}$$

subject to

$$\Re(d[n] - \mathbf{w}^T \mathbf{x}[n]) \leq \varepsilon + \xi_n, \tag{14}$$

$$\Re(-d[n] + \mathbf{w}^T \mathbf{x}[n]) \leq \varepsilon + \xi_n^+, \tag{15}$$

$$\Im(d[n] - \mathbf{w}^T \mathbf{x}[n]) \leq \varepsilon + \zeta_n, \tag{16}$$

$$\Im(-d[n] + \mathbf{w}^T \mathbf{x}[n]) \leq \varepsilon + \zeta_n^+, \tag{17}$$

$$\xi_n, \xi_n', \zeta_n, \zeta_n' \geq 0, \tag{18}$$

where ξ_n (ξ_n^+) stand for positive (negative) errors in the real part of the output, and ζ_n (ζ_n^+) stand for errors in the imaginary part. Parameter C is the usual trade-off between the generalization ability and the empirical risk given the available training data in SVM algorithms. Here we apply a strategy that is slightly different for the one applied in Hill, Wolfe, and Rayner (2001), where the authors apply SVM to speech signal processing.

The optimization of the above problem leads to the dual:

$$L_d = -\frac{1}{2}\psi^H \Re(\mathbf{K} + \frac{\gamma}{2}\mathbf{I})\psi + \Re[\psi^H \mathbf{y}] - (\alpha + \alpha^+ + \beta + \beta^+)\mathbf{1}\varepsilon \tag{19}$$

and to the result

$$\mathbf{w} = \sum_{i=1}^{N}\psi_i^* \mathbf{x}_i^*. \tag{20}$$

The optimization of equation (19) will give a set of parameters $\psi_i = \alpha_i + j\beta_i$, and with the result of equation (20), we can compute the weights of the beamformer. The beamformer output can be expressed as:

$$y[n] = \sum_{i=1}^{N}\psi_i^* \mathbf{x}_i^{*H}\mathbf{x}[n] \tag{21}$$

by combining equation (11) with equation (20).

In order to control the sidelobes the same way equation (7) does, Gaudes, Via, and Santamaría (2004a, 2004b) introduced a variant of the algorithm. The procedure consists of a transformation of the solution provided by the SVM. The optimal solution $\tilde{\mathbf{w}}$ requires the minimization of the quantity $\tilde{\mathbf{w}}^H \mathbf{R}\tilde{\mathbf{w}}$. The squared norm of the SVM solution can be expressed as:

$$\mathbf{w}^H\mathbf{w} = \tilde{\mathbf{w}}^H\mathbf{R}\tilde{\mathbf{w}}. \tag{22}$$

Using the eigenvalue decomposition of the covariance matrix $\mathbf{R} = \mathbf{U}\mathbf{D}\mathbf{U}^H$, where $\mathbf{U}$ is the matrix of eigenvalues of $\mathbf{R}$, and $\mathbf{D}$ is a diagonal matrix containing its eigenvectors, the relationship between the optimal and the SVM solutions can be derived from:

$$\mathbf{w}^H\mathbf{w} = \tilde{\mathbf{w}}^H\mathbf{U}\mathbf{D}\mathbf{U}^H\tilde{\mathbf{w}} \tag{23}$$

as

$$\tilde{\mathbf{w}} = \mathbf{U}\mathbf{D}^{-\frac{1}{2}}\mathbf{w}. \tag{24}$$

Figure 2. BER performance for experiment 1. SVM (cont. line) and regularized LS (dash) beamformers (Reprinted from Martínez-Ramón et al., 2005, copyright 2005, with permission from IEEE)

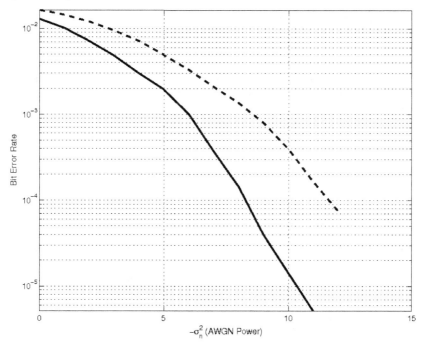

This transformation can be introduced in the solution in order to improve the interference rejection.

Examples

Comparisons of the algorithm against the MVDM (Haykin, 2001) with an array of six elements have been performed. A desired signal coming from a multipath channel consisting of two paths at DOAs -0.1π and 0.25π, and amplitudes 1 and 0.3 has been simulated. Also, three independent interfering signals coming from the DOAs -0.05π, 0.1π, and 0.3π, with amplitude 1, have been added. During the training set, the receiver collects 50 known BPSK binary symbols and trains the beamformer using them. In order to measure the bit error rate, the receiver collects bursts of 10,000 previously unknown symbols.

The cost function is adjusted so that the value of ΔC equals the standard deviation. Here, Δ was set equal to 10^{-6}. Then, most of the errors (due to thermal noise) fall in the quadratic area, whereas the outliers produced by interfering signals will fall in the linear area. Figure 2 shows the BER of MVDR and SVM for different noise levels measured by averaging 100 independent trials. An improvement of 2 to 4 dB is reported in that experiment. This improvement translates into a difference up to a magnitude order between both BER performances.

Figure 3. BER performance for experiment 2. SVM (cont. line) and regularized LS method (dash) beamformers (Reprinted with permission from IEEE)

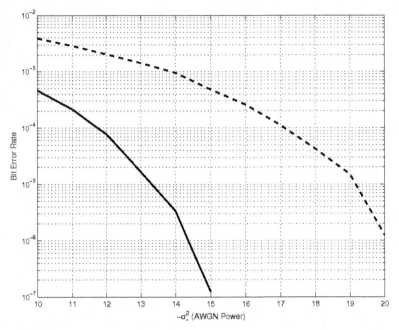

Figure 4. BER performance against the number of training samples. SVM (cont. line) and regularized LS method (dash) beamformers (Reprinted with permission from IEEE)

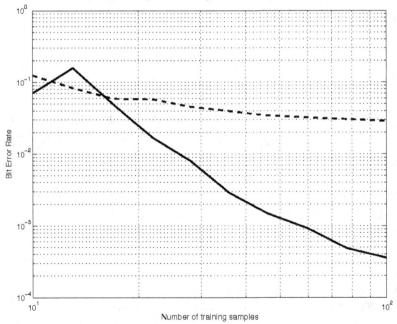

We repeated the same example with the desired signals coming from the DOAs -0.1π and 0.25π, with amplitudes 1 and 0.3, and the interfering signals coming from the DOAs -0.02π, 0.2π, and 0.3π with amplitude 1 (see Figure 3). In this example, the interfering signals are much closer to the desired ones, thus biasing the LS method algorithm. The superior performance of the SVM is due to its better robustness against the non-Gaussian outliers produced by the interfering signals.

The generalization ability is measured by measuring the BER against different numbers of samples from 10 to 50. The results are shown in Figure 4. Here, it can be observed the superior robustness against the overfitting of the SVM approach.

Non-Linear Parameter Estimation of Linear Beamformers

Linear beamformers use a set of training data to estimate the parameters, and they need to solve an optimization problem each time the direction of arrival changes. Instead of this, one may train off line a nonlinear multiregressor with signals coming from different angles of arrival and with their corresponding optimum beamforming parameters. Then, during detection, the network computes the beamformer by performing a nonlinear interpolation and obtains a set of parameters. That way, there is no need for an optimization computation each time the angle of arrival changes, but only to introduce the data into the regressor to produce a solution. This algorithm is adaptive and saves computational burden (Sánchez-Fernández, De Prado-Cumplido, Arenas-García, & Pérez-Cruz, 2004). Here, these ideas are applied to a nonlinear SVM multiregressor.

The idea is, then, to artificially generate a set of pairs $\{\mathbf{X}^l, \mathbf{w}^l\}$ where $\mathbf{X}^l$ is a matrix containing different observations of signals, with a given DOA of interest, and $\mathbf{w}^l$ are the parameters of the optimum linear beamformer computed following the MVDM of equation (10). The set of data pairs must contain examples coming from different DOAs so that there is enough information to train a regressor.

The data set consists of L matrices of the form $\mathbf{X}^l = \{\mathbf{x}_1^l \cdots \mathbf{x}_N^l\}$, $1 < l < L$, and they are generated following equation (4). Each vector is normalized by dividing it by its norm in order to make the network robust to changes in amplitude and to make it less dependent of its kernel parameters. The optimum beamformer can be exactly computed as the autocorrelation matrix is completely known:

$$\mathbf{R}^l = \mathbf{A}^l \mathbf{P}^l (\mathbf{A}^l)^H + (\sigma_g^l)^2 \mathbf{I}. \tag{25}$$

Using equation (10), the optimum beamformer parameters for each example can be computed, and the set of data pairs can be constructed.

Figure 5. Structure of a multiregressor

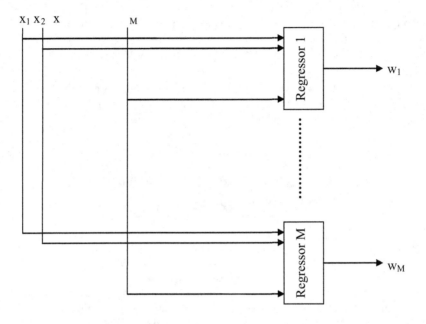

Structure of the Estimator

The estimator consists of a battery of M regressors whose inputs are **X**. The output of regressor m is the parameter $\mathbf{w}_m$. The structure is depicted in Figure 5.

The expression of the output of the multiregressor is:

$$\mathbf{w} = \phi^H(\mathbf{x}_i)\mathbf{V} + \mathbf{b} + \mathbf{e}_i, \tag{26}$$

where

$$\mathbf{V} = [\mathbf{v}_1 \cdots \mathbf{v}_M]$$
$$\mathbf{e}_i = [e_{1,i} \cdots e_{N,i}]^t. \tag{27}$$

Note that here, we intend to minimize the set of parameters **V**. The output of the regressor is the set of beamformer parameters **w**, while in the linear approach presented above, the parameters to be optimized are **w**.

This multiregressor can be trained using a block approach. To use this approach, the ε-insensitivity cost function:

$$\ell(e_i) = \begin{cases} 0 & |e_i| < \varepsilon \\ |e_i| - \varepsilon & |e_i| > \varepsilon \end{cases} \tag{28}$$

must be generalized. That cost function is designed to allow errors less than or equal to ε. Doing this produces a sparse solution in which the used samples are the subset of samples out of the ε band. A first approach to generalize this cost function is to directly apply it to all the components of the regressor output, so the resulting primal functional is an extension of the standard SVR formulation in more dimensions, that is:

$$\begin{aligned} L_p &= \tfrac{1}{2}\sum_{m=1}^{M} \| \mathbf{v}_m \|^2 \\ &+ C\sum_{m=1}^{M}\sum_{n\in I_1}(\xi_{n,m} + \zeta^{+}_{n,m}) + C\sum_{m=1}^{M}\sum_{n\in I_1}(\xi_{n,m} + \zeta^{+}_{n,m}) \\ &+ \tfrac{1}{2\gamma}\sum_{m=1}^{M}\sum_{n\in I_2}(\xi^2_{n,m} + \xi^{+2}_{n,m}) + \tfrac{1}{2\gamma}\sum_{n\in I_2}(\zeta^2_{n,m} + \zeta^{+2}_{n,m}) \end{aligned} \tag{29}$$

subject to

$$\begin{aligned} Re\left(w_{n,m} - \mathbf{v}_m^T \phi^H(\mathbf{x}_{n,m}) - b_m \right) &\le \varepsilon + \xi_{n,m} \\ Re\left(-w_{n,m} + \mathbf{v}_m^T \phi^H(\mathbf{x}_{n,m}) + b_m \right) &\le \varepsilon + \xi'_{n,m} \\ Im\left(w_{n,m} - \mathbf{v}_m^T \phi^H(\mathbf{x}_{n,m}) - b_m \right) &\le \varepsilon + \zeta_{n,m} \\ Im\left(-w_{n,m} + \mathbf{v}_m^T \phi^H(\mathbf{x}_{n,m}) + b_m \right) &\le \varepsilon + \zeta'_{n,m} \\ \xi_{n,m}, \xi'_{n,m}, \zeta_{n,m}, \zeta'_{n,m} &\ge 0 \end{aligned}$$

Care must be exercised if the number M of dimensions of the problem is high, as the ε band turns out to be here a hypercube with M dimensions. The difference between the minimum and maximum distances between the center of the hypercube and its surface is $(\sqrt{M} - 1)\varepsilon$. If M is high, then the errors are not treated evenly.

The solution provided in Sánchez-Fernández et al. (2004) uses a hypersphere, which treats all errors equally. The norm of the vector constructed with all errors as $\| \mathbf{e}_i \| = \sqrt{\mathbf{e}_i^H \mathbf{e}_i}$ is used, and the cost function can be expressed as:

$$\ell(\mathbf{e}_i) = \begin{cases} 0 & \| \mathbf{e}_i \| < \varepsilon \\ (\| \mathbf{e}_i \| - \varepsilon)^2 & \| \mathbf{e}_i \| \ge \varepsilon \end{cases} \tag{30}$$

Then, instead of having an ε hypercube in the cost function, we use a hypersphere. The primal functional is thus expressed as:

$$L_p = \frac{1}{2}\sum_{m=1}^{M} \| \mathbf{v}_m \|^2 + C\sum_{m=1}^{M} \ell(\mathbf{e}_m). \tag{31}$$

This functional cannot be optimized using quadratic programming techniques. The alternate optimization approach consists of an iterative weighted least squares (IWRLS) algorithm. This approach uses a quadratic approximation of the functional of the form:

$$L_p = \frac{1}{2}\sum_{m=1}^{M} \| \mathbf{v}_m \|^2 + \frac{1}{2}\sum_{m=1}^{M} a_m \| \mathbf{e}_m \|^2 + CT, \tag{32}$$

where

$$a_m = \begin{cases} 0 & |e|_{i,m} < \varepsilon \\ \frac{2C(|e|_{i,m})-\varepsilon}{|e|_{i,m}} & |e|_{i,m} \ge \varepsilon. \end{cases} \tag{33}$$

In each recursive step, it is necessary to compute the solution of equation (32). It consists of computing its gradient and setting it to zero. The gradient computation leads to the set of equations:

$$\begin{bmatrix} \boldsymbol{\varphi}^H \mathbf{D}_a \boldsymbol{\varphi} + \mathbf{I} & \boldsymbol{\varphi}^H \mathbf{a} \\ \mathbf{a}^H \boldsymbol{\varphi} & 1'\mathbf{a} \end{bmatrix} \begin{bmatrix} \mathbf{w}_i \\ \mathbf{b}_i \end{bmatrix} = \begin{bmatrix} \boldsymbol{\varphi}^H \mathbf{D}_a \mathbf{y}_i \\ \mathbf{a}^H \mathbf{y}_i \end{bmatrix}, \tag{34}$$

where $1 \le i \le M$, $\boldsymbol{\varphi}$ is a matrix containing all data in the feature space, and $\mathbf{a}$ is a vector containing scalars a_m.

Let us initialize parameters $\mathbf{V}_0$ and $\mathbf{b}_0$ to zero. Define $\mathbf{V}_k$ and $\mathbf{b}_k$ as the values of the parameters at iteration k. The procedure for the optimization has the following steps:

1.   Obtain the solution $\hat{\mathbf{W}}, \hat{\mathbf{b}}$ to the functional of equation (32).

2.   Compute

$$\mathbf{P}_k = \begin{bmatrix} \hat{\mathbf{W}} - \mathbf{W}_k \\ \hat{\mathbf{b}} - \mathbf{b}_k \end{bmatrix}. \tag{35}$$

3.   Compute

$$\begin{bmatrix} \mathbf{W}_{k+1} \\ \mathbf{b}_k \end{bmatrix} = \begin{bmatrix} \mathbf{W}_{k+1} \\ \mathbf{b}_k \end{bmatrix} + \mu \mathbf{P}_k, \tag{36}$$

where μ is an adaptation step.

4.   Compute e_i and a_i for equation (32) and go back to Step 1 until convergence.

Examples

We used the SVM multiregressor described in equations (32) to (36) to train a nonlinear SVM estimator. Fifty different angles of arrival between -80° and 80° have been used. For each SNR and angle of arrival we generate 10 different samples, thus the number of data for training is 1,500.

The results of a test of the estimator using a set of 10 snapshots with DOAs of 0 and 10 degrees are shown in Figures 6 and 7 respectively. The figures also show the optimal beamformer found by applying the MVDM algorithm. The same test with an SNR of 20 dB is shown in Figures 8 and 9. It can be observed that the differences are small and comparable to the result of the application of the MV by estimating the covariance matrix $\mathbf{R}$ from a set of samples.

Figure 6. Beam diagrams for the SVM estimation of the parameters of a linear beamformer of 10 elements, with DOA at 0° and SNR=10dB (cont. line) and optimum MV beamformer (dots)

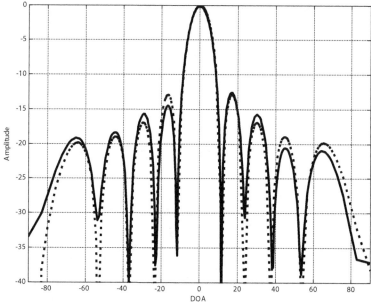

Figure 7. Beam diagrams for the SVM estimation of the parameters of a linear beamformer of 10 elements, with DOA at 10° and SNR=10dB (cont. line) and optimum MV beamformer (dots).

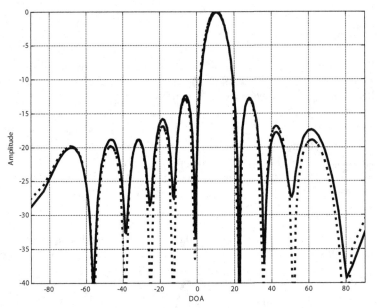

Figure 8. Beam diagrams for the SVM estimation of the parameters of a linear beamformer of 10 elements, with DOA at 0° and SNR=20dB (cont. line) and optimum MV beamformer (dots).

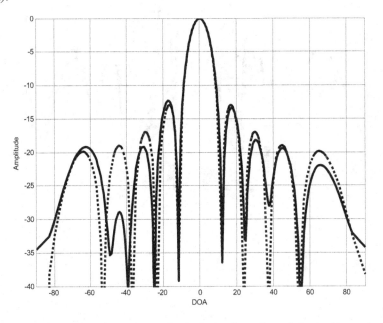

Figure 9. Beam diagrams for the SVM estimation of the parameters of a linear beamformer of 10 elements, with DOA at 10° and SNR=20dB (cont. line) and optimum MV beamformer (dots)

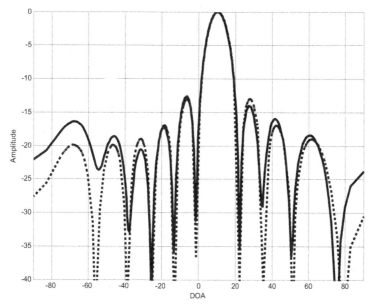

Also, there is no appreciable difference between the results of the data with both SNRs.

Non-Linear SNM Beamformers

Structure of the Estimator

A nonlinear beamformer can be constructed by the simple application of the kernel trick to the algorithm presented earlier. The idea is that, prior to the application of the algorithm, a nonlinear transformation $\varphi(\cdot)$ of the data from the input space to a possibly infinite-dimension Hilbert space is needed. The dot product into the Hilbert space needs to be known since it is a Mercer kernel. Once the data is in the Hilbert space, it is treated linearly.

Two main differences between the linear and the nonlinear beamformers are important to highlight. First, since the function that relates the input and output signals is nonlinear, there is no possibility of drawing a beam shape from the parameters of the beamformer, so all beam shapes will be approximations.

Second, using an adequate nonlinear function, the nonlinear transformation maps the data into an infinite dimensional space in which all vectors are linearly independent. Then, the subspace in which the transformed signal lies has as many dimensions as data. This gives a more powerful structure to process the signal.

The input vector $\mathbf{x}[n]$ is expressed as in equation (4):

$$\mathbf{x}[n] = \mathbf{A}\mathbf{s}[n] + \mathbf{g}[n], \tag{37}$$

where $\mathbf{A}$ is the matrix of the steering vectors of the incoming signals $\mathbf{s}[n]$. The input vector is nonlinearly processed to obtain the output d[n], which is expressed as:

$$y[n] = \mathbf{w}^T \phi(\mathbf{x}[n]) = d[n] + \varepsilon[n], \tag{38}$$

where $d[n]$ is the desired signal at time [n]. We assume that a sequence $d[n]$, $n = 1, \cdots, N$ is known and we will use it to train the beamformer.

Note that here we apply a nonlinear transformation $\phi(\mathbf{x}[n])$. As usual, this nonlinear transformation may not be known and the weight vector $\mathbf{w}$ will possibly have an infinite dimension. So, this formulation is in fact not explicit in the structure of the beamformer, but only an equivalent one that uses the dot product $< \phi(u), \phi(v) = \chi(u,v) >$ in the Hilbert space.

Figure 10. Simulations of the linear and the nonlinear beamformers for three array elements

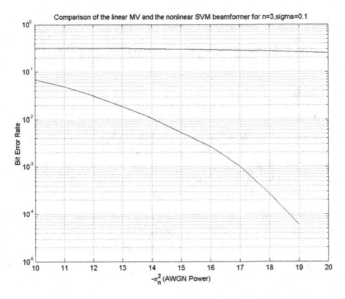

Figure 11. Simulations of the linear and the nonlinear beamformers for 4 array elements

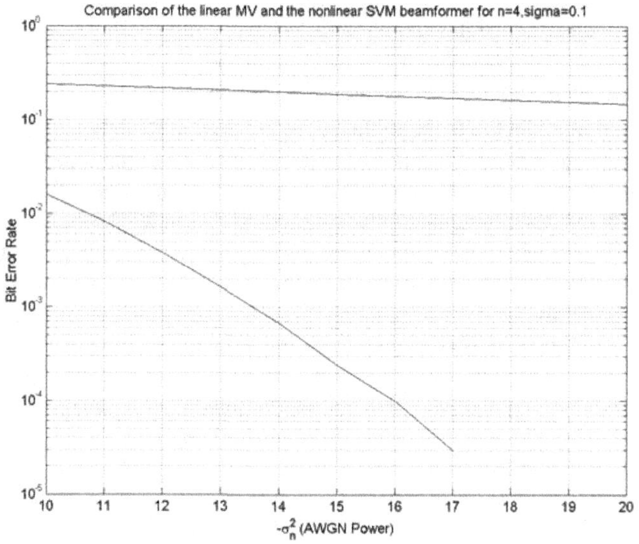

Assuming that a set of N observed samples of $\mathbf{x}[n]$ are available for training and that the desired signal at the output of the receiver is known, we can directly formulate the dual functional:

$$L_d = -\frac{1}{2}\psi^H \Re(\mathbf{K} + \frac{\gamma}{2}\mathbf{I})\psi + \Re[\psi^H \mathbf{d}] - (\alpha + \alpha^+ + \beta + \beta^+)\mathbf{1}\varepsilon, \tag{39}$$

where $\mathbf{d}$ is the vector of all desired signals.

Solving the functional gives the optimum values for parameters ψ_i, and the solution has the same form as that for the linear beamformer except that the dot product between vectors is given by the chosen kernel function $\chi(\cdot,\cdot)$:

$$d[n] = \sum_{i=1}^{N} \psi_i^* \, \chi(\mathbf{x}_i, \mathbf{x}[n]). \tag{40}$$

Here we do not have an explicit solution for the parameters $\mathbf{w}$. As we pointed out earlier, the Fourier transform does not apply here, so we cannot find the beam shape of the beamformer. In other words, where vectors $\mathbf{x} = [1, \exp(\omega_n)..., \exp(k\omega_n)]^T$ are eigenvectors of linear systems, their transformations $\phi(\mathbf{x}) = \phi([1, \exp(\omega_n)..., \exp(k\,\omega_n)])$ into the Hilbert space are not, so the concept of the Fourier transform disappears on them. The implication of this is that the beam shape will depend on the number and amplitude of the arriving sources.

Examples

We compare the performance of the nonlinear SVM beamformer to those of the linear ones in an environment in which there are N signals; one of them is the desired signal and the other $N-1$ are independent for different numbers of sensors in the antenna.

In this example, we simulated five directions of arrival. Two of them belong to the desired user's signal, traveling through a multipath channel. The other three are interfering or nondesired independent signals. All signals have unitary amplitude and different randomly chosen phase shifts, and the used modulation is QAM. The channel shows complex-valued additive Gaussian noise. In order to train the beamformers, we use a burst of 100 symbols, and then we test it during 10,000 symbol times, using previously unseen signals. Assuming that the thermal noise power σ_n is known, we choose $\varepsilon = \sigma_n$ and $C = 1000$, though the results with other parameter choices do not show significant differences.

We compared the performance of the nonlinear beamformer with those of the linear one for different numbers of array elements from two to six and for different values of the SNR.

In Figures 10 and 11, the solid lines correspond to simulations of the nonlinear beamformer for different numbers of array elements, while the dashed lines correspond to the simulations of the linear beamformer. The performance of the linear beamformer degrades rapidly when the number of elements is less than six, as expected. The performance of the SVM beamformer degrades slowly, being able to detect the desired transmitter even when the number of elements is less than the number of angles of arrival.

Conclusion

Three different algorithms for use in array beamforming for linear arrays have been presented. The first algorithm is a SVM counterpart of the classical least squares procedures. This approach shows better performance in situations where the sample set available for training is small. This is due to the superior generalization performance of SVMs. Also, we can observe an improved robustness of the linear support vector beamformer against non-Gaussian noise. The reason for this is that the applied cost function is better than the quadratic error cost function when non-Gaussian noise appears. These two facts together make the SVM approach a good choice in linear beamforming applications. The second algorithm is a completely different approach that is intended to reduce the computation time of the beamforming operation by removing the need for training a linear regressor. The proposed approach consists of a nonlinear multiregressor that is trained with data coming from different directions of arrival, and whose objective is to determine the optimum beamformer parameters. The third approach is an extension of the first linear SVM beamformer to one that is nonlinear, and it shows better performance than its linear counterpart without significantly increasing the computational burden.

References

Benedetto, S., & Biglieri, E. (1999). *Principles of digital transmission with wireless applications* (2nd ed.). Kluwer.

Gaudes, C. C., Via, J., & Santamaría, I. (2004a). An IRWLS procedure for robust beamforming with sidelobe control. *Sensor Array and Multichannel Signal Processing Workshop Proceedings* (pp. 342-346).

Gaudes, C. C., Via, J., & Santamaría, I. (2004b). Robust array beamforming with sidelobe control using support vector machines. *IEEE 5th Workshop on Signal Processing Advances in Wireless Communications* (pp. 258-262).

Haykin, S. (1988). *Digital communications.* Prentice Hall.

Haykin, S. (2001). *Adaptive filter theory* (4th ed.). Englewood Cliffs, NJ: Prentice-Hall.

Hill, S. I., Wolfe, P. J., & Rayner, P. J. W. (2001). Nonlinear perceptual audio filtering using support vector machines. In *Proceedings of the 11th Workshop on Statistical Signal Processing* (pp. 488-491).

Huber, P. J. (1972). Robust statistics: A review. *Ann. Statistics, 43.*

Martínez-Ramón, M., Xu, N., & Christodoulou, C. (2005). Beamforming using support vector machines. *IEEE Antennas and Wireless Propagation Letters, 4,* 439-442.

Proakis, J. G., & Manolakis, D. K. (1995). *Digital signal processing: Principles, algorithms and applications* (3rd ed.). Prentice Hall.

Proakis, J. G., & Salehi, M. (2001). *Communication systems engineering* (2nd ed.). Prentice Hall.

Rojo-Álvarez, J. L., Martínez-Ramón, M., De Prado-Cumplido, M., Artés-Rodríguez, A., & Figueiras-Vidal, A. R. (2004). Support vector method for ARMA system identification. *IEEE Transactions on Signal Processing, 52*(1), 155-164.

Rojo-Álvarez, J. L., Martínez-Ramón, M, Figueiras-Vidal, A. R., García-Armada, A., & Artés-Rodríguez, A. (2003). A robust support vector method for non-parametric spectral analysis. *IEEE Signal Processing Letters, 10*(11), 320-323.

Sánchez-Fernández, M., De Prado-Cumplido, M., Arenas-García, J., & Pérez-Cruz, F., (2004). SVM multiregression for nonlinear channel estimation in multiple-input multiple-output systems. *IEEE Transactions on Signal Processing, 52*(8), 2298-2307.

Tikhonov, A., & Arsenen, V. (1977). *Solution to ill-posed problems.* V. H. Winston & Sons.

Van Trees, H. L. (2002). *Optimum array processing: Vol. 4. Detection, estimation, and modulation theory.* New York: Wiley Interscience.

Vapnik, V. (1995). *The nature of statistical learning theory.* New York: Springer-Verlag.

Zooghby, A. E., Christodoulou, C. G., & Georgiopoulos, M. (1988). Neural network-based adaptive beamforming for one and two dimensional antenna arrays. *IEEE Transactions on Antennas and Propagation, 46*(12), 1891-1893.

Chapter IX

Applications of Kernel Theory to Speech Recognition

Joseph Picone, Mississippi State University, USA

Aravind Ganapathiraju, Mississippi State University, USA

Jon Hamaker, Mississippi State University, USA

Abstract

Automated speech recognition is traditionally defined as the process of converting an audio signal into a sequence of words. Over the past 30 years, simplistic techniques based on the design of smart feature-extraction algorithms and physiological models have given way to powerful statistical methods based on generative models. Such approaches suffer from three basic problems: discrimination, generalization, and sparsity. In the last decade, the field of machine learning has grown tremendously, generating many promising new approaches to this problem based on principles of discrimination. These techniques, though powerful when given vast amounts of training data, often suffer from poor generalization. In this chapter, we present a unified framework in which both generative and discriminative models are motivated from an information theoretic perspective. We introduce the modern statistical approach to speech recognition and discuss how kernel-based methods are used to model knowledge at each level of the problem. Specific methods discussed include kernel PCA for feature extraction and support vector machines for discriminative modeling. We conclude with some emerging research on the use of kernels in language modeling.

Introduction

The goal of a speech-recognition system is to provide an accurate and efficient means of converting an audio signal to text typically consisting of a string of words. The audio signal is often sampled at a rate between 8 and 16 kHz. The signal is converted to a sequence of vectors, known as features, at a rate of 100 times per second. These features, denoted by $O = \{O_1, O_2, ..., O_R\}$, are referred to as observations. The observations are then ultimately mapped to a sequence of words, denoted by $W = \{W_1, W_2, ..., W_t\}$, by integrating knowledge of human language into a statistical modeling framework. The dominant approach to achieving this signal-to-symbol conversion is based on hidden Markov models (HMMs; Jelinek, 1998; Rabiner & Juang, 1993). A speech-recognition system today is typically just one component in an information-retrieval system that can perform a wide range of human-computer interactions including voice mining, dialog, and question answering (Maybury, 2005). Historically, speech recognition has focused on maximizing the probability of a correct word sequence given the observations, denoted by $P(W|O)$, using generative models. However, in this chapter, we will explore a relatively new class of machines that attempt to directly minimize the error rate using principles of discrimination.

There are several subtle aspects of this problem that make it a challenging machine learning problem. First, our goal is to produce a machine that is independent of the identity of the speaker or the acoustic environment in which the system operates. This requires a learning machine to infer characteristics of the signal that are invariant to changes in the speaker or channel, a problem often described as robustness (Hansen, 1994). Second, the duration of a word can vary in length even for the same speaker, which requires a learning machine to be able to perform statistical comparisons of patterns of unequal length. Third, the pronunciation of a word, which is often represented as a sequence of fundamental sound units referred to as phones, can vary significantly based on factors such as linguistic context, dialect, and speaking style (Jurafsky & Martin, 2000). Fourth, and perhaps most importantly, state-of-the-art speech-recognition systems must learn from errorful transcriptions of the words. Systems are typically trained from transcriptions that contain only the words spoken rather than detailed phonetic transcriptions, and often these word transcriptions have error rates ranging from 1% to 10%. Practical considerations such as these often require careful engineering of any learning machine before state-of-the-art performance can be achieved. Nevertheless, in this chapter, we will focus primarily on the core machine learning aspects of this problem.

An Information Theoretic Basis for Speech Recognition

Given an observation sequence, O, a speech recognizer should choose a word sequence such that there is minimal uncertainty about the correct answer (Valtchev, 1995; Vertanen, 2004). This is equivalent to minimizing the conditional entropy:

$$H(W|O) = \sum_{w,o} P(W = w, O = o) \log P(W = w|O = o). \tag{1}$$

The mutual information, $I(W;O)$ between W and O, is equivalent to:

$$I(W;O) = H(W) - H(W|O). \tag{2}$$

A simple rearrangement of terms results in:

$$H(W|O) = H(W) - I(W;O). \tag{3}$$

Therefore, if our goal is to minimize $H(W|O)$, we can either minimize the entropy, $H(W)$, or maximize the mutual information, $I(W;O)$. We refer to the former problem as language modeling since it involves developing machines that can predict word sequences given a history of previous words and knowledge about the domain. The latter problem is known as the acoustic modeling problem since it involves predicting words given observations, which represent information about the original audio, or acoustic, signal. Most of this chapter will be devoted to various forms of acoustic modeling because this is where kernel machines have had the greatest impact. At the end of this chapter, we will briefly discuss emerging research on applications of kernel machines to language modeling since this is a relatively new area in the field.

Brown (1987) demonstrated that maximizing the mutual information over a set of observations is equivalent to choosing a parameter set, λ, that maximizes the function:

$$F_{MMIE} = \sum_{r=1}^{R} \log \left(\frac{P_\lambda(O_r|M_{W_r})P(W_r)}{\sum_{\hat{w}} P_\lambda(O_r|M_{\hat{w}})P(\hat{w})} \right), \tag{4}$$

where M_w represents a statistical model corresponding to a candidate sequence of words, w, describing the input signal, and $P(w)$ is the probability of this word sequence. $P(w)$ is often computed using a language model, which is designed to minimize $H(W)$. The denominator term sums probabilities over all possible word sequences, $\hat{w}$, and involves contributions from both the acoustic and language models.

The decomposition in equation (4) can often be expanded to include a pronunciation model (Jurafsky & Martin, 2000):

$$P_\lambda(O_r|M_{W_r})P(W_r) = P_\lambda(O_r|M_{W_r})P(U_{W_r}|O_r)P(W_r). \tag{5}$$

The pronunciation model, $P(U_{W_r}|O_r)$, typically describes how words are mapped to phones. The simplest form of a pronunciation model is a lexicon, which lists the sequence of phones that are most commonly used to pronounce a given word. More complicated approaches to pronunciation modeling use learning machines such as decision trees (Odell, 1995). The same statistical methods that are popular for acoustic modeling, such as HMMs, can be applied to pronunciation modeling. The details of such approaches are beyond the scope of this chapter. Here, we will focus primarily on fundamental aspects of the statistical modeling problem.

One approach to the maximization of equation (4) is to increase the numerator term. The solution to this problem is well known and typically involves using maximum likelihood estimation (MLE) of the parameters of the models representing the individual terms. A second approach to the maximization of equation (4) is to decrease the denominator term (Valtchev, Odell, Woodland, & Young, 1997), a process known as maximum mutual information estimation (MMIE). This has been a popular approach to introducing notions of discrimination into the traditional hidden Markov model paradigm, and involves making incorrect hypotheses less probable, thereby minimizing the summation in the denominator of equation (4). This process is also known as discriminative training and has produced significant improvements in performance in the last decade. It is a process that is typically introduced after MLE-based models have been estimated. Therefore, let us first focus on the components of a typical MLE-based speech-recognition system.

Elements of a Speech-Recognition System

The MLE approach to speech recognition, which involves the maximization of the numerator term in equation (4), can be viewed as a classic noisy communications-channel problem (Rabiner & Jung, 1993). This well-known formulation of the speech-recognition problem concisely expresses the relationship between various sources of knowledge using Bayes' rule:

$$W = \arg\max_{\hat{w}} \frac{P(O|\hat{W})P(\hat{W})}{P(O)}. \tag{6}$$

This formulation is important for two reasons. First, the term associated with the acoustic model, $P(O|W)$, provides insight into a process whereby statistical models can be trained. An estimation of the probability of an observation sequence O given a word sequence W can be accomplished by creating a database of speech labeled with the correct word sequences, and the use of an expectation maximization (EM) process that guarantees convergence of model parameters to an MLE solution. Second, the denominator term, which represents the probability of the observation sequence, can be ignored during the maximization process.

Therefore, the MLE approach to the speech-recognition problem often is simplified to:

$$W = \arg\max_{\hat{w}} P(O|\hat{W})P(\hat{W}). \tag{7}$$

Figure 1. The four major components of a speech recognition system.

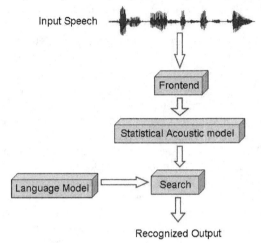

A conceptual block diagram of this approach is shown in Figure 1. There are four major components to the system: feature extraction, acoustic modeling, language modeling, and search. Kernel methods have not been directly applied to the search problem and therefore search will not be discussed here. Comprehensive reviews of this topic are given in Mohri (1997), Zweig, Saon, and Yvon (2002), and Deshmukh, Ganapathiraju, and Picone (1999). Applications of kernel methods in language modeling have only recently emerged and will be discussed at the end of this chapter. Acoustic modeling, the most straightforward application of kernel-based methods, will be discussed. Feature extraction (Picone, 1993) is the process by which the acoustic signal is converted to a sequence of vectors that captures important temporal and spectral information, and is discussed next. The use of kernels for feature extraction is also discussed extensively in Chapter XIV.

Feature Extraction

The general goals of the feature-extraction process are to produce features that model the perceptually meaningful aspects of the signal and to ignore artifacts due to variations in channel, speaker, and other such operational impairments. Traditional speech-recognition features often consist of measurements that are correlated and have unequal variances, and hence require some form of statistical normalization. Early attempts to transform features in a way that could improve discrimination focused on principal components analysis (PCA; Bocchieri & Doddington, 1986) and linear discriminant analysis (Kumar & Andreou, 1998), techniques that operate primarily on the correlation properties of the features.

A typical speech-recognition front end (Young, 2005), as shown in Figure 2, integrates absolute measures of the spectrum computed using a mel frequency-based cepstrum with

Figure 2. A standard speech recognition front end.

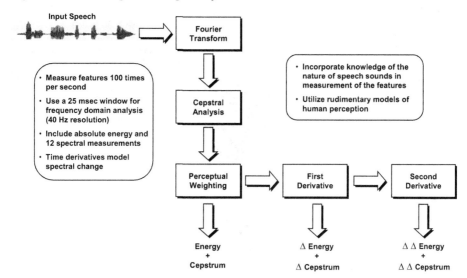

energy (MFCC). Twelve spectral measurements are concatenated with an energy measurement to produce 13 features. These features are then differentiated to measure the rate of change of the spectrum, and then differentiated once again to measure the acceleration. This particular approach produces a feature that contains 39 elements known as mel frequency scaled cepstral coefficients. Since the overall computation involves almost 100 msec of data, and is performed every 10 msec, there is significant overlap of information between two feature vectors that are adjacent in time.

Other approaches to feature extraction compute a much larger number of features, often the result of a fine-grain analysis of the spectrum, and then reduce the dimensionality of the feature set through standard techniques such as linear discriminant analysis. More recently, multistream approaches have become popular as a way to integrate higher levels of knowledge and measurements of asynchronous events into a single feature vector. Since all of these techniques mix heterogeneous measurements, it is easy to see that normalization and decorrelation are essential components of any subsequent processing. The use of linear transformations to decorrelate features has been a part of the speech-recognition systems for the past 30 years.

Kernel-based methods provide a principled way to move beyond simple linear transformations, and to transform the features to a new space in which discrimination is improved. It is important to understand that virtually any low-level measurement of the speech signal is highly ambiguous. This is demonstrated in Figure 3, in which we display the first two MFCC features measured for four vowels extracted from a conversational speech corpus. There are essentially two ways to disambiguate such classes: condition the measurements on more linguistic context or employ nonlinear feature transformations. Though the latter is the focus of a kernel-based approach, in practice it takes a combination of both approaches to achieve high-performance speech recognition.

Figure 3. A scatter plot of the first two cepstral coefficients in an MFCC based front end for two vowels

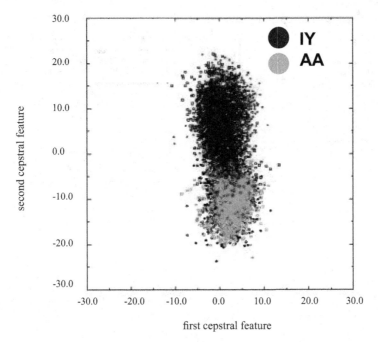

Kernel-based approaches represent a substantial improvement because the use of a nonlinear mapping allows the features to be transformed into high-dimensional spaces that increase the separability of the features. An overview of this approach is shown in Figure 4. These transformations can be computationally expensive. Therefore, any improvements in performance must be weighed against the cost. Feature extraction today typically consumes less than 1% of the overall processing time in a speech-recognition system.

PCA is a well-established technique for statistical normalization dimensionality reduction (Fukunaga, 1990). Here we will focus on the simplest form of PCA in which a single transformation is used to decorrelate all observations. This process is often referred to as class-independent PCA or the pooled covariance approach, since a single covariance method, which mixes measurements on speech and nonspeech (e.g., silence or background noise) is used to model the data. It is relatively straightforward to extend PCA to a class-dependent approach in which individual words, phonemes, or other elements of an acoustic model use a unique transformation. However, the essential advantages of a kernel-based approach can be demonstrated from the simplest form of PCA in which we apply a single linear transformation to the data.

Class-independent PCA on a set of feature vectors, $\mathbf{x}_i \in R^n$, $i = 1,...,M$, begins with the computation of the covariance matrix. Without loss of generality, we will assume the features have a zero mean: $\sum_{i=1}^{M} \mathbf{x}_i = 0$. The covariance matrix is defined as:

Figure 4. A simplified view of KPCA (Lima, et al., 2005).

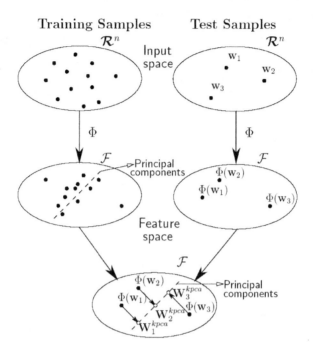

$$\Sigma = \frac{1}{M} \sum_{i=1}^{M} \mathbf{x}_i \mathbf{x}_i^{\mathrm{T}}. \tag{8}$$

We seek a linear transformation of the input vectors that produces decorrelated features. The well-known solution to this problem is a linear transformation derived from an eigenvalue analysis of Σ:

$$y_i = \mathbf{U} \Lambda^{-1/2} \mathbf{x}_i, \tag{9}$$

where Λ is a diagonal matrix consisting of the eigenvalues of Σ, and Y represents a matrix of eigenvectors of Σ. Dimensionality reduction has proven to be a useful way to enhance performance, and can be performed by eliminating the dimensions corresponding to the least significant eigenvalues (Bocchieri & Doddington, 1986). Notions of discrimination were developed initially through the use of simultaneous diagonalization (Fukunaga, 1990), class-dependent transforms (Bocchieri & Doddington), and eventually linear discriminant analysis (Kumar & Andreou, 1998).

Kernel-based PCA (KPCA; Schölkopf et al., 1999) is a technique that applies a kernel function to the PCA process in order to obtain decorrelated feature vectors in the higher dimensional space. The combination of a decorrelation transformation and a nonlinear mapping allows data not separable by a hyperplane decision surface to be more accurately classified. Since speech-recognition features suffer from significant amounts of confusability in the feature space due to, among other things, strong coarticulation in casual speech, classification techniques that can model nonlinear decision surfaces are extremely important.

The nonlinear mapping in KPCA is implemented as a dot product of the mapped variables $\phi(\mathbf{x})$. The kernel matrix, κ, is defined as $\kappa(i,j) = \{(\mathbf{x}_i, \mathbf{y}_j)\}$. Let us define a matrix, $\Phi = \{\phi_i\}$, for $i = 1, .., M$, where ϕ_i represents the mapping of $\mathbf{x}_i$ into a higher dimensional space, D, and $\kappa(\mathbf{x}_i, \mathbf{y}_j) = <\phi_i^t \phi_j>$. We can define a covariance matrix in the transformed feature space in terms of the mapped data:

$$\Sigma = \frac{1}{M} \sum_{j=1}^{M} \varphi_j \varphi_j^T = \frac{1}{M} \Phi\Phi^T. \tag{10}$$

The KPCA representation of $\mathbf{x}$ is given by the projection of $\phi(\mathbf{x})$ onto the eigenvectors of Σ, which can be expressed as:

$$\mathbf{V} = \Phi\mathbf{U}_K\Lambda_K^{-1/2}, \tag{11}$$

where $\mathbf{U}_K$ and Λ_K contain the eigenvectors and eigenvalues of the kernel matrix, κ. The process of transforming input data involves a similar transformation to PCA, but this transformation operates on the mapped data:

$$\mathbf{V}^T\varphi(\mathbf{y}) = \Lambda_K^{-1/2}\mathbf{U}_K^T\mathbf{k}_y^T, \tag{12}$$

where $\mathbf{k}_y$ represents an M-dimensional vector formed by $\kappa(\mathbf{y}, \mathbf{x}_i)$ for $i = 1, ..., M$.

Table 1. Error rate for KPCA using a polynomial kernel

Dim/Kernel	P=1	P=2
8	8.82	7.65
13	7.45	6.71
16	8.19	6.84
32	10.37	**6.53**
64	N/A	8.96
128	N/A	16.31
256	N/A	36.97

Lima, Zen, Nankaku, Miyajima, Tokuda, and Kitamura (2003) initially applied KPCA to a speaker-independent isolated word-recognition experiment consisting of 520 Japanese words spoken by 80 speakers. The experiment consisted of 10,400 training utterances and 31,200 evaluation utterances. A standard MFCC analysis was used for feature extraction. The baseline system achieved a word error rate (WER) of 8.6%. A polynomial kernel function was selected for these experiments.

Performance on speech recognition has not shown a strong dependence on the choice of a kernel. Polynomial and radial basis functions have been popular choices for kernels. First- and second-order polynomial kernels were evaluated in this study. The number of dimensions per kernel was varied from 8 to 256. A summary of the error rates is given in Table 1. A 22% relative reduction in WER was achieved using a second-order polynomial and 32 dimensions.

Though conceptually straightforward, KPCA has a significant drawback that all the training data is required to compute k_y in equation (12). A variety of standard techniques in pattern recognition have been explored to deal with this problem including subsampling (Lima, Zen, Nankaku, Tokuda, Kitamura, & Resende, 2005) and clustering (Lu, Zhang, Du, & Li, 2004).

There are many other variants of PCA that have proven successful in speech recognition. Independent component analysis (ICA; Bell & Sejnowski, 1995) is one of the more promising generalizations of PCA because of its effectiveness at separating speech from noise in applications where little prior information is available about either signal. ICA attempts to minimize the mutual information between its outputs instead of minimizing the correlation, as in PCA. Bach and Jordan (2003) showed that kernel-based ICA provided superior performance on several tasks involving the separation of complex deterministic signals as well as speech signals. Boscolo, Pan, and Roychowdhury (2001) showed that kernel-based ICA performed well on a wide variety of signal-separation tasks in which the a priori statistics of the signals were unknown. Extensions of these approaches to classical problems such as blind deconvolution are an active area of research.

Acoustic Modeling

The acoustic-modeling components of a speech recognizer are based on HMMs (Rabiner & Juang, 1993). The power of an HMM representation lies in its ability to model the temporal evolution of a signal via an underlying Markov process. The ability of an HMM to statistically model the acoustic and temporal variability in speech has been integral to its success. The probability distribution associated with each state in an HMM models the variability that occurs in speech across speakers or phonetic context. This distribution is typically a Gaussian mixture model (GMM) since a GMM provides a sufficiently general parsimonious parametric model as well as an efficient and robust mathematical framework for estimation and analysis.

Widespread use of HMMs for modeling speech can be attributed to the availability of efficient parameter-estimation procedures, such as MLE. One of the most compelling reasons for the success of ML and HMMs has been the existence of iterative methods to estimate the parameters that guarantee convergence. The EM algorithm provides an iterative framework for ML estimation with good convergence properties. The process of estimating parameters is conducted in a supervised learning paradigm in which the recognizer is given large numbers of example utterances along with their transcriptions. These transcriptions typically consist of a sequence of words. Note that segmentation information or speech and nonspeech classification is not required: The supervised learning paradigm allows the statistical models to acquire this information automatically. Hence, a speech-recognition system does a significant amount of self-organization during the training process and has the flexibility to learn subtle distinctions in the training data.

There are, however, problems with an MLE formulation for applications such as speech recognition (Ganapathiraju, 2002). Many promising techniques (Vertanen, 2004) have been introduced for using discriminative techniques to improve the estimation of HMM parameters (McDermott, 1997; Woodland & Povey, 2000). Artificial neural networks (ANNs) represent an important class of discriminative techniques that have been successfully applied to speech recognition. Though ANNs attempt to overcome many of the problems previously described, their shortcomings with respect to applications such as speech recognition are well documented (Bourlard & Morgan, 1994). Some of the most notable deficiencies include the design of optimal model topologies, slow convergence during training, and a tendency to overfit the data. However, it is important to note that many of the fundamental ideas presented here (e.g., soft margin classifiers) have similar implementations within an ANN framework. In most classifiers, controlling a trade-off between overfitting and good classification performance is vital to the success of the approach.

Kernel-based methods, particularly SVMs, are extremely attractive as alternatives to the GMM. SVMs have demonstrated good performance on several classic pattern-recognition problems (*Schölkopf & Smola*, 2002) and have become popular alternatives across a range of human-language technology applications (Wan & Renals, 2005). The primary attraction of these techniques is the way in which they generalize the maximum likelihood and discriminative training paradigms using risk minimization.

SVM Design for Speech Recognition

Since speech-recognition problems suffer from extreme amounts of overlap in the feature space, the use of a soft margin classifier is critical. One particular formulation of the SVM that has been effective in acoustic modeling for speech recognition poses the margin maximization problem as:

$$x_i \bullet w + b \geq +1 - \xi_i, \; for \; y_i = +1, \tag{13}$$

$$x_i \bullet w + b \leq +1 - \xi_i, \; for \; y_i = +1, \tag{14}$$

and

$$\xi_i \geq 0, \qquad \forall i, \tag{15}$$

where y_i are the class assignments, w represents the weight vector defining the classifier, b is a bias term, and the ξ_i are the slack variables. The derivation of an optimal classifier for this nonseparable case exists and is described in detail in Ganapathiraju (2002).

Several approaches for controlling the quality and quantity of support vectors have been studied extensively in recent years (Shawe-Taylor & Cristianini, 2002). Perhaps the most important consideration in speech recognition is the need to be robust to outliers in the data that usually arise from mislabeled training data or anomalous speaker behavior. The linear cost function in equation (13) has proven to be effective in training speech-recognition systems using large amounts of conversational speech-recognition data (Ganapathiraju & Picone, 2000).

Hybrid approaches for speech recognition (Bourlard & Morgan, 1994) provide a flexible paradigm to evaluate new acoustic-modeling techniques such as SVMs. These systems do not entirely eliminate the HMM framework because traditional classification models such as SVMs do not inherently model the temporal structure of speech. Sequence kernels, discussed extensively in Chapter XII, are an emerging technique that overcomes these types of limitations. The process by which we estimate parameters of the models and optimize the number of support vectors for large amounts of acoustic training data is described extensively in Ganapathiraju (2002). In integrating SVMs into more traditional hybrid system approaches, several issues arise: posterior estimation, classifier design, segmental modeling, and N-best rescoring.

The first major concern in using SVMs for speech recognition is the lack of a clear relationship between distance from the margin and the posterior class probability. While newer classifiers have been developed that are more suited to Bayesian classification (Hamaker, Picone, & Ganapathiraju, 2002), for SVMs, unmoderated probability estimates based on ML fitting (Platt, 1999) represent an effective trade-off between computational complexity and error performance. A sigmoid distribution is used to map the output distances to posteriors:

$$p(y = 1 \mid f) = \frac{1}{1 + \exp(Af + B)}, \tag{16}$$

where the parameters A and B can be estimated using a model-trust minimization algorithm (Platt, 1999). In order to avoid biased estimates, a cross-validation set must be used to estimate the parameters of the sigmoid (Ganapathiraju, 2002).

The second major issue relates to classifier design. Frame-level classification in speech recognition has not proven to be a promising approach. The baseline HMM system described here uses an inventory of 8,000 context-dependent phone models to describe the most likely sequences of three consecutive phones. Each phone model uses three states to represent its corresponding sound, arranged in a simple left-to-right topology. Hence, there are approximately 24,000 states in the acoustic models, and it is not practical to train discriminative classifiers for so many states. Instead, for computational efficiency, one-vs.-all classifiers are trained for each phone model, and these classifiers model posteriors for phones rather than states or frames.

A third major issue involves segmental modeling. The acoustic model needs to capture both the temporal and spectral structure of speech that is clearly missing in frame-level classification schemes. HMMs elegantly model such structure using a finite-state machine. Phone durations vary, and learning such duration information is a critical part of the acoustic-modeling problem. Segment durations are correlated with the word choice and speaking rate, but are difficult to exploit in an SVM-type framework. A simple but effective approach motivated by the three-state HMMs used in most systems is to assume that the segments (phones in most cases) are composed of a fixed number of sections. The first and third sections model

Figure 5. A composite feature vector for SVM-based speech recognition

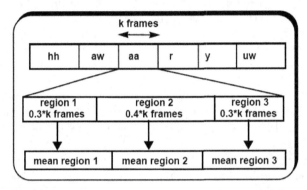

Figure 6. A hybrid SVM/HMM system based on a rescoring paradigm

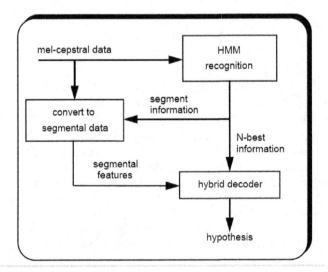

the transition into and out of the segment, while the second section models the stable portion of the segment. Segments composed of three sections are used in all experiments described below. The segment vector is then augmented with the logarithm of the duration of the phone to explicitly model the variability in duration. Figure 5 demonstrates the construction of a composite vector for a phone segment.

A fourth issue relates to the decoding paradigm used in the hybrid system. Though it is highly desirable to embed the SVM classifier within the supervised training process used in HMMs, computationally efficient means for doing this remain elusive. A more standard approach for integrating such classifiers is to use an N-best rescoring paradigm. A conventional HMM system is used to generate a list of sentence hypotheses that includes underlying phone alignments. Segment-level feature vectors are generated from these alignments. These segments are then classified using the SVMs. Posterior probabilities, computed using the sigmoid approximation previously discussed, are then used to compute the utterance likelihood of each hypothesis in the N-best list. The N-best list is reordered based on the likelihood, and the top hypothesis is used to calibrate the performance of the system. An overview of the resulting hybrid system is shown in Figure 6.

Experiments on Conversational Speech

The hybrid SVM-HMM architecture previously described[1] has been extensively analyzed using two relatively simple baselines: the Deterding vowel-recognition task (Deterding, 2000) and the Oregon Graduate Institute (OGI) Alphadigit corpus (Cole, 1997). On the first task, SVMs were shown to outperform many standard classifiers (Ganapathiraju, 2002). On the second task, a radial basis function kernel was shown to provide slightly better performance than a polynomial kernel. An SVM-HMM hybrid system was also shown to provide approximately a 10% decrease in WER over a comparable HMM system. A summary of WERs by the class of sound is shown in Table 2. These word classes have been found to comprise the major error modalities for the data set. These subsets are particularly challenging because they are phonetically very close and can only be disambiguated by the acoustic model since there are no higher level language-modeling constraints applied in this task.

SVMs have also shown encouraging results on a conversational speech task, SWITCHBOARD (SWB; Godfrey, Holliman & McDaniel, 1992). The training set consists of 114,441 utterances while the development test set consists of 2,427 utterances. These utterances have an average length of six words and an average duration of 2 seconds. The test-set vocabulary is approximately 22,000 words while the training-set vocabulary has over 80,000 words. A 42-phone set was used for this task. The baseline HMM system was trained on 60 hours of data from 2,998 conversation sides. The input features were MFCCs that had been normalized to have a zero mean and unit variance. Twelve mixture components per state were used. This baseline system has a WER of 41.6% on the development test set.

The experiments on this task are summarized in Table 3. For this task, 10-best lists with a list error rate of 29.5% were used for all experiments. Segmentations derived from the corresponding HMM hypothesis were used to rescore the N-best list with the SVM classifier. This hybrid approach did improve performance over the baseline, albeit only marginally: a WER of 40.6% compared to a baseline of 41.6%.

Table 2. Comparison of performance of the HMM and SVM systems as a function of word classes for the OGI Alphadigits task.

Data Class	HMM (%WER)	SVM (%WER)	HMM+SVM (%WER)
a-set	13.5	11.5	11.1
e-set	23.1	22.4	20.6
digit	5.1	6.4	4.7
alphabets	15.1	14.3	13.3
nasals	12.1	12.9	12.0
plosives	22.6	21.0	18.9
Overall	**11.9**	**11.8**	**10.6**

Table 3. Summary of recognition experiments using the baseline HMM system and the hybrid system on the Switchboard (SWB) and Alphadigits (AD) tasks.

S. No.	Information Source		HMM		Hybrid	
	Transcription	Segmentation	AD	SWB	AD	SWB
1	N-best	Hypothesis	11.9	41.6	11.0	40.6
2	N-best	N-best	12.0	42.3	11.8	42.1
3	N-best + Ref.	Reference	---	---	3.3	5.8
4	N-best + Ref.	N-best + Ref.	11.9	38.6	9.1	38.1

The use of oracle segmentations and transcriptions in the hybrid system was then explored to gain further insight into the drawbacks of the rescoring paradigm. On the Alphadigits task, using the reference segmentations improved performance of the hybrid system from 11.0% to 7.0% WER (compared to a baseline of 11.9% WER). On the SWB task, the reference segmentation improved the performance of the system from 40.6% to 36.1%. This demonstrates that the mismatch between the HMM segmentations, which are derived using ML training, and the SVM system, trained using a maximum margin classifier, is a source of degradation in performance.

Another set of experiments was conducted to determine the effect of the richness of N-best lists on the performance of the hybrid system. The N-best list error rate was artificially reduced to 0% by adding the reference to the original 10-best lists. Rescoring these new N-best lists using the corresponding segmentations resulted in error rates of 9.1% WER and 38.1%

on Alphadigits and SWB, respectively. This improvement corresponds to a 30% relative improvement in performance on the Alphadigits task. On this task, the HMM system did not improve performance over the baseline even when the reference (or correct) transcription is added to the N-best list.

This result indicated that SVMs are superior to HMMs when they are exposed to accurate segmentations. Unfortunately, the current hybrid approach does not allow the SVM to be trained in a way in which it is exposed to alternate segmentations. Hence, the SVM does not learn to discriminate between alternate segmentations. We hypothesize that this is the reason that introduction of the correct segmentation has such a big impact on performance for the SVM.

Another set of experiments were run to quantify the absolute ceiling in performance improvements the SVM hybrid system can provide. This ceiling can be achieved when we use the hybrid system to rescore the N-best lists that include the reference transcription using the reference-based segmentation. Using this approach, the system gave a WER of 3.3% on the Alphadigits task, and 5.8% on SWB. This huge improvement should not be mistaken for a real improvement for two reasons. First, we cannot guarantee that the reference segmentation is available at all times. Second, generating N-best lists with 0% WER is extremely difficult, if not impossible, for conversational speech. This improvement should rather be viewed as a proof of concept that by using good segmentations to rescore good N-best lists, the hybrid system has a potential to improve performance significantly.

Impact on Language Modeling

Recall from equation (6) that the goal of a language model is to predict the probability of a word sequence, $P(W)$. Methods for computing this quantity have been studied extensively over the years, and ranged from complex, probabilistic finite-state machines (Levinson, 1985) to N-gram analysis (Brown, Della Pietra, de Souza, Lai, & Mercer, 1992). N-gram analysis has proven to be remarkably effective over the years because of its simple formulation and powerful computational properties. In an N-gram approach, the probability of a word is decomposed into a product of its predecessors:

$$P(W) = P(w_1, w_2, ..., w_r)$$
$$= \prod_{k=1}^{n} P(w_1) P(w_2|w_1) P(w_3|w_2, w_1) ... P(w_r|(w_1, w_2, ... w_{r-1}). \tag{17}$$

N-grams orders of three, referred to as a trigram, are commonly used in the first pass of a complex speech-recognition system. Often, longer span models are then applied selectively to improve performance on difficult phrases. Effective ways of encoding the word histories in equation (17) becomes a critical part of the language-modeling problem since there are vast numbers of trigrams possible for a given language.

There are two main drawbacks to the N-gram approach. First, even when trained on large amounts of data, the trigram representation can be sparse and consist of many poorly approximated probabilities. Smoothing techniques based on information theory have been extensively explored to deal with this problem (Jelinek, 1998). Second, these N-grams can become very domain specific and prove difficult to abstract. The ability to predict new phrases is limited when those phrases do not appear in the training data. Many techniques have been explored to improve the generalization ability of the N-gram model (e.g., class-based N-grams). However, the essential problem bears striking similarity to the other problems we have discussed: controlling generalization in a high-dimensional space that is sparsely populated by training data. A computational model that allows mixtures of diverse types of information about word sequences (e.g., semantic tags) to be integrated into a single probabilistic framework and can produce plausible approximations for N-grams previously unseen in the training data is required.

In recent years, the classic probabilistic finite-state machine has been replaced by a neural-network-based language model. In such models, words are represented by points in a continuous multidimensional feature space, and the probability of a sequence of words is computed by means of a neural network. The feature vectors of the preceding words make up the input to the neural network, which then will produce a probability distribution over a given vocabulary (Menchetti, Costa, Frasconi, & Massimiliano, in press).

The fundamental idea behind this model is to simplify the estimation task by mapping words from the high-dimensional discrete space to a low-dimensional continuous one where probability distributions are smooth functions. This is somewhat the reverse of the feature-extraction problem, in which we mapped features from a low-dimensional space to a high-dimensional space. The network achieves generalization by assigning to an unseen word sequence a probability close to a word string seen in the training data. Of course, the main challenge here is whether the network can learn semantically meaningful distances. An added benefit is that the neural network approach is computationally simple and fast, as well as being amenable to parallel processing.

Kernel methods offer similar advantages over neural networks for language-modeling problems as they did for feature extraction and acoustic modeling. Kernel-based algorithms are easier to train because they minimize a convex functional, thus avoiding the difficult problem of dealing with local minima. However, a kernel function usually needs to be adapted to the problem at hand, and learning the kernel function is still an open problem. This is particularly true in the case of the discrete space encountered in the language-modeling problem.

Application of such methods to the language-modeling problem is still a relatively new area of research. Initial experiments with neural network approaches have shown promise. Emami & Jelinek (in press) have shown modest decreases in language model perplexity and recognition error rates on tasks such as the *Wall Street Journal* corpus using a combination of a structured language model and neural network model for probability computation.

Summary

Kernel-based methods are having profound impact on speech processing in general as this research area increasingly embraces machine learning research. Applications of kernel methods are not strictly limited to speech. The use of kernel machines in computational biology was discussed extensively in Chapter III. In Chapter XII, the use of these machines for other speech problems, specifically, speaker verification, is discussed. We did not elaborate on applications of these techniques to diverse problems such as language identification or speaker adaptation.

The speech problem poses some unique challenges for such techniques, however. Though mature approaches such as SVMs have been shown to provide significant improvements in performance on a variety of tasks, there are two serious drawbacks that hamper their effectiveness in speech recognition. First, though sparse, the size of the SVM models (number of nonzero weights) tends to scale linearly with the quantity of training data. For a large speaker-independent corpus such as SWB, this effect causes the model complexity to become prohibitive. Techniques have been developed to overcome these problems, but they typically involve approximations that can only attempt to ensure that the location of the model on the error surface remains reasonably close to optimal. It is much more preferable to examine methods where this sparse optimization is explicit in the training of the model.

Second, SVMs are fundamentally binary classifiers that are only capable of producing a yes-no decision. In speech recognition, this is an important disadvantage since there is significant overlap in the feature space that cannot be modeled by a yes-no decision boundary. Further, the combination of disparate knowledge sources (such as linguistic models, pronunciation models, acoustic models, etc.) requires a method for combining the scores produced by each model so that alternate hypotheses can be compared. Thus, we require a probabilistic classification that reflects the amount of uncertainty in our predictions. Efforts have been made to build posterior probability estimates from the SVM models by mapping the SVM distances to a sigmoid function. While this does build a posterior estimate, Tipping (2001) argues quite effectively that the sigmoid estimate is unreliable and that it tends to overestimate the model's confidence in its predictions.

A promising new area of research is a learning machine that introduces a Bayesian approach into the vector machine concept. MacKay (1995) incorporates an automatic relevance determination (ARD) over each model parameter. This tends to force most of the parameters to zero, leading to a sparse model representation. A kernel-based learning technique termed the relevance vector machine (RVM) is an application of ARD methods. Hamaker et al. (2002) have shown this is a promising technique that provides comparable performance to SVMs, but generates much fewer parameters. ARD techniques are recently being explored in conjunction with many of the learning machines previously introduced (Van Gestel, Suykens, De Moor, & Vandewalle, 2001).

Finally, what tends to be lacking in all these approaches is a tightly integrated closed-loop paradigm for training the parameters of these kernel machines within the supervised learning framework of a speech-recognition system. MLE methods excel in speech recognition because of the supervised learning paradigm. Despite the strong fundamental structure of the classifier, the data input into a speech-recognition system is becoming increasingly imperfect as research systems strive to process tens of thousands of hours of speech data. The MLE process forces models to reorganize information as necessary to reach some sort of optimal state. This process is robust to imperfect data, model topologies, and so forth, and delivers surprisingly good performance on training data with high error rates (Sundaram, 2003). Techniques that combine the robustness and computational efficiency of MLE-based supervised learning with the ability to maintain good generalization will continue to be an active area of research over the next 10 years.

Note that many of the algorithms, software, and recognition systems described in this work are available at http://www.cavs.msstate.edu/hse/ies/projects/speech.

References

Bach, F., & Jordan, M. (2003). Kernel independent component analysis. *Journal of Machine Learning, 3*, 1-48.

Bell, A. J., & Sejnowski, T. J. (1995). An information maximisation approach to blind separation and blind deconvolution. *Neural Computation, 7*(6), 1129-1159.

Bengio, Y., Ducharme, R., & Vincent, P. (2001). A neural probabilistic language model. *Advances in Neural Information Processing Systems*, 932-938.

Bocchieri, E., & Doddington, G. (1986). Frame-specific statistical features for speaker independent speech recognition. *IEEE Transactions on Acoustics, Speech, and Signal Processing, 34*(4), 755-764.

Boscolo, R., Pan, H., & Roychowdhury, V. (2004). Independent density analysis based on nonparametric density estimation, *IEEE transactions on Neural Networks, 15*(1), 55-65.

Bourlard, H. A., & Morgan, N. (1994). *Connectionist speech recognition: A hybrid approach.* Boston: Kluwer Academic Publishers.

Brown, P. (1987). *The acoustic modeling problem in automatic speech recognition.* Unpublished doctoral dissertation, Carnegie Mellon University, Pittsburgh, PA.

Brown, P. F., Della Pietra, V. J., de Souza, P. V., Lai, J. C., & Mercer, R. L. (1992). Class-based n-gram models of natural language. *Computational Linguistics, 18*(4), 467-479.

Cole, R. (1997). *Alphadigit corpus.* Center for Spoken Language Understanding, Oregon Graduate Institute. Retrieved from http://.cse.ogi.edu/CSLU/corpora/alphadigit

Deshmukh, N., Ganapathiraju, A., & Picone, J. (1999). Hierarchical search for large vocabulary conversational speech recognition. *IEEE Signal Processing Magazine, 16*(5), 84-107.

Deterding, D. (2000). *Vowel recognition.* Retrieved from http://.ics.uci.edu/pub/machine-learning-databases/undocumented/connectionist-bench/vowel/

Emami, A., & Jelinek, F. (in press). A neural syntactic language model. *Journal of Machine Learning.*

Fukunaga, K. (1990). *Introduction to statistical pattern recognition.* New York: Academic Press.

Ganapathiraju, A. (2002). *Support vector machines for speech recognition.* Unpublished doctoral dissertation, Mississippi State University.

Ganapathiraju, A., Hamaker, J., & Picone, J. (2004). Applications of support vector machines to speech recognition. *IEEE Transactions on Signal Processing, 52*(8), 2348-2355.

Ganapathiraju, A., & Picone, J. (2000). Support vector machines for automatic data cleanup. In *Proceedings of the International Conference of Spoken Language Processing* (pp. 210-213).

Godfrey, J., Holliman, E., & McDaniel, J. (1992). SWITCHBOARD: Telephone speech corpus for research and development. *International Conference on Acoustics, Speech and Signal Processing, 1*, 517-520.

Hamaker, J., Picone, J., & Ganapathiraju, A. (2002). A sparse modeling approach to speech recognition based on relevance vector machines. *International Conference of Spoken Language Processing* (pp. 1001-1004).

Hansen, J.H.L. (ed.) (1994). Special Issue on Robust Recognition, *IEEE Transactions on Speech & Audio Processing, 2*(4).

Jelinek, F. (1998). *Statistical methods for speech recognition*. Boston: MIT Press.

Jurafsky, D., & Martin, J. H. (2000). *Speech and language processing: An introduction to natural language processing, computational linguistics, and speech recognition.* Englewood Cliffs, NJ: Prentice-Hall.

Kumar, N., & Andreou, A. G. (1998). Heteroscedastic discriminant analysis and reduced rank HMMs for improved speech recognition. *Speech Communication, 26*, 283-297.

Levinson, S. E. (1985). Structural methods in automatic speech recognition. *IEEE Proceedings, 73*(11), 1625-1650.

Lima, A., Zen, H., Nankaku, C., Tokuda, K., Kitamura, T. & Resende, F. G. (2005). Sparse KPCA for feature extraction in speech recognition. *International Conference on Acoustics, Speech and Signal Processing* (pp. 353-356).

Lima, A., Zen, H., Nankaku, Y., Miyajima, C., Tokuda, K., & Kitamura, T. (2003). On the use of kernel PCA for feature extraction in speech recognition. *European Conference on Speech Communication and Technology* (pp. 2625-2628).

Lu, C., Zhang, T., Du, X., & Li, C. (2004). Robust kernel PCA algorithm. *International Conference on Machine Learning and Cybernetics* (pp. 3084-3087).

MacKay, D. J. C. (1995). Probable networks and plausible predictions: A review of practical Bayesian methods for supervised neural networks. *Network: Computation in Neural Systems, 6*, 469-505.

Maybury, M. (Ed.). (2005). *New directions in question answering.* Menlo Park, CA: AAAI Press.

McDermott, E. (1997). *Discriminative training for speech recognition.* Unpublished doctoral dissertation, Waseda University, Japan.

Menchetti, S., Costa, F., Frasconi, P., & Massimiliano, P. (in press). Wide coverage natural language processing using kernel methods and neural networks for structured data. *Pattern Recognition Letters.*

Mohri, M. (1997). Finite-state transducers in language and speech processing. *Computational Linguistics, 23*(2), 269-311.

Odell, J. J. (1995). *The use of context in large vocabulary speech recognition.* Unpublished doctoral dissertation, University of Cambridge, UK.

Picone, J. (1993). Signal modeling techniques in speech recognition. *IEEE Proceedings, 81*(9), 1215-1247.

Platt, J. (1999). Probabilistic outputs for support vector machines and comparisons to regularized likelihood methods. In *Advances in large margin classifiers,* (pp.61-74). Cambridge, MA: MIT Press.

Rabiner, L. R., & Juang, B. H. (1993). *Fundamentals of speech recognition.* Englewood Cliffs, NJ: Prentice Hall.

Schölkopf, B., & Smola, A. J. (2002). *Learning with kernels.* Cambridge: MIT Press.

Schölkopf, B., Mika, S., Burges, C., Knirsch, P., Müller, K.-R., Rätsch, G., et al. (1999). Input space vs. feature space in kernel-based methods. *IEEE Transactions on Neural Networks, 10,* 1000-1017.

Shawe-Taylor, J., & Cristianini, N. (2002). On the generalization of soft margin algorithms. *IEEE Transactions on Information Theory, 48*(10), 2721-2735.

Sundaram, R. (2003). *Effects of transcription errors on supervised learning in speech recognition.* Unpublished master's thesis, Mississippi State University.

Tipping, M. (2001). Sparse Bayesian learning and the relevance vector machine. *Journal of Machine Learning, 1,* 211-244.

Valtchev, V. (1995). *Discriminative methods in HMM-based speech recognition.* Unpublished doctoral dissertation, University of Cambridge, UK.

Valtchev, V., Odell, J. J., Woodland, P. C., & Young, S. J. (1997). MMIE training of large vocabulary speech recognition systems. *Speech Communication, 22,* 303-314.

Van Gestel, Suykens, A. K., De Moor, B., & Vandewalle, J. (2001). Automatic relevance determination for least squares support vector machine regression. *International Joint Conference on Neural Networks* (pp. 2416-2421).

Vertanen, K. (2004). *An overview of discriminative training for speech recognition.* Cambridge, UK: University of Cambridge.

Wan, V., & Campbell, W. M. (2000). *Support vector machines for speaker verification and identification.* Proceedings of the IEEE International Workshop on Neural Networks for Signal Processing, Sydney, Australia.

Wan, V., & Renals, S. (2005). Speaker verification using sequence discriminant support vector machines. *IEEE Transactions on Speech and Audio Processing, 13*(2), 203-210.

Woodland, P., & Povey, D. (2000). *Very large scale MMIE training for conversational telephone speech recognition.* Proceedings of the NIST Speech Transcription Workshop, College Park, MD.

Young, S. J. (2005). *HTK: Hidden Markov model toolkit V3.3.* Cambridge, UK: Cambridge University.

Zweig, G., Saon, G., & Yvon, F. (2002). Arc minimization in finite state decoding graphs with cross-word acoustic context. *International Conference on Spoken Language Processing* (pp. 389-392).

Endnote

[1]   Note that traditional MFCC features were used for all experiments described in this section.

Chapter X

Building Sequence Kernels for Speaker Verification and Word Recognition

Vincent Wan, University of Sheffield, UK

Abstract

This chapter describes the adaptation and application of kernel methods for speech processing. It is divided into two sections dealing with speaker verification and isolated-word speech recognition applications. Significant advances in kernel methods have been realised in the field of speaker verification, particularly relating to the direct scoring of variable-length speech utterances by sequence kernel SVMs. The improvements are so substantial that most state-of-the-art speaker recognition systems now incorporate SVMs. We describe the architecture of some of these sequence kernels. Speech recognition presents additional challenges to kernel methods and their application in this area is not as straightforward as for speaker verification. We describe a sequence kernel that uses dynamic time warping to capture temporal information within the kernel directly. The formulation also extends the standard dynamic time-warping algorithm by enabling the dynamic alignment to be computed in a high-dimensional space induced by a kernel function. This kernel is shown to work well in an application for recognising low-intelligibility speech of severely dysarthric individuals.

Introduction

In recent years, support vector machines (SVMs) have become an important tool in speaker verification and speech recognition. This chapter describes the development of sequence kernels in these domains. The following paragraphs introduce the speaker verification techniques established prior to the advent of sequence kernels. We then assess the impact of sequence kernels in speaker and speech recognition.

In text-independent speaker verification, the aim is to determine from a sample of speech whether a person's asserted identity is true or false; this constitutes a binary classification task well suited to SVM discriminative training and generalisation. The robust classification of speech signals of variable duration comprises one of the principal challenges in this area. Classifiers such as *multilayer perceptrons*, *Gaussian mixture models* (GMMs), and *vector quantisers* do not process variable-length sequences directly. Traditionally, speaker verification applications depended on modeling the distribution of cepstral input vectors (e.g., mel frequency cepstral coefficients) using GMMs; variable-length sequence scoring was achieved by computing the average log likelihood score of the input vectors over the length of the test utterance.

The GMM (see Bishop, 1995) is a well-known modeling technique that was applied to speaker verification by Reynolds (1992). Let $f(x_A)$ denote the score for an utterance of speech x_A that is represented as a sequence of L frames $x_A = \{x_{A1}, \dots, x_{AL}\}$ where x_{Ai} is a vector of cepstral features and A enumerates the utterances. In speaker verification, each frame x_{Ai} is scored separately by the GMM of the asserted speaker, and the utterance score is the mean of the frame log likelihood scores:

$$f(x_A) = \frac{1}{L} \sum_{i=1}^{L} \log P(x_{Ai} \mid M_{ml}),\qquad(1)$$

where M_{ml} is the model of the asserted speaker created using the maximum likelihood criterion. If $f(x_A)$ is greater than a predetermined threshold, then the speaker's asserted identity is confirmed. An improvement on this approach incorporates a (Gaussian mixture) universal background model (UBM), U, which is trained on a large number of speakers. The improved scores are the ratio of the speaker model's likelihood to the UBM's likelihood:

$$f(x_A) = \frac{1}{L} \sum_{i=1}^{L} \log P(x_{Ai} \mid M_{ml}) - \log P(x_{Ai} \mid U).\qquad(2)$$

A further refinement replaces M_{ml} with a better model M_{ad} created by adapting U to the speaker using Maximum a Posteriori Probability (MAP) adaptation (Reynolds, 1995):

$$f(x_A) = \frac{1}{L} \sum_{i=1}^{L} \log P(x_{Ai} \mid M_{ad}) - \log P(x_{Ai} \mid U).\qquad(3)$$

Early SVM approaches by Schmidt and Gish (1996) and then by Wan and Campbell (2000) replaced the GMM estimate of the log likelihood in equation (1) with the raw output of polynomial and Radial Basis Function (RBF) kernel SVMs. The success of this approach, however, was limited since it proved difficult to train SVMs on a large set of cepstral input vectors: Using all available data resulted in optimisation problems requiring significant computational resources that were unsustainable. Employing clustering algorithms to reduce the data also, unfortunately, reduced the accuracy. Furthermore, this type of training ignores the concept of an utterance: This is important since discriminative training may discard information that is not considered useful for classification, thus training discriminatively on the (frame-level) input vectors may inadvertently discard information that could prove useful for classifying the sequence.

The solution was to map each complete utterance onto one point in the *feature space* using sequence kernels (Campbell, 2002; Fine, Navratil, & Gopinath, 2001; Wan & Renals, 2002) described in the next section. They enable SVMs to classify variable-length sequences directly, simultaneously incorporating the notion of an utterance, enabling sequence-level discrimination, and effectively reducing the number of input vectors (now sequence-level input vectors) by several orders of magnitude compared to the frame-level approach. Sequence kernels have been so effective in reducing error rates that they are now incorporated into many state-of-the-art speaker verification systems.

Other recent advances in kernel methods for speaker verification include Shriberg, Ferrer, Kajarekar, Venkataraman, and Stolcke (2005) and Campbell, Campbell et al. (2004) for processing high-level stylistic or lexical features. Those approaches include the adaptation of word and *n*-gram vector space kernels that were developed for document classification (Dumais, Platt, Heckerman, & Sahami, 1998). However, we limit this chapter to the description of sequence kernels and to their application to low-level acoustic features, even though sequence kernels have also been applied to high-level features.

There have been many attempts to apply SVMs and its principles to improve existing speech recognition engines. Research in this domain has been quite extensive, thus mention is made of only a small number of such approaches to give the reader an appreciation of recent developments in the field. The approach described in Chapter IX and by Ganapathiraju (2002) uses SVMs to estimate HMM (hidden Markov model) state likelihoods instead of GMMs in a manner similar to hybrid speech recognition (Bourlard & Morgan, 1994). Venkataramani, Chakrabartty, and Byrne (2003) applied SVMs to refine the decoding search space; Gales and Layton (2004) use SVMs to train augmented statistical models for large-vocabulary continuous speech recognition.

Later in this chapter, we extend the use of sequence kernels to isolated-word speech recognition. Smith, Gales, and Naranjan (2001) first applied sequence kernels to speech recognition by exploiting HMMs in much the same way that GMMs were exploited for speaker verification. In the section devoted to speech recognition, we describe a sequence kernel based on dynamic time warping (DTW) for the recognition of isolated-word dysarthric speech in a command and control application for disabled people. We also outline how the same formulation can extend the standard dynamic time-warping algorithm by enabling the dynamic alignment to be computed in a high-dimensional space induced by a kernel function.

Sequence Kernels

A sequence kernel is a function that operates on two sequences and computes their inner product even if these sequences have different durations. They enable SVMs to perform discriminative scoring at the sequence level directly. This contrasts with traditional approaches where sequences are divided into frames and the discrimination is applied only at frame level, potentially resulting in the loss of information useful for sequence-level classification. The SVM's advantage lies in the ability to derive a kernel that can correctly process vector sequences of unequal length.

There has been a significant amount of research on sequence kernels, particularly in the field of bioengineering (Chapter III) where the Fisher kernel (Jaakkola & Haussler, 1999) and dynamic alignment or pair HMM kernel (Watkins, 1999) were first applied. Other examples of sequence kernels include generalised linear discriminant sequence (GLDS) kernels (Campbell, 2002) and score-space kernels (Smith et al., 2001).

Fisher, score-space, and GLDS kernels are closely related: They each define a function φ such that $\varphi(x_A)$ is a column vector (in feature space) with fixed dimensionality N irrespective of the utterance length L, where N is greater than one. The corresponding kernels are derived by computing the inner product:

$$\kappa\,(x_A, x_B) = \varphi(x_A)\Gamma\varphi(x_B)^T,$$

(4)

which will always satisfy Mercer's condition (Chapter I and Vapnik, 1998). The matrix Γ is defined by the metric of the feature space induced by φ and is the inverse Fisher information matrix. It may be estimated by the inverse covariance matrix of the set $\{\varphi(x_A)$ for all $A\}$. However, since the feature space dimensionality may be arbitrarily large, a full covariance matrix may be impractical to invert. Diagonal approximations of the covariance matrix are often used to improve efficiency. An equivalent solution is to set Γ to be the identity matrix and instead normalise the feature space vectors to have zero mean and unit diagonal covariance. In the context of SVM processing, it is important to normalise the vector components because SVM solutions are not invariant to affine transformations in the feature space: The decision boundaries obtained both with and without applying an affine transformation to the feature vectors cannot usually be mapped to each other by the same transformation.

In principle, the function φ may be chosen arbitrarily, provided the feature space dimensionality is fixed. One possible solution is to construct the feature vector using a set of N equations, each yielding a scalar. However, it is more meaningful to define the mapping using a less arbitrary approach. We first describe polynomial sequence kernels, then the Fisher and score-space sequence kernels that are derived from GMMs.

Polynomial Sequence Kernels

The approach adopted by Campbell (2002) is simple and efficient, and has yielded good results in the annual National Institute of Standards and Technology (NIST) speaker recognition evaluations (Doddington, Przybocki, Martin, & Reynolds, 2000). It uses an explicit polynomial expansion involving the terms of a pth order polynomial expansion:

$$\varphi(x_A) = \frac{1}{L}\sum_{i=1}^{L}[x_{Ai,1},...,x_{Ai,n},x_{Ai,1}x_{Ai,2},...,x_{Ai,1}x_{Ai,n},...],\tag{5}$$

where $x_{Ai,j}$ is the jth component of the vector x_{Ai}. This expansion is analogous to the standard polynomial kernel and can be derived by expanding the terms in $(1+\langle x_{Ai},x_{Bi}\rangle)^p$. The advantage of an explicit expansion is that it enables some terms to be removed, which is known to improve the accuracy of the resulting classifier (Campbell, Reynolds, & Campbell, 2004). It also enables the summation over the different lengths of x_A and x_B and the estimation of Γ, which is not possible when the explicit mapping is unknown. Note that equation (5) also requires the normalisation of the individual cepstral vectors, x_{Ai}, to zero mean and unit diagonal covariance, otherwise a bias toward cepstral coefficients with greater absolute magnitudes and variances may be introduced.

Interestingly, there is a close relationship between the binomial expansion and a Gaussian process. If the likelihood in equation (1) is modeled by a normal distribution, parameterised by mean μ and full covariance matrix Σ, then the utterance score is:

$$f(x_A) = \frac{1}{L}\sum_{i=1}^{L}-\frac{1}{2}(x_{Ai}-\mu)^T\Sigma^{-1}(x_{Ai}-\mu)+b,\tag{6}$$

where b is a constant from the normalisation factor of the normal distribution. Expanding the right-hand side of equation (6) allows it to be written as an inner product of two vectors:

$$f(x_A) = \langle\varphi_{p=2}(x_A), w\rangle + b.\tag{7}$$

The first vector, $\varphi_{p=2}(x_A)$, is an explicit binomial expansion defined by equation (5) augmented with a bias. The second vector, w, is a parameter vector dependent upon μ and Σ. Thus, in the special case of a binomial sequence kernel, the SVM's utterance score formula is effectively identical to that obtained using the log likelihood of a normal distribution. The difference between the two methods lies in the way that parameters are estimated.

Fisher and Score-Space Kernels

Score-space kernels were introduced by Smith et al. (2001) and generalises Jaakkola and Haussler's Fisher kernel (1999). The Fisher kernel was applied to speaker verification by Fine et al. (2001) and score-space kernels by Wan and Renals (2002). In these kernels, each component of the feature vector is a derivative of a function, such as equations (1) to (3), with respect to one of the models' parameters:

$$\varphi(x_A) = \nabla f(x_A).\tag{8}$$

The likelihoods in equations (1) to (3) are estimated using the GMMs of a traditional system so the gradients in equation (8) are computed with respect to the parameters of the GMMs M_{ml}, M_{ad}, and U. Substituting f in equation (8) with equation (1) results in the Fisher kernel (Jaakkola & Haussler, 1999). Substituting equations (2) and (3) results in special cases of score-space kernels that are equivalent to the concatenation of the feature spaces of the two Fisher kernels obtained using each GMM separately (Wan & Renals, 2005). In fact, any combination of Fisher kernels derived from M_{ml}, M_{ad}, and U may be used as kernels. The equations for computing these derivatives and full details of the score-space kernel implementation are presented in Wan and Renals (2005).

A Speaker Verification Example

The sequence kernels described have been shown to work well for speaker verification by improving the traditional GMM approaches. In terms of complexity, the score-space sequence kernel is not as simple to implement as its polynomial counterpart. It is computationally more demanding and its solutions occupy more memory because it is dependent upon a set of GMMs. The principal advantage of the score-space approach, however, is its ability to exploit a UBM trainable on a much larger collection of speakers than the SVM could process directly. This indirect access to a bigger speaker corpus could potentially lead to greater accuracy.

As mentioned previously, SVMs already feature prominently in many state-of-the-art speaker recognition systems tested in the annual NIST speaker recognition evaluations. To provide a simple demonstration of these kernels, we choose the (relatively) small PolyVar database (Chollet, Cochard, Constantinescu, Jaboulet, & Langlais, 1996), which has well-defined training and testing sets for 38 client speakers and an additional 952 utterances from impostor speakers.

The speech was encoded as 12th-order perceptual linear prediction (PLP) cepstral coefficients, computed using a 32-ms window and a 10-ms frame shift. The 12 cepstral coefficients were augmented with an energy term, and first and second derivatives were estimated, resulting in vectors of 39 dimensions. Silence frames within each utterance were removed using an automatic detector.

Two baseline systems based on the traditional GMM approaches were used. The first, labeled GMM (M_{ml}/U), employs 400-component GMM client models trained using maximum likelihood (M_{ml}) and a 1,000-component UBM (U) trained using maximum likelihood on the 952 impostor utterances. The second, labeled GMM (M_{ad}/U), replaces M_{ml} in the first baseline with M_{ad}, a client model MAP adapted from U using the formulation by Mariéthoz and Bengio (2001) for updating the Gaussian means (a single iteration of adaptation was used with an update factor of 0.05).

The polynomial sequence kernel used the monomial terms of a third-order polynomial expansion to map each utterance to a feature space of 9,880 dimensions. The score-space sequence kernel used the three GMMs (M_{ml}, M_{ad}, and U) to map to a feature space of 149,600 dimensions. Linear SVMs were trained on 85 client utterances and 952 impostor utterances, and tested on data not used during training (which resulted in 36,186 individual tests in total).

Table 1. Equal error rates of the classifiers and their fusion

Classifiers	EER (%)	Min HTER (%)
GMM (M_{ml}/U)	6.4	5.8
GMM (M_{ad}/U)	3.9	3.5
Polynomial sequence kernel SVM	4.0	3.7
Score-space (M_{ml}, M_{ad}, U) kernel SVM	3.6	3.3
Fusion of GMM (M_{ad}/U) with polynomial	3.5	3.2
Fusion of GMM (M_{ad}/U) with score-space	3.4	3.1
Fusion of GMM (M_{ad}/U) with polynomial & score-space	3.3	3.0

Figure 1. The detection error trade-off curve for GMMs and sequence kernel SVMs on the PolyVar database. The score fusion curve is the T-norm combination of the GMM (M_{ad}/U) with the polynomial and score-space SVMs.

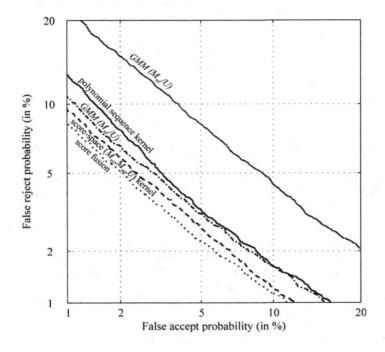

Since the dimensionality of the feature spaces exceed the number of training utterances, the linearly separable formulation of the SVM may be used. The polynomial sequence kernel SVMs typically contained around 200 support vectors while the score-space kernel approach yielded solutions with over 1,000 support vectors. However, since the feature space expansion is explicit and a linear SVM is used, the solution can be simplified by computing the resultant decision boundary from the weighted sum of the support vectors.

Figure 1 shows a detection error trade-off curve (Martin, Doddington, Kamm, Ordowski, & Przybocki, 1997), which is a receiver operating curve with a nonlinear scale. The equal error rate, or EER (defined as the error rate when the false accept probability is equal to the false reject probability), and minimum half total error rate, or HTER (defined as the minimum value of the false accept probability plus the false reject probability), results are tabulated in Table 1. The graph shows that the individual SVM results are close to the GMM (M_{ad}/U) baseline system and better than the GMM (M_{ml}/U) baseline. On this particular data set, the polynomial sequence kernel has a slightly lower accuracy than the GMM (M_{ad}/U) system while the score-space kernel has a slightly better accuracy. However, this ranking may change if a different database is used. Specifically, the score-space (M_{ml}, M_{ad}, U) kernel was developed on PolyVar, so any attempt to draw definitive conclusions from these results would be premature as further testing on another data set is necessary.

Further gains may be achieved by fusing the scores of the classifiers. This is achieved by normalising each classifier so that the output scores of a set of unseen impostor speakers have common mean and variance. The scores for each utterance are fused by summing the normalised output scores of each classifier, known as T-norm fusion (Auckenthaler, Carey, & Lloyd-Thomas, 2000; Navrátil & Ramaswamy, 2003). Fusion of the GMM (M_{ad}/U) system with either the polynomial or score-space sequence kernel SVMs yields similar results as shown in Table 1. Fusion of the GMM (M_{ad}/U) with both SVM systems produces the best result. Other researchers have also independently demonstrated the benefits of SVM using other sequence kernels (e.g., Louradour & Daoudi, 2005) on the traditional GMM approach.

Toward a Better Sequence Kernel

The sequence kernels described in the preceding sections have worked well for text-independent speaker verification. Unfortunately, although labeled *sequence kernels*, these functions do not encode the ordering within the sequence: They merely compute an average over time across a given sequence. If two sequences x_A and x_B are such that one is the reverse of the other, then the above sequence kernels will map both sequences to the same point in feature space. This lack of *temporal discrimination* makes these kernels unsuitable for text-dependent applications including speech recognition.

To address this problem of temporal ordering, it is possible to conceive a set of N equations that retain the temporal information in the resulting feature space. The Fisher and score-space kernels may be adapted to encode some temporal information by replacing the GMMs with hidden Markov models. The formulae for constructing such kernels were derived by Smith et al. (2001). However, HMMs (and also GMMs) require an abundance of data to reliably estimate their parameters (a speech corpus may contain more than 100 hours of recordings), whereas SVMs generalise well given sparse data and are difficult to optimise on large training sets. This makes the pairing of SVMs with HMMs for speech applications nontrivial.

The implementation of speech user interfaces for dysarthric speakers to control assistive technology devices (Green, Carmichael, Hatzis, Enderby, Hawley, & Parker, 2003) is a task usually hampered by sparse training corpora. Persons affected by dysarthria, a family of speech disorders characterised by loss of articulator control resulting in low-intelligibility speech, often exhibit speech impairments so individual specific and dissimilar to normal speech that it is not feasible to adapt the pretrained models of commercial HMM-based speech recognisers. Depending upon the severity of the disability, the dysarthric individual may display a high degree of variability when producing utterances representing the same word and, over time, articulatory competence may degrade if the individual suffers from a progressive form of the disease. It is often not practical, therefore, to collect large quantities of speech samples under such circumstances. Given such data constraints, traditional HMMs may not generalise well and an SVM implementation may be the better solution if it is possible to realise an appropriate sequence kernel that enables temporal discrimination.

Watkins (1999) proposed the dynamic alignment kernel based on pair HMMs (Durbin, Platt, Heckerman, & Sahami, 1998). A pair HMM is, essentially, a statistical version of dynamic time warping (Rabiner & Juang, 1993) and an extension of an HMM that emits into two sequences (A and B) simultaneously. It is a finite-state automaton consisting of three states: one state that inserts symbols into both A and B, one that inserts into A only, and one that inserts into B only. It was proven that a valid kernel can be derived under the assumption that the joint probability distribution of inserting simultaneously into both A and B is conditionally symmetrically independent (Watkins, 1999). However, estimating such a distribution for speech is not trivial, particularly when constrained by limited data. We thus look toward the original nonparametric formulation of DTW for our solution.

Basic DTW

DTW defines a global distance between two sequences. Broadly speaking, the global distance between two sequences is analogous to the distance between two points in space. Let us examine the simplest form of symmetric DTW that maintains the temporal ordering within the two sequences and does not allow omission of vectors.

Let the local distance be the Euclidean distance between the points defined by two vectors, $D_{local}(x_{Ai}, x_{Bj}) = \| x_{Ai} - x_{Bj} \|_2$. Let $D_{global}(x_A, x_B)$ denote the global distance between two sequences. Since the two sequences may not be of equal length, an alignment must be defined so that each vector in x_A is matched with a corresponding vector in x_B. Define the alignment using $a(v)$ and $b(v)$, which are indices to vectors within the sequences x_A and x_B respectively. The alignment index $v = \{ 1, \dots, V \}$ enumerates the pairings between frames within the two sequences, and V is the length of the alignment. Using this notation, $x_{Aa(v)}$ is matched with $x_{Bb(v)}$.

The DTW alignment distance is determined for a given alignment by summing the local distances between matched vectors:

$$D_{\text{align}}(x_A, x_B) = \sum_{v=1}^{V} D_{\text{local}}(x_{Aa(v)}, x_{Bb(v)}).\tag{9}$$

The global distance is the alignment distance along the Viterbi alignment defined by:

$$D_{\text{global}}(x_A, x_B) = \frac{1}{V} \min \left\{ D_{\text{align}}(x_A, x_B) \right\},\tag{10}$$

which has been normalised by the length of the Viterbi alignment. A dynamic programming beam search is used to compute the global distance efficiently.

DTW Kernel

The global distance estimated by DTW may be used to derive sequence kernels. Bahlmann, Haasdonk, and Burkhardt (2002) substituted the global distance between two sequences into the RBF kernel, replacing the term corresponding to the distance between two points in space, thereby creating a radial basis function DTW kernel. Bahlmann et al. recognised that this particular kernel architecture does not satisfy Mercer's condition (Chapter 1 and Vapnik, 1998) for a valid kernel by finding specific cases for which the kernel matrix was negative definite.

Another approach by Shimodaira, Noma, Nakai, and Sagayama (2001) substituted the local distance in the DTW algorithm with a similarity measure defined by the RBF kernel, and then used a modified DTW alignment criterion to maximise the global similarity. However, the resulting alignment path found by this method differs from that obtained when using the standard DTW formulation involving the Euclidean local distance metric.

We describe another method of exploiting DTW inside a kernel (Wan & Carmichael, 2005) that uses a different mathematical formulation. It makes use of the spherical normalisation mapping (Wan & Campbell, 2000), which is closely related to feature space normalisation (Graf & Borer, 2001). The mapping enables distance measures to be converted to inner products and vice versa. Spherical normalisation is a fixed reversible mapping from the input space X, in nD space, to X', in $(n+1)$D space. The mapping projects X onto the surface, a unit hypersphere embedded in X'. A simple aid to understanding this mapping is to imagine

Figure 2. Spherical normalisation mapping

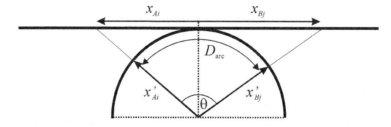

wrapping a flat piece of elastic material over the surface of a ball. The specific mapping used to project to the sphere is shown in Figure 2, and the explicit mapping from x_{Ai} to x'_{Ai} is:

$$x_{Ai} :\rightarrow x'_{Ai} = \frac{1}{\left\| \begin{bmatrix} x_{Ai} \\ 1 \end{bmatrix} \right\|_2} \begin{bmatrix} x_{Ai} \\ 1 \end{bmatrix}. \tag{11}$$

In X', the inner product equals the cosine of the angle between the vectors since each vector has unit length:

$$\langle x'_{Ai}, x'_{Bj} \rangle = \cos\theta. \tag{12}$$

Since the angle between two vectors equals the length of the arc measured along the surface of the unit sphere, $\theta = D_{\text{arc}}$, then $\langle x'_{Ai}, x'_{Bj} \rangle = \cos D_{\text{arc}}$. We have thus derived a simple formula for converting between distances and inner products.

The DTW kernel may now be formulated as follows. The vectors of each sequence are first mapped to the sphere using the spherical normalisation mapping defined in equation (11). The DTW local distances are the arc lengths on the surface of the hypersphere calculated using:

$$D_{\text{local}} = D_{\text{arc}} = \arccos (\langle x'_{Ai}, x'_{Bj} \rangle), \tag{13}$$

where the inner product is computed between the spherically normalised vectors. Standard symmetric DTW is then performed using D_{local} as defined by equation (13), to get D_{global} via equations (9) and (10). Since the local distances are equal to the *local angles*, the DTW global distance is merely the average angle along the Viterbi path between the two sequences. To revert to an inner product, we take the cosine of D_{global}.

Thus the DTW sequence kernel is:

$$\kappa_{\text{SphDTW}}(x_A, x_B) = \cos\left(\frac{1}{V} \sum_{v=1}^{V} \arccos (\langle x'_{Aa(v)}, x'_{Bb(v)} \rangle)\right), \tag{14}$$

computed along the Viterbi alignment. Higher order solutions may be obtained by substituting equation (14) into another kernel such as a polynomial kernel:

$$\kappa_{\text{pSphDTW}}(x_A, x_B) = \cos^p\left(\frac{1}{V} \sum_{v=1}^{V} \arccos (\langle x'_{Aa(v)}, x'_{Bb(v)} \rangle)\right). \tag{15}$$

Note that equation (14) can only be a valid kernel if the symmetric form of DTW is used. Moreover, in addition to symmetry, the function must satisfy Mercer's condition (Chapter 1; Vapnik, 1998) or be proven by alternative means to be a valid inner product. By definition, the cosine of the angle between two unit vectors is an inner product. In this formulation, the global distance is the mean (computed along the Viterbi path) of the angles between the pairs of vectors from the two sequences. However, it may be disputed whether the cosine of such a mean is still an inner product. Our simulations have not encountered any negative Hessian matrices that would indicate an invalid kernel. A naïve exhaustive search for a counterexample that leads to a negative definite kernel matrix can be time consuming and somewhat counterproductive. An analytical proof that indicates the precise conditions under which the kernel is valid would be more useful. For example, Burges (1998) provided analytic proof that the tanh kernel is only valid for certain parameters. Also, there are ways of learning with nonpositive semidefinite kernels, and such methods are discussed by Ong, Mary, Canu, and Smola (2004).

Kernel DTW

One of the features of earlier sequence kernels was their ability to incorporate dependencies between input vector components by computing cross-terms such as presented in equation (5). Since equation (14) is expressed entirely in terms of inner products, it is straightforward to incorporate cross-component dependencies by applying an explicit polynomial expansion to the frame-level input vectors prior to spherical normalisation and dynamic alignment. Indeed, kernels for which there is no known explicit expansion may also be used since the spherical normalisation mapping can be kernelised and expressed as a function of other kernels by computing the inner product of equation (11) with itself:

$$\kappa_{\text{spnorm}}\left(x_{Ai}, x_{Bj}\right) = \frac{\kappa\left(x_{Ai}, x_{Bj}\right) + 1}{\sqrt{\left(\kappa\left(x_{Ai}, x_{Ai}\right) + 1\right)\left(\kappa\left(x_{Bj}, x_{Bj}\right) + 1\right)}}. \tag{16}$$

This extension enables DTW to be performed in a kernel-induced space, resembling the extension of principal component analysis (PCA) to kernel PCA (Chapters XI and XV, and Schölkopf et al., 1998) in which PCA is performed in a kernel-induced space to extract nonlinear components.

Isolated-Word Dysarthric Speech Recognition

Speaker-dependent, isolated-word speech recognition simulations were performed using speech collected from both normal and dysarthric speakers (Green et al., 2003). Since dysarthric speech can differ enormously between speakers depending upon the severity of their disability, it is necessarily a speaker-dependent task. The challenges specific to recognising dysarthric speech have been outlined already. The speech data originated from seven dysarthric and seven normal speakers, each uttering between 30 and 40 examples of each of the words *alarm, lamp, radio, TV, channel, volume, up, down, on,* and *off.*

An experiment was conducted to determine how effective the DTW kernel SVM would be under limited quantities of training data compared to a traditional HMM system and a simple one-nearest-neighbour DTW system. Training set sizes were varied from 3 to 15 exemplars per word. Due to the lack of available data, N-fold cross-validation was used to increase the number of tests performed in order to obtain statistically significant results. For a given training set size, that number of exemplars per word was randomly selected for model building, and the remaining utterances were used for testing. This process was repeated to include only exemplars that were not previously part of a training set so that, eventually, every utterance was used once. This yielded over 17,000 individual tests when training sets were at the three-sample minimum and approximately 1,700 tests when training on 15 exemplar utterances per word.

The speech was parameterised using 12 mel frequency cepstral coefficients and energy computed using a 32-ms window with a 10-ms frame shift, augmented with their first-order derivatives and normalised to zero mean and unit diagonal covariance resulting in vectors of 26 dimensions. A Gaussian mixture silence detector, employing smoothing techniques, was used to remove all frames representing silence or containing short bursts of nonspeech noise.

The one-nearest-neighbour DTW system used all the utterances in the training selection as its templates and classified a test utterance according to the single closest matching template. The training utterances were manually end-pointed to contain only the relevant speech. During testing, this system required the use of a detector to remove frames of silence.

The HMM system was implemented by Hatzis et al. (2003). It employs a silence-word-silence grammar and uses a continuous density, "straight-through" model topology, and 11-state HMM with three Gaussians per state. The system was based on the Hidden Markov Model Toolkit (HTK) (Young, 1993) using a multipass reestimation strategy bootstrapped

Figure 3. Recognition error rate as a function of the training set size for normal and dysarthric speech (Adapted from Wan & Carmichael, 2005)

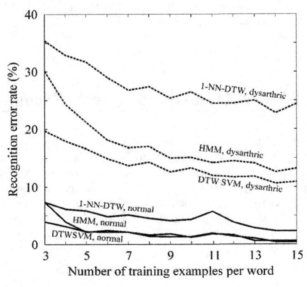

from manually end-pointed speech. The silence models also captured any other nonspeech noises in the audio.

A DTW kernel SVM was implemented using equation (15). Testing showed that the best accuracy was obtained with $p = 3$ and the linearly separable formulation of the SVM. Multiclass classification was achieved using the directed acyclic graphs approach by Platt, Cristianini, and Shawe-Taylor (2000). In that approach, an SVM trained to discriminate between two classes is used to eliminate one of them. The process is repeated until one class remains. Using the same procedures as for the standard DTW system, the training utterances were manually end-pointed and the test utterances were stripped of silence frames using an automatic detector. The average Lagrange multiplier value in the resulting SVMs was of the order 0.1 with maximum values in the range of 1 to 5. Due to the paucity of training data, the SVM solutions, save a few exceptions, used all of the training data for support vectors.

A summary of the results is shown in Figure 3. The standard DTW system returned the highest error rate across all conditions. On dysarthric speech, when trained on three examples per word, the DTW-SVM system had a 19.7% error rate and the HMM 30.1%, a relative reduction of 35% by the SVM. When training corpus size ranged from 6 to 15 samples per model, the SVM continued to outperform the HMM, with the difference in respective error rates remaining roughly constant at about 2% absolute. For isolated-word speaker-dependent dysarthric speech recognition, the DTW sequence kernel SVM approach is clearly better than the standard HMM approach.

Results for isolated-word speaker-dependent normal speech showed no significant difference between the DTW sequence kernel SVM and HMM approaches except when training sets were reduced to three examples per word: The SVMs' error rate was 4.0% compared to the HMMs' 7.4%, a 46% relative reduction by the SVM. These results may be explained by the fact that, for normal speech, variability within a given word is small, so the HMM is able to generalise with just four utterances per word.

Conclusion

This chapter described the use of sequence kernel SVMs for speaker verification and speech recognition. The highly successful use of support vector machines for text-independent speaker verification has been attributed to the development of sequence kernels that enable discriminative classification of sequences irrespective of length differences. Those sequence kernels map each frame of the sequence to some high-dimensional space before computing the average vector in feature space to represent the whole sequence. This approach, however, resulted in large feature spaces. Louradour and Daoudi (2005) have shown that it is possible to obtain SVMs with better accuracy using a smaller feature-space dimensionality by choosing a different kernel expansion. This is hardly surprising considering that performance usually benefits from the judicious selection of a few high-relevance features as opposed to lots of indiscriminately chosen ones. It suggests that a better understanding of kernel mappings in relation to speech is needed.

The averaging step in speaker verification sequence kernels made them text independent and thus suitable for that task. However, they lacked temporal discrimination and so are unsuitable for speech recognition. DTW and spherical normalisation were used to derive a sequence kernel incorporating this property. Although that kernel has not been shown to satisfy Mercer's condition for validity, it has proven highly effective in the classification of isolated-word dysarthric speech for controlling assistive technology devices, outperforming an HMM approach. The formulation not only has temporal discrimination, but also enables DTW to be performed in some high-dimensional, kernel-induced space. This latter property was not exploited in this work and may be of interest for future research effort in this area.

Acknowledgments

The author would like to thank Steve Renals, Mohamed Alkanhal, James Carmichael, William Campbell, and Roger Moore for their contributions that have made this chapter possible.

References

Auckenthaler, R., Carey, M., & Lloyd-Thomas, H. (2000). Score normalization for text-independent speaker verification systems. *Digital Signal Processing, 10*, 42-54.

Bahlmann, C., Haasdonk, B., & Burkhardt, H. (2002). On-line handwriting recognition with support vector machines: A kernel approach. In *Proceedings of the 8th International Workshop on Frontiers in Handwriting Recognition* (pp. 49-54).

Bishop, C. M. (1995). *Neural networks for pattern recognition.* Oxford University Press.

Bourlard, H., & Morgan, N. (1994). *Connectionist speech recognition: A hybrid approach.* Kluwer Academic Publishers.

Burges, C. (1998). Geometry and invariance in kernel based methods. In B. Schölkopf, C. Burges, & A. Smola (Eds.), *Advances in kernel methods: Support vector learning.* MIT Press.

Campbell, W. M. (2002). Generalised linear discriminant sequence kernels for speaker recognition. In *Proceedings of IEEE International Conference on Audio Speech and Signal Processing* (pp. 161-164).

Campbell, W. M., Campbell, J. P., Reynolds, D. A., Jones, D. A., & Leek, T. R. (2004). High-level speaker verification with support vector machines. In *Proceedings of IEEE International Conference on Audio Speech and Signal Processing* (pp. 73-76).

Campbell, W. M., Reynolds, D. A., & Campbell, J. P. (2004). Fusing discriminative and generative methods for speaker recognition: Experiments on switchboard and NFI/TNO field data. *Proceedings of Odyssey: The Speaker and Language Recognition Workshop* (pp. 41-44).

Chollet, G., Cochard, L., Constantinescu, A., Jaboulet, C., & Langlais, P. (1996). *Swiss French PolyPhone and PolyVar: Telephone speech databases to model inter- and intra-speaker variability* (Tech. Rep. No. 96-01). IDIAP.

Doddington, G., Przybocki, M., Martin, A., & Reynolds, D. (2000). The NIST speaker recognition evaluation: Overview, methodology, systems, results, perspective. *Speech Communication, 31*(2), 225-254.

Dumais, S., Platt, J., Heckerman, D., & Sahami, M. (1998). Inductive learning algorithms and representations for text categorisation. In *Proceedings of 7th International Conference on Information and Knowledge Management,* (pp. 229-237).

Durbin, R., Eddy, S., Krogh, A., & Mitchison, G. (1998). *Biological sequence analysis.* Cambridge University Press.

Fine, S., Navratil, J., & Gopinath, R. A. (2001). A hybrid GMM/SVM approach to speaker identification. In *Proceedings of IEEE International Conference on Audio Speech and Signal Processing* (pp. 417-420).

Gales, M., & Layton, M. (2004). SVMs, generative kernels and maximum margin statistical models. *Beyond HMM Workshop on Statistical Modelling Approach for Speech Recognition.* Retrieved on October 9, 2006 from http://svr-www.eng.cam.ac.uk/~mjfg/BeyondHMM.pdf

Ganapathiraju, A. (2002). *Support vector machines for speech recognition.* Unpublished doctoral dissertation, Mississippi State University.

Graf, A. B. A., & Borer, S. (2001). Normalization in support vector machines. In *Lecture notes in computer science: (Vol. 2191). Pattern recognition (DAGM)* (pp. 277-282). Springer.

Green, P., Carmichael, J., Hatzis, A., Enderby, P., Hawley, M., & Parker, M. (2003). Automatic speech recognition with sparse training data for dysarthric speakers. In *Proceedings of Eurospeech* (pp. 1189-1192).

Hatzis, A., Green, P., Carmichael, J., Cunningham, S., Palmer, R., Parker, M., et al. (2003). An integrated toolkit deploying speech technology for computer based speech training to dysarthric speakers. In *Proceedings of Eurospeech* (pp. 2213-2216).

Jaakkola, T. S., & Haussler, D. (1999). Exploiting generative models in discriminative classifiers. *Advances in Neural Information Processing Systems, 11.*

Louradour, J., & Daoudi, K. (2005). Conceiving a new sequence kernel and applying it to SVM speaker verification. In *Proceedings of Interspeech 2005* (pp. 3101-3104).

Mariéthoz, J., & Bengio, S. (2001). *A comparative study of adaptation methods for speaker verification* (Tech. Rep. No. IDIAP-RR 01-34). IDIAP.

Martin, A., Doddington, G., Kamm, T., Ordowski, M., & Przybocki, M. (1997). The DET curve in assessment of detection task performance. In *Proceedings of Eurospeech 1997* (pp. 1895-1898).

Navrátil, J., & Ramaswamy, G. N. (2003). The awe and mystery of T-Norm. In *Proceedings of Eurospeech 2003* (pp. 2009-2012).

Ong, C. S., Mary, X., Canu, S., & Smola, A. (2004). Learning with non-positive kernels. *ACM International Conference Proceeding Series:* In *Proceedings of 21st International Conference on Machine Learning, 69*, 81.

Platt, J., Cristianini, N., & Shawe-Taylor, J. (2000). Large margin DAGs for multiclass classification. *Advances in Neural Information Processing Systems, 12, 547-553.*

Rabiner, L., & Juang, B. (1993). *Fundamentals of speech recognition.* Prentice Hall.

Reynolds, D. A. (1992). *A Gaussian mixture modelling approach to text-independent speaker identification.* Unpublished doctoral dissertation, Georgia Institute of Technology.

Reynolds, D. A. (1995). Speaker identification and verification using Gaussian mixture speaker models. *Speech Communication, 17,* 91-108.

Schmidt, M., & Gish, H. (1996). Speaker identification via support vector classifiers. In *Proceedings of IEEE International Conference on Audio Speech and Signal Processing* (pp. 105-108).

Schölkopf, B., Smola, A., & Muller, K. (1998). Nonlinear component analysis as a kernel eigenvalue problem. *Neural Computation, 10*(5), 1299-1319.

Shimodaira, H., Noma, K., Nakai, M., & Sagayama, S. (2001). Support vector machine with dynamic time-alignment kernel for speech recognition. In *Proceedings of Eurospeech* (pp. 1841-1844).

Shriberg, E., Ferrer, L., Kajarekar, S., Venkataraman, A., & Stolcke, A. (2005). Modelling prosodic feature sequences for speaker recognition. *Speech Communication, 46,* 455-472.

Smith, N., Gales, M., & Niranjan, M. (2001). *Data-dependent kernels in SVM classification of speech patterns* (Tech. Rep. No. CUED/F-INFENG/TR.387). Cambridge University Engineering Department.

Vapnik, V. N. (1998). *Statistical learning theory.* Wiley.

Venkataramani, V., Chakrabartty, S., & Byrne, W. (2003). Support vector machines for segmental minimum Bayes risk decoding of continuous speech. In *Proceedings of IEEE Automatic Speech Recognition and Understanding Workshop,* (pp. 13-18).

Wan, V. (2003). *Speaker verification using support vector machines.* Unpublished doctoral dissertation, University of Sheffield.

Wan, V., & Campbell, W. M. (2000). Support vector machines for speaker verification and identification. In *Proceedings of Neural Networks for Signal Processing X* (pp. 775-784).

Wan, V., & Carmichael, J. (2005). Polynomial dynamic time warping kernel support vector machines for dysarthric speech recognition with sparse training data. In *Proceedings of Interspeech* (pp. 3321-3324).

Wan, V., & Renals, S. (2002). Evaluation of kernel methods for speaker verification and identification. In *Proceedings of IEEE International Conference on Audio Speech and Signal Processing* (pp. 669-672).

Wan, V., & Renals, S. (2005). Speaker verification using sequence discriminant support vector machines. *IEEE Transactions on Speech and Audio Processing, 13*(2), 203-210.

Watkins, C. (1999). *Dynamic alignment kernels* (Tech. Rep. No. CSD-TR-98-11). London: Royal Holloway College, University of London.

Young, S. J. (1993). *The HTK HMM toolkit: Design and philosophy* (Tech. Rep. No. CUED/F-INFENG/TR.152). University of Cambridge, Department of Engineering.

Chapter XI

A Kernel Canonical Correlation Analysis for Learning the Semantics of Text

Blaž Fortuna, Jožef Stefan Institute, Slovenia

Nello Cristianini, University of Bristol, UK

John Shawe-Taylor, University of Southampton, UK

Abstract

We present a general method using kernel canonical correlation analysis (KCCA) to learn a semantic of text from an aligned multilingual collection of text documents. The semantic space provides a language-independent representation of text and enables a comparison between the text documents from different languages. In experiments, we apply the KCCA to the cross-lingual retrieval of text documents, where the text query is written in only one language, and to cross-lingual text categorization, where we trained a cross-lingual classifier.

Introduction

The ideas of using statistical techniques from communication theory to translate text from one natural language to another have been around for many years. Literally, computational text analysis is as old as computers (which were introduced as part of UK decryption efforts in World War II).

A pioneer of information theory, Warren Weaver suggested automatic approaches to cross-language analysis as early as 1949, but efforts in this direction were soon abandoned for various technical and theoretical reasons (Weaver, 1955). The idea of automatically detecting relations between languages has not been abandoned, however. Today, state-of-the art methods in automatic translation rely on statistical modeling.

In the mid-'30s a statistical technique had been introduced to find correlations between two sets of vectors: canonical correlation analysis (CCA). Various computational and conceptual limitations made a statistical analysis of bilingual text based on CCA impractical (Hoteling, 1936). For one, the vector space model of text documents became popular in information retrieval (IR) only in the 1970s. The recent combination of CCA with kernel methods (Bach & Jordan, 2002; Lai & Fyfe, 2000; Shawe-Taylor & Cristianini, 2004) paved the way to a number of statistical, computational, and conceptual extensions. Various kernels were used to represent semantic relations, dual representation to speed up computations, and regularization-theory ideas to avoid discovering spurious correlations.

We present in this chapter a method based on kernel CCA to extract correlations between documents written in different languages with the same content. Given a paired bilingual corpus (a set of pairs of documents, each pair being formed by two versions of the same text in two different languages), this method defines two embedding spaces for the documents of the corpus, one for each language, and an obvious one-to-one correspondence between points in the two spaces. KCCA then finds projections in the two embedding spaces for which the resulting projected values are highly correlated. In other words, it looks for particular combinations of words that appear to have the same co-occurrence patterns in the two languages. Our hypothesis is that finding such correlations across a paired cross-lingual corpus will locate the underlying semantics since we assume that the two languages are conditionally independent, or that the only thing they have in common is their meaning.

The directions would carry information about the concepts that stood behind the process of the generation of the text and, although expressed differently in different languages, are, nevertheless, semantically equivalent. A preliminary version of this study appeared in Vinokourov, Shawe-Taylor, and Cristianini (2002).

Other methods exist to analyze statistically relations within bilingual text, such as cross-lingual latent semantic indexing (LSI; Littman, Dumais, & Landauer, 1998). LSI (Deerwester, Dumais, Furnas, Landauer, & Harshman, 1990) has been used to extract information about the co-occurrence of terms in the same documents, an indicator of semantic relations, and this is achieved by singular value decomposition (SVD) of the term-document matrix. The LSI method has been adapted to deal with the important problem of cross-language retrieval, where a query in a language is used to retrieve documents in a different language. Using a paired corpus, after merging each pair into a single document, we can interpret frequent co-occurrence of two terms in the same document as an indication of cross-linguistic correlation (Littman et al.). In this framework, a common vector space, including words from both languages, is created in which the training set is analyzed using SVD. This method, termed CL-LSI, will be briefly discussed in the next section.

In order to gain a first insight about the kind of knowledge produced by this system, it may be useful to consider subsets of words as concepts, and to assume that we are looking for a subset of words in the English version of the corpus whose occurrence in the documents is highly correlated with the occurrence of a subset of words in the corresponding French documents. This information can capture semantic relations both within and between such subsets. Since this problem can be computationally very expensive, we relax it to finding soft membership functions that represent such subsets by means of a real-valued (not Boolean) characteristic function. In this way, concepts are represented by weight vectors over the entire dictionary, and a concept in English is related to the corresponding concept in French when some measure of correlation between the two is satisfied. Notice finally that since we are representing documents in a space spanned by words, concepts represented in this way can also be considered as directions in the vector space. The CL-LSI method embeds all documents—French and English—in the same space, and then looks for sets of words that have high internal correlation. The KCCA method we present here will keep the two spaces separate and will consider subsets of words in each space that have high correlation between sets across the languages.

Such directions can then be used to calculate the coordinates of the documents in a language-independent way, and this representation can be used for retrieval tasks, providing better performance than existing techniques, or for other purposes such as clustering or categorization. Of course, particular statistical care is needed for excluding spurious correlations. We introduce a new method for tuning the relevant regularization parameters, and show that the correlations we find are not the effect of chance, and that the resulting representation significantly improves the performance of retrieval systems.

We find that the correlation existing between certain sets of words in English and French documents cannot be explained as a random correlation. Hence, we need to explain it by means of relations between the generative processes of the two versions of the documents, which we assume to be conditionally independent given the topic or content. Under such assumptions, such correlations detect similarities in content between the two documents, and can be exploited to derive a semantic representation of the text. We then use this representation for retrieval tasks, obtaining a better performance than with existing techniques.

We first apply the KCCA method to cross-lingual information retrieval, comparing performance with a related approach based on LSI described below (Littman et al., 1998). Second, we apply the method to text categorization where we compare the performance of KCCA trained on either a human-generated paired cross-lingual corpus or a corpus created using machine translation. From the computational point of view, we detect such correlations by solving an eigen problem, that is, avoiding problems like local minima, and we do so by using kernels.

We will give a short introduction to the vector space model and cross-lingual LSI. The KCCA machinery will be discussed afterward, and then we will show how to apply KCCA to cross-lingual retrieval and text categorization. Finally, results will be presented.

Related Work

Vector Space Representation of Text

The classic representation of a text document in information retrieval (Salton, 1991) is a bag of words (a bag is a set where repetitions are allowed), also known as the vector space model, since a bag can be represented as a (column) vector recording the number of occurrences of each word of the dictionary in the document at hand. In this chapter we will work with translations of the same document in English and in French, and we will represent them as two vectors, one in the English space and the other in the French space (of dimension equal to the number of entries in the respective dictionary).

Definition 1. *A document is represented, in the vector space model, by a vertical vector d indexed by all the elements of the dictionary (ith element from the vector is the frequency of the ith term in the document TF_i). A corpus is represented by a matrix D, whose columns are indexed by the documents and whose rows are indexed by the terms, $D = (d_1, ..., d_\ell)$. We also call the data matrix D the **term-document matrix**.*

In the information-retrieval experiment, we will need a similarity measure between documents. The classic similarity measure in IR is cosine similarity (Salton, 1991):

$$\text{sim}(d_i, d_j) = \frac{d'_i d_j}{\| d_i \| \cdot \| d_j \|} = \cos\alpha, \tag{1}$$

where α is the angle between the two vectors.

Since not all terms are of the same importance for determining similarity between the documents, we introduce term weights. A term weight corresponds to the importance of the term for the given corpus, and each element from the document vector is multiplied with the respective term weight. The most widely used weighting is called TFIDF (term frequency/inverse document frequency) weighting.

Definition 2. *An **IDF weight** for term i from the dictionary is defined as $w_i = \log(\ell/DF_i)$, where DF_i is the number of documents from the corpora that contain word i. A document's **TFIDF vector** is a vector with elements $w_i = TF_i \log(\ell/DF_i)$.*

We will consider linear combinations of terms as concepts. The magnitude of the coefficients of a term in a given combination could be interpreted as the level of membership of that given term to the concept. For the application point of view, these could be interpreted as generalized versions of sets of terms. Geometrically, we will interpret them as directions in the term space.

In order to introduce some semantic information to the document representation, we can consider linear transformations (feature mapping) of the document vectors of the type:

$$\Phi(d) = Ad,$$

where A is any matrix. If we view the rows of the matrix A as concepts, then the elements of the new document vector $\Phi(d)$ are similarities to these concepts. We can define a kernel using feature mapping Φ as:

$$K(x_i, x_j) = x_i AA'x'_j.$$

Recall that, for two vectors x_i and x_j, and for any linear mapping denoted by the matrix A, the function $K(x_i, x_j) = x_i AA'x'_j$ is always a kernel. The feature space defined by the mapping $\Phi(d) = Ad$ is called the **semantic space**.

Given two sets of documents in two different languages, we will see them as sets of points in two different spaces provided with a one-to-one relation. We will exploit correlations between the two sets in order to learn a better embedding of the documents into a space, where semantic relations are easier to detect. By detecting correlated directions between the two spaces, we will detect groups of terms (concepts) that have a similar pattern of occurrence across the two corpora, English and French, and hence can be considered as semantically related.

Kernels for Text Documents

We will introduce a dual version of canonical correlation analysis known as kernel CCA, which accesses the data only through the kernel matrix. This enables the use of kernels developed for comparing variable-length sequences, which were already introduced in Chapters II and X. Different types of string kernels can by naturally applied to text documents by viewing them as a sequence of characters, syllables, or words (Lodhi, Saunders, Shawe-Taylor, Cristianini, & Watkins, 2002; Saunders, Shawe-Taylor, & Vinokourov, 2002; Saunders, Tschach, & Shawe-Taylor, 2002).

String kernels also significantly improve the performance of information-retrieval and text-categorization methods on highly inflected languages (Fortuna & Mladenic, 2005), where the same word can have many different forms. This comes from the fact that string kernels are not so sensitive about prefixes and suffixes. Therefore, string kernels can also improve the performance of the KCCA when dealing with such languages.

Cross-Lingual Latent Semantic Indexing

The use of LSI for cross-language retrieval was proposed by Littman et al. (1998). LSI uses a method from linear algebra, singular value decomposition, to discover the important associative relationships. An initial sample of documents is translated by human or, perhaps, by machine, to create a set of dual-language training documents $D_x = \{\mathbf{x}_i\}_{i=1}^{\ell}$ and $D_y = \{\mathbf{y}_i\}_{i=1}^{\ell}$. After preprocessing the documents, a common vector space, including words from both languages, is created, and the training set is analyzed in this space using SVD:

$$D = \begin{pmatrix} D_x \\ D_y \end{pmatrix} = U\Sigma V', \tag{2}$$

where the ith column of D corresponds to the ith document with its first set of coordinates giving the first language features and the second set giving the second language features. To translate a new document (query) d to a language-independent representation, one projects (folds in) its expanded (components related to another language are filled up with zero) vector representation d into the space spanned by the k first eigenvectors U_k: $\Phi(d) = U'_k d$. The similarity between two documents is measured as the inner product between their projections. The documents that are the most similar to the query are considered to be relevant.

Regularized Kernel CCA

In order to carry on our analysis, we will use a form of regularized kernel canonical correlation analysis. We will choose directions in each space such that the projections of the data on them give rise to maximally correlated scores. We will do it in a document-by-document (i.e., dual) setting for computational reasons and will add some regularization, that is, a bias toward shorter solutions in the two-norm sense. This will enable us to extract features from the English (or French) space in a way that is supervised (by the other language) and hence more likely to be effective. In a way, we could see the French documents as very rich labels for the English ones, or alternatively we could consider this as an unsupervised cross-language task.

In the rest of this section, we will provide some basic definitions from statistics and use them to formulate the CCA. Then we well derive dual formulations of the CCA (KCCA) and introduce regularization in order to avoid overfitting.

Definition 3. *For two zero-mean univariate random variables x and y, we define their **covariance** as cov(x, y)=E[xy] and their **correlation** as:*

$$\mathrm{corr}(x, y) = \frac{E[xy]}{\sqrt{E[xx]E[yy]}} = \frac{\mathrm{cov}(x, y)}{\mathrm{var}(x)\mathrm{var}(y)}.$$

Given a sample of ℓ points from the distribution underlying the random variables, we can write down the empirical estimation of those quantities as follows:

$$\text{cov}(x, y) = \frac{1}{\ell-1}\sum_i x_i y_i \; , \quad \text{corr}(x, y) = \frac{1}{\ell-1}\frac{\sum_i x_i y_i}{\sqrt{\sum_i x_i x_i \sum_i y_i y_i}} \; .$$

Definition 4. *For zero-mean multivariate random variables $x \in \mathbb{R}^N$ and $y \in \mathbb{R}^M$, we define the* ***covariance*** *matrix as* $C_{xy} = E[\mathbf{xy}']$. *We will also use the* ***empirical*** *form of* $C_{xy} = \frac{1}{\ell}\sum x_i \mathbf{y}'_i$ *where x_i and y_i are vectors. In general, given two sets of vectors x_i and y_i, in a bijection, we can define the matrix:*

$$C = \begin{pmatrix} C_{xx} & C_{xy} \\ C_{yx} & C_{yy} \end{pmatrix} = E\left[\begin{pmatrix} x \\ y \end{pmatrix}\begin{pmatrix} x \\ y \end{pmatrix}'\right] \tag{3}$$

where C_{xx} and C_{yy} are the within-class covariances, and C_{xy} and C_{yx} are the between-class covariances.

We can extend the notions of covariance and correlation to multivariate variables. For two zero-mean multivariate random variables, $x \in \mathbb{R}^N$ and $y \in \mathbb{R}^M$, we consider the correlation and the covariation between their projections respectively onto the directions w_x and w_y, where $||w_x|| = ||w_y|| = 1$. These new random variables are univariate and linear combinations of the previous ones. The covariance of the multivariate random variables x and y along directions w_x and w_y is the quantity:

$$\text{cov}(w'_x x, \; w'_x y).$$

Correlation can be extended to the multivariate variables in a similar way.

Semantic Directions

For us, the multivariate random variables will correspond to document vectors (in the bag-of-words representation) in English and French, and there will be a one-to-one relation between them corresponding to documents that are translations of each other. We will now consider sets of words that are correlated between the two languages (sets of words in the two languages that have a correlated pattern of appearance in the corpus). We will assume that such sets approximate the notion of concepts in each language, and that such concepts are the translation of each other. Rather than considering plain sets, we will consider terms to have a degree of membership to a given set. In other words, the term t_j will be assigned a weight ω_j for each concept we consider, and every concept will correspond to a vector $\omega^{(x)} \in \mathbb{R}^N$ in English, and a vector $\omega^{(y)} \in \mathbb{R}^M$ in French. To illustrate the conceptual representation, we have printed a few of the most probable (most typical) words in each language for first few components found for the bilingual 36th Canadian Parliament corpus (Hansard; first row is

Box 1.

ENGLISH	health, minister, quebec, prime, he, we, federal, hepatitis, provinces, not, victims, they, care, are, people, resources, development, their, canadians, what
FRENCH	sante, ministre, quebec, nous, premier, federal, provinces, hepatite, ils, pas, developpement, il, canadiens, dollars, leur, ont, victimes, avons, dit, qu
ENGLISH	motion, house, agreed, standing, bill, adams, members, commons, order, parliamentary, leader, peter, consent, petitions, division, secretary, pursuant, response, unanimous, committee
FRENCH	motion, chambre, leader, voix, adams, communes, loi, accord, parlementaire, peer, reglement, conformement, secretaire, consentement, petitions, adoptee, projet, comite, vote, honneur
ENGLISH	motion, bill, division, members, act, declare, paired, nays, deferred, no, yeas, vote, stage, reading, c, carried, proceed, motions, recorded, read
FRENCH	motion, loi, vote, deputes, projet, no, paires, consentement, adoptee, o, voix, unanime, votent, motions, rejetee, lecture, differe, nominal, declare, lu
ENGLISH	petitions, standing, response, parliamentary, languages, honour, secretary, pursuant, adams, official, table, report, both, committee, order, peer, procedure, commons, affairs, committees
FRENCH	petitions, honneur, reponse, langues, officielles, parlementaire, reglement, deposer, secretaire, paragraphe, adams, conformement, rapport, comite, affaires, peter, permanent, procedure, ai, leader

English space and second row is French space) (see Box 1). The words are sorted by their weights ω_j.

Searching for correlated linear functions of the random variables leads us to the algorithm known in multivariate analysis as CCA. We will discuss the primal and the dual form of such an algorithm, one based on a terms view and the other based on a documents view. Each will contribute to our cross-linguistic analysis. For computational reasons, we will work in the document-based view, where the dimensionality is typically lower. We will call this the dual representation so that the terms view will be called the primal representation. Ultimately, we will focus on obtaining high-level (semantic) descriptions $\Phi(d)$ of a document vector d as $\Phi(d)=A'd$. Each column of A will be some concept vector ω.

Canonical Correlation Analysis

The goal of CCA is to find pairs of directions, w_x and w_y, along which the multivariate random variables x and y are maximally correlated. This can be formulated as an optimization problem:

$$\rho = \max_{w_x, w_y} \mathrm{corr}(w'_x x, w'_y y) = \max_{w_x, w_y} \frac{E[w'_x xy' \, w_y]}{\sqrt{E[w'_x xx' \, w_x] E[w'_y yy' w_y]}}.$$

We can rewrite this by using equation (3):

$$\rho = \max_{w_x, w_y} \frac{w'_x C_{xy} w'_y}{\sqrt{w'_x C_{xx} w_x \cdot w'_y C_{yy} w_y}}. \tag{4}$$

This can be further simplified by observing that the value of ρ is invariant to the norm of vectors w_x and w_y. After removing this degree of freedom by imposing:

$$w'_x C_{xx} w_x = w'_y C_{yy} w_y = 1,$$

we have arrived to the primal form of CCA

$$\max_{w_x, w_y} \quad w'_x C_{xy} w_y$$

subject to $\quad w'_x C_{xx} w_x = w'_y C_{yy} w_y = 1. \tag{5}$

Applying the Lagrange multiplier technique to the optimization of equation (5) gives us a generalized eigenvalue problem that has directions of maximal correlation for eigenvectors:

$$\begin{pmatrix} 0 & C_{xy} \\ C_{yx} & 0 \end{pmatrix} \begin{pmatrix} w_x \\ w_y \end{pmatrix} = \lambda \begin{pmatrix} C_{xx} & 0 \\ 0 & C_{xy} \end{pmatrix} \begin{pmatrix} w_x \\ w_y \end{pmatrix}.$$

Such a solution has a number of important properties. If λ is an eigenvalue, so is $-\lambda$ (the opposite direction is anticorrelated), thus the spectrum is:

$$\{\lambda_1, -\lambda_1, ..., \lambda_\ell, -\lambda_\ell, 0, 0, ..., 0\}.$$

Dualization of the Problem and Regularization

One can easily consider the dual representation of these problems by substituting in equation (4) $w_x = D_x \alpha_x$ and $w_y = D_y \alpha_y$, where D_x and D_y are respectively the term-document matrices of the training corpus of two feature spaces. After substitution, we get the dual form of CCA:

$$\rho = \max_{\alpha_x,\alpha_y} \frac{\alpha'_x K_x K_y \alpha_y}{\sqrt{\alpha'_x K_x^2 \alpha_x \cdot \alpha'_y K_y^2 \alpha_y}} = \max_{\alpha_x,\alpha_y} \frac{\alpha'_x K_x K_y \alpha_y}{\| \alpha'_x K_x^2 \alpha_x \| \cdot \| \alpha'_y K_y^2 \alpha_y \|} . \tag{6}$$

Here, $K_x = D'_x D_x$ and $K_y = D'_y D_y$ are respectively the *kernels* of the two feature spaces, that is, matrices of the inner products between images of all the data points (Cristianini & Shawe-Taylor, 2000).

Once we have moved to a kernel-defined feature space, the extra flexibility introduced means that there is a danger of overfitting. By this we mean that we can find spurious correlations by using large-weight vectors to project the data so that the two projections are completely aligned. For example, if the data are linearly independent in both feature spaces, we can find linear transformations that map the input data to an orthogonal basis in each feature space. It is now possible to find ℓ perfect correlations between the two representations. Using kernel functions will frequently result in linear independence of the training set, for example, when using Gaussian kernels. It is clear, therefore, that we will need to introduce a control on the flexibility of the maximal correlation directions. One way of doing this is by penalising their two-norm in the primal space (Shawe-Taylor & Cristianini, 2004). The formulation of equation (4) changes to:

$$\rho = \max_{w_x,w_y} \frac{w'_x C_{xy} w_y}{\sqrt{((1-\kappa)w'_x C_{xx} w_x + \kappa \| w_x \|^2) \cdot ((1-\kappa)w'_y C_{yy} w_y + \kappa \| w_y \|^2)}} . \tag{7}$$

Note that the regularization parameter κ interpolates smoothly between the maximization of the correlation (for $\kappa = 0$) and the maximization of the covariance (for $\kappa = 1$).

Again, by substituting $w_x = D_x \alpha_x$ and $w_y = D_y \alpha_y$, this time in equation (7), we derived the dual regularized CCA:

$$\max_{\alpha_x,\alpha_y} \quad \alpha'_x K_x K_y \alpha_y$$

$$\text{subject to} \quad (1-\kappa)\alpha'_x K_x^2 \alpha_x + \kappa \alpha'_x K_x^2 \alpha_x = 1$$
$$(1-\kappa)\alpha'_y K_y^2 \alpha_y + \kappa \alpha'_y K_y^2 \alpha_y = 1 \tag{8}$$

After applying the Lagrangian technique for solving equation (8), we arrive to the following generalized eigenvalue problem:

$$\begin{pmatrix} 0 & K_x K_y \\ K_y K_x & 0 \end{pmatrix} \begin{pmatrix} \alpha_x \\ \alpha_y \end{pmatrix} = \lambda \begin{pmatrix} (1-\kappa)K_x^2 + \kappa K_x^2 & 0 \\ 0 & (1-\kappa)K_y^2 + \kappa K_y^2 \end{pmatrix} \begin{pmatrix} \alpha_x \\ \alpha_y \end{pmatrix}.$$

The standard approach to the solution of a generalized eigenvalue problem of a form $Ax = \lambda Bx$ in the case of a symmetric B is to perform incomplete Cholesky decomposition (Bach & Jordan, 2002; Cristianini, Lodhi, & Shawe-Taylor, 2002) of the matrix B: $B = C'C$ and define $y = Cx$, which allows us, after simple transformations, to rewrite it as a standard eigenvalue problem:

$$(C')^{-1} A\, C^{-1} y = \lambda\, y.$$

The regularization parameter κ is chosen experimentally and will be discussed later.

Applications of KCCA to Information-Retrieval and Text-Categorization Tasks

The kernel CCA procedure identifies a set of projections from both languages into a common semantic space, where documents can be represented in a language-independent way described only by semantic dimensions. This provides a natural framework for performing cross-language information retrieval and text categorization.

To form a map from the English or French space into the common semantic space, we first select a number k of semantic dimensions, $1 \leq k \leq \ell$, with the largest correlation values ρ. To translate a new document, we first transform it to a TFIDF vector for its language d. The semantic directions obtained by solving equation (8) are represented in the dual space (document view) and therefore we have to move the new document into the dual space by $D'd$, and only then project it onto the selected semantic dimensions: $\Phi(d) = A'D'd$. Here, A is an $\ell \times k$ matrix whose columns are the first solutions of equation (8) for the given language, sorted by eigenvalue in descending order, and D is the training corpus for the given language: D_x or D_y.

Note that in the dual form of CCA (equation (8)), training documents are accessed only through kernel matrices (K_x and $K_{x \to y}$). This allows the KCCA to run on data that are not explicitly available as feature vectors, however, there is a kernel function defined on that data (Cristianini & Shawe-Taylor, 2000). String kernels come as natural candidates when dealing with text documents.

Table 1. Hansard's paired cross-lingual corpora

	TRAIN	TEST1
TEXT CHUNKS	495,022	42,011
DOCUMENTS	9,918	896
EN. WORDS	38,252	16,136
FR. WORDS	52,391	21,001

Experiments

Implementations of algorithms used in the experiments, KCCA and SVM, are part of the Text Garden text-mining library (Grobelnik & Mladenic, in press).

Information-Retrieval Experiment

The first part of experiments was done on the Hansard corpus. This corpus contains around 1.3 million pairs of aligned text chunks from the official records of the 36th Canadian Parliament. The raw text was split into sentences with Adwait Ratnaparkhi's MXTERMINATOR (Reynar & Ratnaparkhi, 1997) and aligned with I. Dan Melamed's GSA tool (Melamed, 1996). The corpus is split into two parts, House Debates (around 83% of text chunks) and Senate Debates. These parts are than split into a training part and two testing parts. For our experiments, we used the House Debates part from which we used only the training part and first testing part. The text chunks were split into paragraphs based on delimiters represented by three stars (***), and these paragraphs were treated as separate documents. We only used documents that had the same number of lines in both their English and French version. Some statistics on the corpora used in this experiment can be found in Table 1.

From the training parts, we randomly selected five subsets of 910 documents, and all results presented here were averaged over these five subsets. As parameters for KCCA, we set the regularization parameter κ to 0.5 and the threshold for the incomplete Cholesky decomposition of the kernel matrices to 0.4.

Figure 1. Quantities $\|j - KCCA_\kappa (E, rand(E))\|$, $\|j - KCCA_\kappa (E, F)\|$, *and*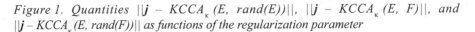
$\|j - KCCA_\kappa(E, rand(F))\|$ *as functions of the regularization parameter*

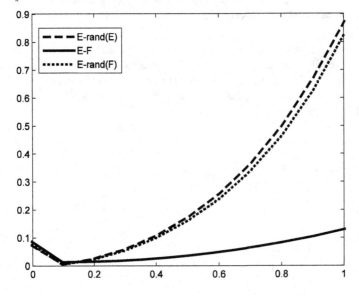

For the information-retrieval task, the entire first testing part of the Hansard corpus was projected into the language-independent semantic space learned with KCCA or CL-LSI, as described previously. Each query was treated as a text document and its TFIDF vector was also projected into the semantic space. Documents from the testing part, which were the nearest to the query document in the semantic space, were retrieved and ranked according to the cosine similarity equation (1) in the semantic space. Experiments were carried out for different dimensionalities of the semantic space: 100, 200, 300, 400, and 800 dimensions.

Selecting the Regularization Parameter

The regularization parameter κ in equation (8) not only makes equation (6) well posed numerically, but also provides control over the capacity of the function space where the solution is being sought. The larger the values of κ are, the less sensitive the method to the input data is, therefore, the more stable (less prone to finding spurious relations) the solution becomes. We should thus observe an increase in the reliability of the solution. We measure the ability of the method to catch useful signals by comparing the solutions on original input and random data. The random data is constructed by random reassociations

Table 2. Pseudo query test's baseline Top1 and Top10 results for the queries with five keywords on the left side and 10 keywords on the right side

n	1 [%]	10 [%]	1 [%]	10 [%]
Eɴ - Eɴ	96	100	99	100
Fʀ - Fʀ	97	100	100	100

Table 3. Pseudo query test Top1 and Top10 results for the queries with five keywords for the KCCA (top) and CL-LSI (bottom). The numbers represent the ratio of Top1/Top10.

	Eɴ – Eɴ	Eɴ – Fʀ	Fʀ – Eɴ	Fʀ – Fʀ
dim	1/10	1/10	1/10	1/10
100	49/86	38/78	37/77	47/85
200	64/94	47/86	46/86	61/93
300	71/96	53/89	51/89	69/96
400	75/97	56/90	53/90	72/97
800	82/99	59/92	58/92	79/99
100	42/83	29/72	30/71	41/82
200	52/90	37/81	39/80	54/91
300	60/94	41/85	43/84	60/93
400	65/96	44/86	46/86	64/95
800	73/98	52/91	52/89	73/98

Table 4. Pseudo query test Top1 and Top10 results for the queries with 10 keywords for the KCCA (top) and CL-LSI (bottom). The numbers represent the ratio of Top1/Top10.

	Eɴ – Eɴ	Eɴ – Fʀ	Fʀ – Eɴ	Fʀ – Fʀ
dim	1/10	1/10	1/10	1/10
100	74/96	58/90	56/89	70/95
200	86/99	68/95	68/94	83/99
300	90/100	73/97	73/96	88/99
400	92/100	75/97	75/97	90/100
800	96/100	77/98	77/97	94/100
100	63/93	43/85	43/83	62/94
200	75/98	55/91	53/91	75/97
300	83/99	61/95	59/95	81/99
400	86/99	64/96	62/96	83/99
800	91/100	70/98	68/98	90/100

of the data pairs, for example, $(E, \text{rand}(F))$ denotes an English-French parallel corpus that is obtained from the original English-French aligned collection by reshuffling the French (equivalently, English) documents. Let $KCCA_\kappa(D_1, D_2)$ denote the correlations of the KCCA directions on the paired data set (D_1, D_2). If the method is overfitting the data, it will be able to find perfect correlations and hence $||j - KCCA_\kappa(D_1, D_2)|| \approx 0$, where j is the all-one vector. We therefore use this as a measure to assess the degree of overfitting. Three graphs in Figure 1 show the quantities $||j - KCCA_\kappa(E, \text{rand}(E))|| \approx 0$, $||j - KCCA_\kappa(E, F)|| \approx 0$ and $||j - KCCA_\kappa(E, \text{rand}(F))|| \approx 0$ as functions of the regularization parameter κ.

For small values of κ, the correlations of all the tests is close to the all-one correlations (the correlations $||j - KCCA_\kappa(E, E)||$). This indicates overfitting since the method is able to find correlations even in randomly associated pairs. As κ increases, the correlations of the randomly associated data become far from all one, while that of the paired documents remain closer to all one. This observation can be exploited for choosing the optimal value of κ. From the graph in Figure 1, this value could be derived as lying somewhere between 0.4 and 0.8. For lower values of regularization parameter κ we risk overfitting, while for larger values we risk getting directions that give little correlation on the input data.

Mate Retrieval

In the first experiment, each English document was used as a query and only its mate document in French was considered relevant for that query. The same was done with French documents as queries and English documents as test documents. We measured the number of times that the relevant document appeared in the set of the top *n* retrieved documents (Top*n*). The Top1 results for KCCA averaged around 99% for all dimensions, while the results for CL-LSI started at only around 77% for 100 dimensions and than grew up to 98% when

Table 5. English-French and English-German paired cross-lingual corpora from the Reuters Corpus

	En-Fr	En-Gr
PARAGRAPHS	119,181	104,639
DOCUMENTS	10,000	10,000
ENGLISH WORDS	57,035	53,004
FRENCH WORDS	66,925	—
GERMAN WORDS	—	121,193

using all the dimensions. The Top10 results were 100% for the KCCA and around 98% for CL-LSI. As one can see from the results, KCCA seems to capture most of the semantics in the first few components, achieving 98% accuracy with as little as 100 components when CL-LSI needs all components for a similar figure.

Pseudo Query Test

For the next experiment, we extracted 5 or 10 keywords from each document, according to their TFIDF weights, and used the extracted words to form a query. Only the document from which the query was extracted and its mate document were regarded as relevant. We first tested queries in the original bag-of-words space, and these results can serve as a baseline for the experiments done in the KCCA- and CL-LSI-generated semantic spaces. Baseline results are shown in Table 2. All queries were then tested in a similar way as before, the only difference is that this time we also measured the accuracy for cases where the language of the query and the relevant document were the same. Results for the queries with 5 keywords are presented in Table 3, and the queries with 10 keywords in Table 4.

Machine Translation and Text-Categorization Experiments

In the second set of experiments, we applied KCCA to the categorization of multilingual text documents. This was done by using the SVM classifier (Joachims, 1998) in the language-independent semantic space learned with KCCA.

Two data sets are needed for this: a bilingual corpus of paired documents for the KCCA and a training corpus of annotated documents for training the SVM classifier. The problem with this approach is that in practice, it is often hard to get two such corpora that contain documents both from similar domains and with similar vocabulary. In this experiment, we test two different combinations.

In both combinations, we used Reuters' RCV2 multilingual corpus (Reuters, 2004) as a training set for the SVM classifier. The difference was in the paired corpus used for the KCCA. In the first combination, we used the Hansard corpus, which was already described and used in the previous experiments. In the second combination, we used machine translation (MT; e.g., *Google Language Tools*[1]) for generating artificial paired cross-lingual corpora, generated from the documents of the Reuters RCV2 corpus. We will refer to the paired corpora generated with machine translation as *artificial corpora*.

By using MT for generating paired corpus for the KCCA, we can ensure a close similarity between the vocabulary and topics covered by the paired and annotated corpora. As it will be shown in the experiments, this reflects a better performance of the second combination.

Data Set

The experiments for text categorization were done on the Reuters multilingual corpora (Reuters, 2004), which contain articles in English, French, German, Russian, Japanese, and other languages. Only articles in English, French, and German were used for this experiment. Articles for each language were collected independently, and all articles were annotated with categories.

For this experiment, we picked 5,000 documents for each of the three languages from the Reuters corpus. Subsets of these documents formed the training data sets for the classifiers. These same documents were also used for generating artificial aligned corpora in the same way as in the first part of the experiments. Google Language Tools were used to translate English documents to French and German, and the other way around. In this way, we generated English-French and English-German paired cross-lingual corpora. We used the

Table 6. Categorization baseline average precision (%) for classifiers trained in original vector space models

	CCAT	MCAT	ECAT	GCAT
ENGLISH	85%	80%	62%	86%
FRENCH	83%	85%	63%	94%
GERMAN	85%	86%	62%	91%

Table 7. Categorization average precision (%) for classifiers trained in KCCA semantic space through Hansard and artificial corpus. The results are for the semantic spaces with 400 (top) and 800 (bottom) dimensions.

	CCAT	MCAT	ECAT	GCAT
EN-EN	59/79	40/76	25/51	51/78
EN-FR	41/78	21/81	18/54	75/89
FR-EN	55/80	30/76	22/50	40/77
FR-FR	40/78	24/82	19/54	77/89
EN-EN	67/80	61/82	38/54	67/79
EN-FR	47/79	32/82	27/55	80/90
FR-EN	60/80	43/76	30/52	51/78
FR-FR	53/79	59/83	38/56	85/89

Table 8. Categorization average precision (%) for classifiers trained in KCCA semantic space through artificially generated English-German aligned corpus

	CCAT	MCAT	ECAT	GCAT
En-En	75	77	49	81
En-Gr	72	82	46	87
Gr-En	70	75	43	78
Gr-Gr	67	83	44	86
En-En	76	78	52	82
En-Gr	73	82	47	88
Gr-En	71	75	46	79
Gr-Gr	68	83	47	86

Figure 2. Average precision (%) for the classification of English and French documents in the 800 dimensional semantic space

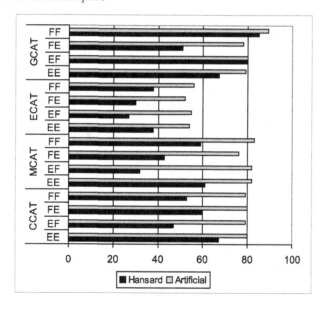

training part of the Hansard corpus as English-French human-generated aligned corpora. Some statistics on the corpora used in this experiment can be found in Table 5.

Experiment

The text-categorization experiment was done in the following way. To provide baseline results, we first trained and tested classifiers in the original bag-of-words spaces. Then we used KCCA to learn a language-independent semantic space from the paired cross-lingual corpora and mapped the documents from the Reuters data set into this semantic space. Classifiers were trained and tested in the semantic space for the following categories from the Reuters data set: CCAT (corporate/industrial), MCAT (markets), ECAT (economics), and GCAT (government/social). This was repeated for the Hansard (English-French) and artificial (English-French and English-German) paired cross-lingual corpora.

The parameters used for KCCA were the same as for the information-retrieval task, and subsets of 1,000 documents from the paired corpus were used for learning. These subsets were selected randomly, and the results presented were averaged over five runs.

A linear SVM (Joachims, 1998) was used as a classification algorithm with cost parameter C set to 1. All the classifiers were trained on subsets of 3,000 documents from the training set, and the results were averaged over five runs. This means that the presented results, together with five different subsets used for KCCA, are averaged over 25 runs. The classifiers were tested on a subset of 50,000 documents, and average precision was measured. Baseline results are shown in Table 6.

The results for the human-generated Hansard corpus and for the artificial English-French corpus (generated using machine translation) are presented in Table 7 and in Figure 2. The results obtained with the artificial corpus were in all cases significantly better than the results obtained with the Hansard corpus, and they are close to the baseline results for single-language classification. Note that the results for the artificial corpus only slightly improve when the dimensionality of semantic space increases from 400 to 800, while the results for the human-generated corpus increase by 10 or more percent. This shows that the first 400 dimensions learned from the artificial corpus are much richer at capturing the semantics of news articles than the ones learned from the Hansard corpus.

Results for classification based on English-German artificial aligned corpus are shown in Table 8. Surprisingly, in some cases, the cross-lingual classifications do better than a straight German classifier.

Conclusion

We have presented a novel procedure for extracting semantic information in an unsupervised way from a bilingual corpus, and we have used it in text-retrieval and categorization applications. Our main findings are that the correlation existing between certain sets of words in English and French documents cannot be explained as random correlations. Hence, we need to explain it by means of relations between the generative processes of the two versions of the documents. The correlations detect similarities in content and can be exploited to derive a semantic representation of the text. The representation is then used for cross-lingual text-mining tasks, providing better performance than existing techniques such as CL-LSI.

References

Bach, F. R., & Jordan, M. I. (2002). Kernel independent component analysis. *Journal of Machine Learning Research, 3*, 1-48.

Cristianini, N., Lodhi, H., & Shawe-Taylor, J. (2002). Latent semantic kernels. *Journal of Intelligent Information Systems (JJIS), 18*(2), 66-73.

Cristianini, N., & Shawe-Taylor, J. (2000). *An introduction to support vector machines and other kernel-based learning methods.* Cambridge University Press.

Deerwester, S., Dumais, S. T., Furnas, G. W., Landauer, T. K., & Harshman, R. (1990). Indexing by latent semantic analysis. *Journal of the American Society for Information Science, 41*, 391-407.

Fortuna, B., & Mladenic, D. (2005). Using string kernels for classification of Slovenian Web documents. In *Proceedings of 29th Annual Conference of the German Classification Society (GfKl),* 366-373.

Germann, U. (2001). *Aligned Hansards of the 36th Parliament of Canada* (Release 2001-1a). Retrieved from http://www.isi.edu/natural-language/download/hansard

Grobelnik, M., & Mladneic, D. (in press). *Text mining recipes.* Berlin, Germany: Springer-Verlag.

Hoskuldsson, A. (1988). Partial least squares regression method. *Journal of Chemometrics, 2*, 211-228.

Hoteling, H. (1936). Relations between two sets of variates. *Biometrika, 28*, 321-377.

Joachims, T. (1998). Text categorization with support vector machines: Learning with many relevant features. In *Proceedings of ECML-98, 10th European Conference on Machine Learning* (pp. 137-142).

Lai, P. L., & Fyfe, C. (2000). Kernel and nonlinear canonical correlation analysis. *International Journal of Neural Systems, 10*(5), 365-377.

Littman, M. L., Dumais, S. T., & Landauer, T. K. (1998). Automatic cross-language information retrieval using latent semantic indexing. In G. Grefenstette (Ed.), *Cross language information retrieval,* (pp.57-62). Kluwer.

Lodhi, H., Saunders, C., Shawe-Taylor, J., Cristianini, N., & Watkins, C. (2002). Text classification using string kernels. *Journal of Machine Learning Research, 2*, 419-444.

Mardia, K. V., Kent, J. T., & Bibby, J. M. (1979). *Multivariate analysis.* Academic Press.

Melamed, I. D. (1996). A geometric approach to mapping bitext correspondence. In *Proceedings of the First Conference on Empirical Methods in Natural Language Processing,* (pp. 1-12).

Reuters. (2004). *RCV1-v2/LYRL2004: The LYRL2004 distribution of the RCV1-v2 text categorization test collection.* Retrieved from http://jmlr.csail.mit.edu/papers/volume5/lewis04a/lyrl2004_rcv1v2_README.htm

Reynar, J. C., & Ratnaparkhi, A. (1997). A maximum entropy approach to identifying sentence boundaries. In *Proceedings of the Fifth Conference on Applied Natural Language Processing* (16-19).

Salton, G. (1991). Developments in automatic text retrieval. *Science, 253*, 974-979.

Saunders, C., Shawe-Taylor, J., & Vinokourov, A. (2002). String kernels, Fisher kernels and finite state automata. *Advances of Neural Information Processing Systems, 15,* 633-640.

Saunders, C., Tschach, H., & Shawe-Taylor, J. (2002). Syllables and other string kernel extensions. *Proceedings of Nineteenth International Conference on Machine Learning,* 530-537.

Shawe-Taylor, J., & Cristianini, N. (2004). *Kernel methods for pattern analysis.* Cambridge University Press.

Vinokourov, A., Shawe-Taylor, J., & Cristianini, N. (2002). Inferring a semantic representation of text via cross-language correlation analysis. *Advances of Neural Information Processing Systems, 15,* (1473-1480).

Weaver, W. (1949). Translation. In *Machine translation of languages,* (pp. 15-23). MIT Press.

Endnote

[1]   http://www.google.com/language_tools

Section III

Image Processing

Chapter XII

On the Pre-Image Problem
in Kernel Methods

Gökhan H. Bakır, Max Planck Institute for Biological Cybernetics, Germany

Bernhard Schölkopf, Max Planck Institute for Biological Cybernetics, Germany

Jason Weston, NEC Labs America, USA

Abstract

In this chapter, we are concerned with the problem of reconstructing patterns from their representation in feature space, known as the pre-image problem. We review existing algorithms and propose a learning-based approach. All algorithms are discussed regarding their usability and complexity, and evaluated on an image denoising application.

Introduction

In kernel methods, the feature map induced by the kernel function leads to a possibly non-linear embedding of the input data into a high-dimensional linear space. In this chapter we are interested in inverting this map. Thus, given a kernel function k and its feature map ϕ, does the map ϕ^{-1} exist and how can it be evaluated (see Figure 1)? Calculating this inverse feature map ϕ^{-1} is of wide interest in kernel methods.

Applications cover, for example, *reduced set methods* by Burges (1996), *denoising* by Mika, Schölkopf, Smola, Müller, Scholz, and Rätsch (1999), *hyperresolution* using kernels in Kim et al. (2005), and structured prediction in Weston, Chapelle, Elisseeff, Schölkopf, and Vapnik (2003). Let us give a definition of the pre-image problem.

Problem P1: The Pre-Image Problem

Given a point ψ in a reproducing kernel Hilbert space (RKHS) F_z, find a pattern z^* in the set $\mathcal{Z}$ such that the feature map ϕ_z maps z^* to ψ, that is:

$$\psi = \phi_z(z^*). \tag{1}$$

A special case of the problem **P1** is the case when ψ is given by a linear expansion of patterns mapped into the feature space.

Problem P2: The Pre-Image Problem for Expansions

Given a point ψ in an RKHS F_z expressed by a linear combination of patterns $\{x_1, ..., x_N\} \subset \mathcal{Z}^N$, that is, $\psi = \sum_{i=1}^{N} \alpha_i \phi_z(x_i)$, find a pattern z^* in space $\mathcal{Z}$ such that:

$$\psi = \sum_{i=1}^{N} \alpha_i \phi_z(x_i) = \phi_z(z^*)$$

Figure 1. Feature map leads to a linear embedding in some high-dimensional space. Here, it is illustrated for a two-dimensional point set and the Gaussian Kernel.

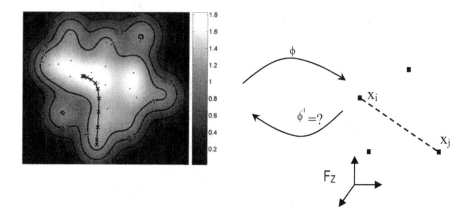

Obviously, solving pre-image problems corresponds to an inverse problem since ideally:

$$z^* = \phi_z(\psi)^{-1},$$ (2)

and thus solving a pre-image problem requires one to invert the used feature map. Unfortunately, in the most common cases, it turns out that the problem of inverting ϕ_z belongs to the class of *ill-posed* problems. Roughly speaking, an inversion problem as in equation (2) is said to be *ill posed* if the solution is not unique, does not exist, or is not a continuous function of the data, that is, if a small perturbation of the data can cause an arbitrarily large perturbation of the solution. For an introduction to ill-posed problems, see Vogel (2002).

It turns out that for pre-images, the most critical property is existence, and thus we will focus our discussion on the existence property.

The Pre-Image Problem

Let us consider first the case that ψ is given by an expansion. One can show (see Schölkopf & Smola, 2002; chapter 18) that if the kernel can be written as $\kappa(x,x')=f_\kappa(x^\top x')$ with an invertible function f_κ (e.g., polynomial kernels with $\kappa(x,x')=(x^\top x')^d$ with odd d), and if an exact pre-image exists, then one can compute it analytically as:

$$z = \sum_{i=1}^{m} f_\kappa^{-1}\left(\sum_{j=1}^{N} \alpha_j \kappa(x_j, e_i)\right) e_i,$$ (3)

where $\{e_1, ..., e_N\}$ is any orthonormal basis of the input space. Unfortunately, this is rather the exception than the rule. One reason is that the span of the data points does not need to coincide with the image of the feature map ϕ_κ, and thus for many points in the feature space, there is no exact pre-image. In fact, for the most widely used radial basis function kernel, *any* nontrivial linear combination of mapped points will leave the image of ϕ_κ, and this guarantees that there does not exist any exact pre-image.

Summarizing, we see that inverting the feature map is likely to be an ill-posed problem. Thus, to overcome the ill-posed formulation, Burges (1996) suggested relaxing the original pre-image problem.

Relaxation of the Pre-Image Problem

A straightforward relaxation of the inversion problem is to drop the requirement on the pattern z^* to be the exact pre-image, but to be as close as possible to an ideal pre-image. Thus, we consider the following approximate pre-image problem.

Figure 2. The approximate pre-image problem involves searching for a pre-image z^* of a point ψ, given in feature space F_z, that corresponds to finding the nearest point $\phi(z^*)$ on a nonlinear manifold.

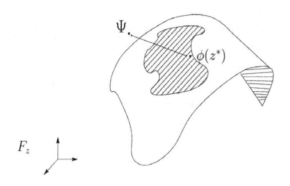

Problem P3: The Approximate Pre-Image Problem

Given a point ψ in F_z, find a corresponding pattern $z^* \in Z$, such that:

$$z^* = \arg\min_{x \in Z} \| \phi_z(x) - \psi \|^2_{F_z} =: \arg\min_{x \in Z} \mathcal{L}(x) \tag{4}$$

We will denote henceforth the objective function by: $\mathcal{L} : \mathcal{Z} \to \mathbb{R}$.

Note that Problem **P3** is an optimization problem and not an inversion problem. In the case where the inverse map ϕ_z^{-1} exists, $\phi_z(\psi)^{-1}$ equals the optimal solution z^* of equation (4) in **P3**. Otherwise, the found z^* is a solution with minimal defect $\| \phi_z(x) - \psi \|^2_{F_z}$. Furthermore, note that the new problem is formulated:

- in a high and possibly infinite-dimensional feature space (illustrated in Figure 2),
- and the optimization is over an arbitrary set in the input space.

It is not straightforward to see that a tractable algorithm-solving Problem **P3** should exist. Fortunately, for some interesting sets $\mathcal{Z}$, we can formulate algorithms that can be used to solve Problem **P3**, and this is the subject of this chapter. These algorithms are not applicable in general cases for $\mathcal{Z}$, but are always going to be *tailored* specifically to $\mathcal{Z}$ by using special properties inherent to the set $\mathcal{Z}$. In this chapter, we will focus on the case that $\mathcal{Z}$ is a subset of a real vector space $\mathbb{R}^d$. Discrete pre-image problems, that is, if the set $\mathcal{Z}$ is discrete, is a matter of current research. For the case of graphs, see, for example, Bakır et al. (2004). We will review existing pre-image techniques that are applicable in this case and propose a new pre-image algorithm based on learning. Furthermore, we will focus on feature mappings that are induced by a Gaussian kernel since it is the most widely used kernel in practice. Thereafter, we will compare the introduced algorithms on the problem of signal enhancement via kernel PCA denoising.

Pre-Images by Smooth Optimization

In this section, we review several existing approaches to solve the *approximate* pre-image problem and propose new techniques. We will start with pure optimization-based approaches and continue with strategies based on learning that can take advantage of additional prior information on the pre-image.

Gradient Descent

The most straightforward approach is to use nonlinear optimization techniques to solve the approximate pre-image problem. In the case that ψ is given by an expansion:

$$\sum_{i=1}^{N} \alpha_i \phi_k(x_i),$$

one can express the objective function in equation (4) directly by using the kernel trick itself

$$\mathcal{L}(x) = || \phi_k(x) - \psi ||_{F_z}^2 = \kappa(x,x) - 2\sum_{I=1}^{N} \alpha_i \kappa(x_i, x) + C, \tag{5}$$

where C denotes some constant independent of x. Taking the derivatives of equation (5) is straightforward as long as the kernel function is smooth and continuous in its argument.

The problem with a plain gradient-descent approach is that equation (5) is mostly not linear and not convex. For this reason, one has to use multiple starting values to initialize the gradient descent in the hope that one of the found minima is good enough. People therefore considered speeding up pre-image techniques, for example, by taking advantage of special properties of the used kernel function. One such example is the fixed-point iteration method introduced by Schölkopf, Smola, Knirsch, and Burges (1998), which we discuss next.

The Fixed-Point Iteration Method

For kernels with the property $k(z,z) = 1$, for example, the Gaussian kernel, one can reformulate Problem **P3** as follows:

$$z^* = \arg\min_{x \in \mathcal{Z}} || \phi_z(x) - \psi ||_{F_z}^2 = \arg\max_{x \in \mathcal{Z}} \phi_z(x)^\top \psi. \tag{6}$$

The reformulation is possible since all points have the same distance to the origin,[1] and therefore the dot product contains all relevant information. For example, for kernels of the form $\kappa(x, z) = \kappa(\| x - z \|^2)$ and the case that ψ is given as an expansion, it is possible to derive an efficient fixed-point algorithm as follows:

$$0 = \frac{\partial}{\partial z} \phi_z(z)^\top \psi = \sum_{i=1}^{N} \frac{\partial}{\partial z} \phi_z(z)^\top \phi_k(x_i)$$

$$= \sum_{i=1}^{N} \alpha_i \kappa'(x_i, z)(x_i - z)$$

which leads to the relation

$$z = \frac{\sum_{i=1}^{N} \alpha_i \kappa'(x_i, z) x_i}{\sum_{i=1}^{N} \alpha_i \kappa'(x_i, z)} \ .$$

This identity does not hold for an arbitrary z_0 but only for the solution z^*. The idea is now to construct a sequence $z_1, z_2, \ldots$ via:

$$z_{t+1} = \frac{\sum_{i=1}^{N} \alpha_i \kappa'(x_i, z_t) x_i}{\sum_{i=1}^{N} \alpha_i \kappa'(x_i, z_t)} \tag{7}$$

such that ideally z_t converges to the fixed point in equation (6). Since one does not need to perform any line search, which is typically needed in gradient-descent methods, fixed-point-based techniques are generally faster than gradient-descent methods. However, the method suffers similar to gradient-descent techniques from evaluating all kernel functions for each optimization step, though it needs overall much less kernel evaluations than plain gradient descent does.

Unfortunately, the fixed-point technique tends to be numerically instable in practice if initialized randomly. This phenomenon might be due to (a) the fact that the denominator can get too small for an arbitrarily chosen start point z_0 during the iteration, and (b) the fact that there exist several regions of attraction that can influence each other and thus might lead to oscillation or even divergence. A common recipe in this case is to restart the iteration with different starting points z_0 often, and choose the best candidate of the converged runs. We present the fixed-point algorithm in A1.

Algorithm A1: Fixed-Point Pre-Image Calculation.

Given data $D_N = \{ x_i \}_{i=1}^{N}$, a feature map ϕ_κ from a kernel k, the expansion $\psi = \sum_{i=1}^{N} \alpha_i \phi_z(x_i)$, and the number of desired restarts n:

1. choose randomly an initial value z_0 from D_N

2. until convergence: $z = \dfrac{\sum_{i=1}^{N}\alpha_i\kappa'(x_i,z)x_i}{\sum_{i=1}^{N}\alpha_i\kappa'(x_i,z)}$.

If the denominator is smaller than some ε, restart at 1.

Repeat n times the pre-image computation and take the best z from n trials.   □

An interesting fact about the fixed-point method is that the pre-image obtained is in the span of the data points x_i. This is a major difference from a pure optimization-based technique like gradient descent where the full input space is explored. Thus, in the fixed-point method, the pre-image is constructed using data points explicitly. For example, the fixed-point algorithm can never generate a pre-image that is orthogonal to the span of the training data, being in contrast to the gradient-descent method. Nevertheless, the fixed-point algorithm shows that in principle, one can relate the pre-image not only to a single point ψ in feature space, but to a complete set of points D_N and thus use side information provided by these additional data. In the next section, we discuss a classical technique from statistics that is used for pre-image calculation and that is entirely based on such a strategy.

Multidimensional Scaling Based Technique

Multidimensional scaling (MDS) deals in particular with the problem of finding a lower dimensional representation $x_1, ..., x_N \in \mathbb{R}^{d2}$ of a set of points $x_1, ..., x_N \in \mathbb{R}^{d1}$ where $d_1 >> d_2$ and ideally the distances are preserved, that is:

$$d_{\mathbb{R}^{d1}}(x_1, x_2) = d_{\mathbb{R}^{d2}}(x_1, x_2).$$

Often, such a set of points does not exist, and one solves the optimization problem:

$$\{x_1, ..., x_N\} = \arg\min_{x_1,...,x_N}\sum_{i=1}^{N}\sum_{j=1}^{N}\left(d_{\mathbb{R}^{d1}}(\mathbf{x}_i, \mathbf{x}_j) - d_{\mathbb{R}^{d2}}(x_i, x_j)\right)^2.$$

In contrast to the standard MDS setting, in pre-image computation, we are just interested in finding the lower dimensional representation of a single point, namely, the pre-image z^* only. The basic idea behind the MDS method for pre-image computation is to declare that the distance from the point ψ to each point $\mathbf{x}_i$ of a reference set $\mathbf{x}_i, ..., \mathbf{x}_N$ should be related to the distance from the pre-image z^* to the pre-images $\mathbf{x}_i, ..., \mathbf{x}_N$ of the reference set. This is insofar a reasonable assumption since the feature map is usually considered to be smooth. Obviously, these distances will not be the same and we need to obtain the input distance from the feature map. In the following, we will describe the necessary steps to obtain the input distances for the Gaussian and polynomial kernel, and we will discuss how a pre-image can be obtained using least squares minimization leading to a closed-form solution of the optimal approximate pre-image. Let us consider the used distance for the Gaussian kernel $\kappa(x,y) = e^{-\gamma\|x-y\|^2} = e^{-\gamma d_{\mathcal{Z}}^2(x,y)}$:

$$d_{\mathcal{Z}}(x,y) = \sqrt{-\frac{\log \kappa(x,y)}{\gamma}}\ .$$

Given the distance among two points in feature space:

$$d_{F_k}(\mathbf{x},\mathbf{y})^2 = \|\ \phi(x) - \phi(y)\ \|_{\mathcal{F}_z}^2 = 2 - 2\kappa(x,y),$$

it is possible to obtain the squared input distance as

$$d_{\mathcal{Z}}(x,y)^2 = -\frac{1}{\gamma}\log\left(1 - \frac{1}{2}d_{\mathcal{F}_k}(\mathbf{x},\mathbf{y})^2\right). \tag{8}$$

Thus, we see that, given just the expression of the kernel function, we can retrieve the distance of two points in input space. Now, let us consider the Euclidean distance in feature space. As we noted above, the distance between two points $\mathbf{x}$ and ψ can be calculated without their input representation. In the case that ψ is given as an expansion, the Euclidean distance between ψ and a point $\mathbf{x}$ in feature space is given by:

$$d_{F_\kappa}(\mathbf{x},\psi)^2 = \kappa(x,x) - 2\sum_{i=1}^{N}\kappa(x_i,x) + \sum_{i=1}^{N}\sum_{j=1}^{N}\alpha_i\alpha_j\kappa(x_i,x_j).$$

Now calculating the input space distances between the point of interest ψ and each reference point in some training data D_N via equation (8), we obtain a distance vector $d^2 = [d_1^2,...d_N^2]$ of size N.

This vector can be used to pose an optimization problem similar to the original MDS optimization problem:

$$z^* = \arg\min_{z \in \mathcal{Z}} \sum_{i=1}^{N}\left(d_{\mathcal{Z}}^2(z,x_i) - d_i^2\right)^2.$$

Unfortunately, this is as hard to optimize as optimizing the distance in feature space directly. However, considering the term $d_{\mathcal{Z}}^2(z^*,x_i) - d_i^2$, we see that:

$$d_{\mathcal{Z}}^2(z^*,x_i) - d_i^2 = x_i^\top x_i + z^{*\top}z^* - 2x_i^\top z^* - d_i^2,$$

and thus for the ideal case $d_Z^2(z^*, x_i) - d_i^2 = 0$, we obtain the identities

$$2x_i^\top z^* = x_i^\top x_i + z^{*\top} z^* - d_i^2, \text{for all } 1 \le i \le N. \tag{9}$$

Let us write all N equations in matrix form as:

$$2X^\top z^* = d_0^2 - d^2 + 1_N z^{*\top} z^*, \tag{10}$$

where $d_0^2 = \left[x_1^\top x_1, \dots, x_N^\top x_N \right]^N$ and $X = [x_1, \dots, x_N] \in \mathbb{R}^{d \times N}$, and $1_N = [1, \dots, 1] \in \mathbb{R}^d$. It seems that we did not gain anything since the desired and unknown pre-image z^* appears also on the right side. But note that from equation (10) and the definition of d_0, we can get yet another relationship:

$$z^{*\top} z^* = 2x_i^\top z^* + d_i^2 - d_{0_i}^2, \text{for all } 1 \le i \le N. \tag{11}$$

If we average both sides of equation (11) over all used N points and require that the points in D^N are centered, that is, $\sum_{i=1}^{N} x_i = 0$, we can rewrite the unknown quantity $z^{*\top} z^*$ as:

$$z^{*\top} z^* = \frac{1}{N} \sum_{i=1}^{N} 2x_i^\top z^* + d_i^2 - d_{0_i}^2 = \frac{1}{N} \sum_{i=1}^{N} (d_i^2 - d_{0_i}^2) + 2\frac{1}{N} \underbrace{\left[\sum_{i=1}^{N} x_i \right]^\top}_{=0} z^* = \frac{1}{N} \sum_{i=1}^{N} (d_i^2 - d_{0_i}^2),$$

and we obtain the new equation

$$2X^\top z^* = d_0^2 - d^2 + \frac{1}{N} 1_N 1_N^\top (d^2 - d_0^2). \tag{12}$$

The pre-image z^* can now be obtained by the least squares solution of equation (12):

$$z^* = \frac{1}{2}(XX^\top)^\dagger X (d_0^2 - d^2) + \frac{1}{N}(XX^\top)^\dagger X 1_N 1_N^\top (d^2 - d_0^2),$$

where $(XX^\top)^\dagger$ denotes the pseudo-inverse of $XX^\top$. Note that this can be simplified further because we required the N data points in D_N to be centered. Thus, the second term:

$$\frac{1}{2}(XX^\top)^{-1} X 1_N 1_N^\top (d^2 - d_0^2)$$

equals zero since $X 1_N = \sum_{i=1}^{N} x_i = 0$ by construction. Therefore, the optimal pre-image reconstruction is given by:

$$z^* = \frac{1}{2}\left(XX^\top\right)^\dagger X\left(d^2 - d_0^2\right).$$ (13)

Note that the nature of the kernel function entered only in the calculation of the input distance vector in d^2, thus in a similar manner, one can get pre-images for any kernel by replacing the calculation in equation (8). For example, for the polynomial kernel $\kappa(x_1, x_2) = \left(x_1^\top x_2\right)^q$, we would have:

$$d_Z^2(x, y) = \sqrt[q]{\kappa(x, y)} + \sqrt[q]{\kappa(y, y)} - 2\sqrt[q]{\kappa(x, y)}.$$ (14)

The MDS-based pre-image calculation was pioneered by Kwok and Tsang (2004), in which the original formulation required one to calculate a singular value decomposition of the data beforehand. This is indeed not necessary, and our introduced version is easier and faster.

MDS uses the distances to some other points as side information to reconstruct an approximate pre-image. Note that this generalizes the exact pre-image approach of equation (3): There, we were computing the dot product in the input domain from the dot product in the feature space (i.e., from the kernel), and reconstructing a pattern from these dot products.

The MDS method is noniterative in contrast to fixed-point methods but still needs to solve a least squares problem for each prediction. Furthermore, Kwok and Tsang (2004) suggested using only n nearest neighbors instead of all N points, which gives a further speedup. We give a summary of the MDS-based pre-image algorithm in A2.

Algorithm A2: Pre-image Calculation with Multidimensional Scaling.

Given data $D_N = \{x_i\}_{i=1}^N$, a feature map ϕ_κ from a kernel k, and n as the number of nearest neighbors in D_N of ψ:

1. Choose the n nearest neighbor coordinates $\{x_{i_1}, \ldots, x_{i_n}\}$ of ψ.
2. Center the nearest neighbors via:

$$\bar{x} = \sum_{i=1}^n x_i, \quad x_i = x_i - \bar{x} \text{ to ensure } \sum_{i=1}^n x_i \overset{!}{=} 0.$$

3. Calculate the Euclidean distances $d_{\mathcal{F}_k}(\phi(x_i), \psi)^2$ using equation (8).
4. Calculate the squared input space distance vector $d^2 = [d_1^2, \ldots, d_n^2]$.
5. Calculate the matrix $XX^\top$ of the nearest neighbors $X = \{x_{i_1}, \ldots, x_{i_n}\}$ and the squared input space norm vector $d_0 = \text{diag}\left(XX^\top\right)$.

The optimal pre-image z^* is given by $z^* = \frac{1}{2}\left(XX^\top\right)^\dagger X\left(d_0^2 - d^2\right) + \bar{x}.$ □

Pre-Images by Learning

Unfortunately, all techniques introduced so far suffer from one of the following points. They are:

- formulated as a difficult nonlinear optimization problem with local minima requiring restarts and other numerical issues,

- computationally inefficient, given that the problem is solved individually for each new point, and

- not the optimal approach depending on the task (e.g., we may be interested in minimizing a classification error rather then a distance in feature space).

Consider an application where we would like to use a pre-image technique. For each new presented point x, we have to solve a possibly nonconvex optimization problem. This is clearly a disadvantage since it does not allow the application of pre-image computation in a time-critical scenario. A further aspect shared by all the methods discussed so far is that they do not explicitly make use of the fact that we have labeled examples of the unknown pre-image map: Specifically, if we consider any point in $z^* \in \mathcal{Z}$, we know that the pre-image of is simply. It may not be the only pre-image, but this does not matter as long as it minimizes the value of Problem **P3**. Bakır et al. (2004) proposed a method that makes heavy use of this information and can resolve all the mentioned difficulties: The simple idea is to estimate a function Γ by learning the map $\psi \to z^*$ from examples $\{\phi_z(x_i), x_i\}_{i=1}^N$. Depending on the learning technique used, this means that after estimating the map Γ, each use of this map can be computed very efficiently since pre-image computation equals evaluating a (possibly nonlinear) function. Thus, there are no longer issues with complex optimization code during the testing phase. Note that this approach is unusual in that it is possible to produce an infinite amount of training data (and thus expect to get good performance on the set $\phi(\mathcal{Z})$ by generating points in $\mathcal{Z}$ and labeling them using the identity $\phi_z(z) = z$. Furthermore, it is often the case that we have knowledge about the distribution over the possible pre-images. For example, when denoising digits with kernel principal components analysis, one expects as a pre-image something that looks like a digit, and an estimate of this distribution is actually given by the original data. Taking this distribution into account, it is conceivable that a learning method could outperform the naive method, that of Problem **P3**, by producing pre-images that are subjectively preferable to the minimizers of Problem **P3**.

Details of the Learning Approach

We seek to estimate a function $\Gamma : F_\kappa \to \mathcal{Z}$ with the property that, at least approximately, $\Gamma(\phi_z(x_i)) \approx x_i$, $1 \leq i \leq N$. Assume now that the input $\mathcal{Z}$ is the d-dimensional real vector space $\mathbb{R}^d$. If we were to use regression using the kernel k corresponding to F_κ, then we would simply look for weight vectors $\mathbf{w}_j \in F_\kappa$, $j = 1,...,d$ such that $\Gamma_j(\psi) := \mathbf{w}_j^\top \psi$, and use the kernel trick to evaluate Γ. However, in general, we might want to use a *different* kernel κ, and thus we cannot perform our computations implicitly by the use of the original kernel function anymore. Fortunately, we can use the fact that although the mapped data may live in an infinite-dimensional space F_{κ}, any finite data set spans a subspace of the finite dimension. A convenient way of working in that subspace is to choose a basis and to work in coordinates $\mathbf{V}r$. This basis could be, for instance, obtained by kernel principal components analysis (kPCA). Let $R_N = [\gamma_1,...,\gamma_N] \in \mathbb{R}^{r \times N}$ denote the coordinate matrix of the data D_N with regard to the orthogonal basis $\mathbf{V}_r$. Given $\mathbf{V}_r$, we can decompose Γ into the concatenation of $\hat{\Gamma} : \mathbb{R}^r \to \mathbb{R}^d$ and $\mathbf{V}_r$, such that $z^* = \Gamma(\psi) = \hat{\Gamma}\left(\mathbf{V}_r^\top \psi\right)$. Note that the task is now to find the pre-image map $\hat{\Gamma}_j : \mathbb{R}^r \to \mathbb{R}$, $j = 1...d$ from feature space coordinates $\mathbf{V}_r^\top \psi \in \mathbb{R}^r$ to the input space $\mathbb{R}^d$. This is a standard regression problem for the N training points x_i. Thus, we can use any arbitrary regression method, for example, kernel ridge regression with a kernel κ_2 different from the kernel κ. The map $\hat{\Gamma}_j$ would be then completely given once the ridge regression weights $\{\beta_1,...\beta_d\} \in \mathbb{R}^{N \times d}$ are specified. To find the regression coefficients in ridge regression, we would have to solve the following optimization problem:

$$\beta_j = \arg\min_{\beta \in \mathbb{R}^N} \sum_{i=1}^{N} \mathrm{L}\left(x_i^j, \Gamma_j\left(x_i \mid \beta^j\right)\right) + \lambda \parallel \beta^j \parallel^2.$$

Here, L denotes some loss function used for pre-image learning and λ denotes the ridge parameter. Let us give a detailed example.

Example 1: Pre-Image Map for the Squared Reconstruction Error. *Consider the estimation of the reconstruction map for the squared reconstruction error* $\parallel x - \Gamma(\phi(x)) \parallel^2$. *A nonlinear map from feature space coordinates* $\mathbf{V_r}^\top \phi(x)$ *to the ith input dimension Z can be obtained by collecting all ith dimensions of all patterns in D_N. Thus, we obtain a vector $y \in \mathbb{R}^N$ where the ith entry of y contains the jth entry of the sample $x_i \in D_N$, that is, $y_i = x_i^j$. The coefficients β_j can now be obtained by:*

$$\beta_j = \arg\min \sum_{i=1}^{N}\left(y_i - \sum_{s=1}^{N}\beta_j^s \kappa\left(\mathbf{V}_r^\top \phi(x_i), \mathbf{V}_r^\top \phi_\kappa(x_s)\right)\right)^2 + \lambda \parallel \beta_i \parallel^2.$$

The optimal coefficient vector β_j is obtained by $\beta_j = (\mathbf{K}+\lambda\mathbf{I})^{-1}y$, where $\mathbf{K} = [\kappa(\mathbf{V}_r^\top\phi(x_s), \mathbf{V}_r^\top\phi(x_t))]_{s,t}$ and $1 \leq s, t \leq N$ denotes the kernel matrix on D_N with kernel κ. Given some coordinates $\mathbf{V}_r^\top \psi$, the i-th entry of the pre-image z^* can now be predicted as:

$$z^{*i} = \sum_{j=1}^{N}\beta_i^j y_j \kappa(\mathbf{V}_r^\top\phi(x_j), \mathbf{V}_r^\top \psi).$$

Note that the general learning setup allows for using any suitable loss function, incorporating invariances and a priori knowledge. For example, if the pre-images are (natural) images, a psychophysically motivated loss function such as in Gutiérrez, Gómez-Perez, Malo, and Camps-Valls (Chapter XIII) and Malo, Epifanio, Navarro, and Simoncelli (2006) could be used that would allow the algorithm to ignore differences that cannot be perceived. Note that the learning-based pre-image algorithm requires additional data to learn the reconstruction map similar to MDS and the fixed-point pre-image method. However, this is the only method that does not need any optimization during a testing stage and that has an adaptable loss function.

Pre-Images Using A Priori Information

The definition of the pre-image Problem **P3** can be reformulated in a probabilistic setting such that prior information can be incorporated. Assume that we are given a distribution $P(x)$, which gives high probability to patterns x, which we assume to be likely. Given this prior distribution, we can reformulate Problem **P3** in a probabilistic way as:

$$z^* = \arg\max_{x \in Z} \ P(\psi \mid \phi_z(x)) \cdot P(x). \tag{15}$$

Here we choose our likelihood function $P(\psi \mid \phi_z(x))$ to be a Gaussian using the Euclidian distance between the pre-image and the point ψ in feature space, that is:

$$P(\psi \mid \phi_z(x)) = \exp^{-\frac{1}{2\sigma^2}\|\phi_z(x)-\psi\|^2}.$$

The best pre-image could then be found by minimizing the negative **log** of the probability on the right hand side of equation (15). This would yield the new optimization problem:

$$z^* = \text{argmin}_{x \in Z} \left(\|\ \phi_z(x) - \psi\ \|^2_{F_\kappa} - 2\sigma^2 \log P(x) \right). \tag{16}$$

In the simplest case, we know a priori that the solution should be close to a single prototype x^*. In this case, we can set the prior distribution function to be Gaussian using the Euclidian distance in the input space. Thus, our new approximate pre-image problem assuming a Gaussian uncertainty model in the input and output space follows:

$$z^* = \arg\min_{x \in Z} \left(\|\ \phi_z(x) - \psi\ \|^2_{F_\kappa} + \lambda\ \|\ x - x^*\ \|^2 \right). \tag{17}$$

The influence of the a priori knowledge can be controlled via the scalar weight λ.

Applications: Pre-Images for Signal Enhancement

In the following experiment, we will demonstrate the use of pre-image techniques for the case of image denoising, which aims to reduce the amount of noise in an image. Image denoising is mostly a necessary postprocessing step in imaging since noise is simply om-nipresent when working with typical imaging devices. For example, a camera must use a finite exposure time that introduces stochastic noise due to the random arrival of photons. Further noise can be introduced by instrumentation noise and/or communication errors and compression. Thus, in a typical camera recorded image, there exist various noise sources of different nature. These different noises can be modeled as additive and multiplicative mathematical operations. Assume that the true image pixel $\bar{x}_{ij}$ is corrupted by the noise term η. Then, we finally observe the corrupted image pixel x_{ij} as $x_{ij} = \bar{x}_{ij} + \eta$ and/or $x_{ij} = \bar{x}_{ij}\eta$ per pixel. Classical denoising methods build an explicit probabilistic model of the image and aim to denoise by, for example, Bayesian inference. For the application of such meth-ods, see, for example, Simoncelli and Adelson (1996) and Portilla, Strela, Wainwright, and Simoncelli (2003). In contrast to these parametric methods, nonparametric methods aim to build a statistical model of the image by considering special features extracted from the image. The simplest features one can extract are image patches and for our discussion we will restrict ourselves to these.

One approach for image denoising is kernel principal components analysis denoising, where one first represents each image patch x by its principal components $v_i \in F_k$ in some feature space F_κ, that is:

$$\phi(x) = \sum_{i=1}^{N} \phi(x)^\top v_i v_{i.}$$ (18)

If we assume that the noise only contaminates kernel principal components corresponding to small eigenvalues, denoising can be achieved by truncation of the kernel principal com-ponents analysis representation in equation (17), that is:

$$\psi = \sum_{i=1}^{M} \psi^\top v_i v_i,$$

with $M < N$. However, since this truncated representation is an element of the feature space F_κ we need to calculate the pre-image of ψ to retrieve the denoised image patch. For details on kernel principal components analysis and its interpretations, see Schölkopf, Smola, and Müller (1998).

We will follow the experimental setting described in Kim et al. (2005), which used the MDS approach to get a pre-image that was then used as the initialization for the gradient-descent pre-image computation. In contrast, we will only use a single-step pre-image computation to compare our introduced pre-image techniques. Kernel principal components analysis parameters are chosen as in Kim et al. (2005).

All experiments were performed using the Lena image, which is a standard image-processing test image. In our experiment, we used a 200x200 sized window showing the face of Lena only. We added two types of noise (first additive and then multiplicative) to the original Lena image and obtain a new noise-corrupted image with a signal-to-noise ratio of 1.37dB (see Figure 3).

For denoising, we randomly extract 1,000 patches $x_i \in \mathbb{R}^{10 \times 10}, 1 \leq i \leq 1000$ and express

Figure 3. The original Lena image and the corrupted noisy image with an SNR 1.37dB

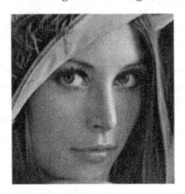 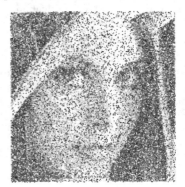

them by their kernel principal components. For each patch x_i, this leads to a 1,000-dimensional feature vector where feature j describes the coordinate of x_i regarding v_j. We will report, if possible, the reconstruction of patches using 2, 5, and 10 kernel principal components.[2] Reconstructed patches are averaged whenever they overlap. All experiments are done in MATLAB on a 2.2 Ghz Pentium 4 processor with 1 GB RAM using the SPIDER[3] machine learning library for kernel methods.

A1: The Fixed-Point Algorithm

For the fixed-point algorithm, we only report the reconstruction using 10 kernel principal components. Since the fixed-point algorithm can get stuck, we have to perform multiple restarts. To this end, we perform two experiments with different numbers of restarts and report the result in Figure 4. In the first experiment (Figure 4, left), we have used a randomly

Figure 4. Denoising using the fixed-point algorithm with 5 restarts (left, SNR 2.52 dB) and 50 restarts (right, SNR 7.93 dB)

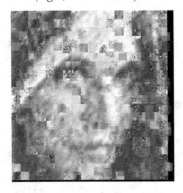 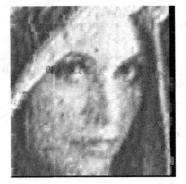

selected patch of the noisy image as a starting point. The final pre-image is then the best of five trials. Note that using the fixed-point algorithm, the number of trials is crucial for the quality of the pre-image. This yields a reconstruction with SNR 2.52 dB and took overall 141 seconds.

As one can see, the denoising still has a lot of artefacts. A repetition of the experiment with 50 restarts led to a more successful pre-image computation and better SNR rate of 7.93 dB. Unfortunately, the pre-image computation time now took $18.75 \cdot 10^3$ seconds, thus over a factor of 100 longer.

A2: The MDS Algorithm

The advantage of the MDS approach is that it uses only standard linear algebra for pre-image computation. As suggested by Kwok and Tsang (2004), we use a fraction of all available patches for pre-image computation. In our experiments, we have used five nearest neighbors. Thus, in a first step, the MDS algorithm requires us to search five nearest neighbors for each patch to denoise. This is effectively as expensive as sorting an array, that is, O(N log N). Since we have 1,000 patches to choose from, we have $N = 1,000$. After this step, we have to effectively invert a 5×5 matrix for each patch. Thus, the complexity of the MDS approach is effectively $O(N^2 \log N + Nk^3)$, where k equals 5 in our case. If k is small then one can expect MDS to be quite fast. Indeed, in our case, we yield an average run time of 40 seconds for each of the three denoising experiments. The resulting pre-images are shown in Figure 5. As one can see, the denoising performance is quite acceptable for 5 (Figure 5, middle) and 10 (Figure 5, right) principal components (SNR 5.37 dB and 6.22 dB). Using only two principal components (Figure 5, left) leads already to an increase of the SNR to 3.11 dB.

Better pre-images are possible as we have seen from the previous denoising experiments using the fixed-point algorithm. However, the MDS approach is appealing since it gives fast initial starting values for a postprocessing based on pure optimization. This was the strategy performed in Kim et al. (2005).

Finally we can speculate about why any improvement is possible at all. Note that the MDS algorithm assumes distances in the feature space to be related to the distances in the input space. This assumption does not need to hold for arbitrary pre-image settings, and a possible increase of the pre-image quality seems to be due to this restriction.

Figure 5. Denoising using the MDS algorithm and using different numbers of kernel principal components (left, SNR 3.11 dB; middle, SNR 5.37 dB; right, SNR 6.22 dB).

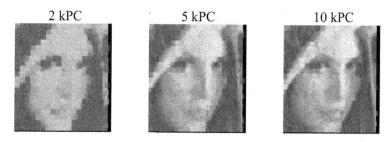

| 2 kPC | 5 kPC | 10 kPC |

Figure 6. Denoising using the learning algorithm and using different numbers of kernel principal components (left, SNR 3.9 dB; middle, 6.78 dB; right, 8.60 dB)

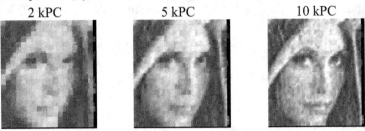

A3: The Learning Approach

For the learning approach, we perform kernel ridge regression as explained in example 1 using the squared loss function. Thus, we build a regression model Γ that maps a feature vector to the grayscale pixel values. Note that using a squared loss, we explicitly train the model to perform predictions that are expected to maximize the signal-to-noise ratio. To apply kernel ridge regression, we have to choose a kernel function with kernel parameter σ and a ridge parameter λ. As a kernel function, we choose the Gaussian kernel with kernel parameter σ. The model parameters (σ and λ) were chosen by a five-fold cross-validation on the grid $(\lambda, \sigma) \in [10^{-8}, 10^{-7}, ..., 10^{-2}] \times [0.5, 1, 5]$ using 500 randomly selected patches from the noisy image.

As we can see in Figure 6, the pre-images found by prediction perform consistently better than the MDS approach and better than the optimization-based approach. Furthermore, the evaluation's overall run time was on average 29 seconds (including cross-validation and training). In general, the learning-based approach is very well suited if one has to repeatedly perform pre-image computation since the most time-expensive operation is searching for parameters and training the model. Once the model is taught, the complexity of finding a single pre-image is linear in the number of training patterns (in our case it equals evaluating a kernel expansion). On the other hand, this can be a drawback if the size of the training data set is large and one is only interested in evaluating the model once.

Conclusion and Outlook

The pre-image problem in kernel methods deals with the problem of pattern reconstruction from their feature space representation. In this chapter we have discussed different algorithms for pre-image computation when the input patterns are elements of some vector space. As a conclusion, we saw that algorithms that are based on optimization such as the fixed-point algorithm place the smallest number of assumptions into the pre-image reconstruction, but on the other hand, they are computationally the most demanding ones. In contrast, algorithms that explicitly use side information, such as the MDS method and the learning-based technique, are often substantially faster for pre-image computation. Learning-based techniques are especially interesting for applications where one has to repeatedly compute pre-images. In such a situation learning-based techniques build a model of the pre-image map in a training phase that then can be repeatedly used for pre-image computation by evaluating a map. Using kernel techniques to learn the pre-image map results in pre-images that can be computed in linear time. In the experiments section, we also showed that if we know the criteria to judge the quality of the pre-image beforehand, we can use learning to build models that are optimized for the criteria at hand. We gave an example based on the signal-to-noise ratio for images that corresponds to using a squared loss for image comparison. In this case, we showed empirically that using a least squares regression technique for learning a pre-image map leads to better results than the general assumptions encoded in the MDS algorithm.

Future research will cover the design of techniques that integrate prior knowledge and the use of specialized application-dependent loss functions for learning pre-image models. For example, including additional statistical or perceptual information in the signal enhancement task might be done by a loss function that exploits the local frequency domain.

References

Bakır, G., Weston, J., & Schölkopf, B. (2004). Learning to find pre-images. *Advances in Neural Information Processing Systems, 16*, 449-456.

Bakır, G., Zien, A., & Tsuda, K. (2004). Learning to find graph pre-images. Pattern Recognition: *In Proceedings of the 26th DAGM Symposium*, 253-261.

Burges, C. J. C. (1996). Simplified support vector decision rules. In *Proceedings of the 13th International Conference on Machine Learning*, 71-77.

Fletcher, R. (1987). *Practical methods of optimization.* Wiley.

Kwang. (2005). Iterative kernel principal component analysis for image modeling. *IEEE Transactions on Pattern Analysis and Machine Intelligence, 27*(9), 1351-1366.

Kwok, J. T., & Tsang, I. W. (2004). The pre-image problem in kernel methods. *IEEE Transactions on Neural Networks, 15*(6), 1517-1525.

Malo, J., Epifanio, I., Navarro, R., & Simoncelli, E. P. (2006). Non-linear image representation for efficient perceptual coding. *IEEE Transactions of Image Processing, 15*(1).

Mika, S., Schölkopf, B., Smola, A. J., Müller, K.-R., Scholz, M., & Rätsch, G. (1999). Kernel PCA and de-noising in feature spaces. *Advances in Neural Information Processing Systems, 11*, 536-542.

Portilla, V., Strela , M., Wainwright, E. P., & Simoncelli. (2003). Image denoising using scale mixtures of Gaussians in the wavelet domain. *IEEE Transactions on Image Processing, 12*(11), 1338-1351.

Schölkopf, B., & Smola, A. (2002). *Learning with kernels.* Cambridge, MA: MIT Press.

Schölkopf, B., Smola, A., Knirsch, P., & Burges, C. (1998). Fast approximation of support vector kernel expansions, and an interpretation of clustering as approximation in feature spaces. In *Proceedings of the 20ᵗʰ DAGM-Symposium*, 125-132.

Schölkopf, B., Smola, A., & Müller, K.-R. (1998). Nonlinear component analysis as a kernel eigenvalue problem. *Neural Computation, 10*, 1299-1319.

Simoncelli, E. P., & Adelson, E. H. (1996). Noise removal via Bayesian wavelet coring. In *Proceedings of the 3ʳᵈ International Conference on Image Processing*, 379-382.

Vogel, C. R. (2002). *Computational methods for inverse problems*. Philadelphia: Society for Industrial & Applied Mathematics (SIAM).

Weston, J., Chapelle, O., Elisseeff, A., Schölkopf, B., & Vapnik, V. (2003). Kernel dependency estimation. *Advances in Neural Information Processing Systems, 15*.

Endnotes

[1] $\left\| \varphi_\kappa(z) \right\| = \sqrt{\kappa(z,z)} = 1$ by construction.

[2]   Note that Kim et al. (2005) were using larger numbers of components in their experiments.

[3]   http://www.kyb.tuebingen.mpg.de/bs/people/spider/

Chapter XIII

Perceptual Image Representations for Support Vector Machine Image Coding

Juan Gutiérrez, Universitat de València, Spain

Gabriel Gómez-Perez, Universitat de València, Spain

Jesús Malo, Universitat de València, Spain

Gustavo Camps-Valls, Universitat de València, Spain

Abstract

Support vector machine (SVM) image coding relies on the ability of SVMs for function approximation. The size and the profile of the ε-insensitivity zone of the support vector regression (SVR) at some specific image representation determines (a) the amount of selected support vectors (the compression ratio), and (b) the nature of the introduced error (the compression distortion). However, the selection of an appropriate image representation is a key issue for a meaningful design of the ε-insensitivity profile. For example, in image coding applications, taking human perception into account is of paramount relevance to obtain a good rate-distortion performance. However, depending on the accuracy of the considered perception model, certain image representations are not suitable for SVR training.

In this chapter, we analyze the general procedure to take human vision models into account in SVR-based image coding. Specifically, we derive the condition for image representation selection and the associated ε-insensitivity profiles.

Introduction

Nowadays, the volume of imaging data increases exponentially in a very wide variety of applications, such as remote sensing, digital and video camera design, medical imaging, digital libraries and documents, movies, and videoconferences. This poses several problems and needs for transmitting, storing, and retrieving images. As a consequence, digital image compression is becoming a crucial technology. However, compressing an image is significantly different than compressing raw binary data given their particular statistical properties, and thus the application of general-purpose compression methods would be far from optimal. Therefore, statistical knowledge about the problem becomes extremely important to develop efficient coding schemes. Another critical issue in visual communications to be judged by human observers is introducing perception models in the algorithm design procedure.

The efficient encoding of images relies on understanding two fundamental quantities, commonly known as *rate* and *distortion*. The rate expresses the cost of the encoding (typically in bits) and the distortion expresses how closely the decoded signal approximates the original image. Extensive literature has shown that the problem can be made much more tractable by transforming the image from an array of pixels into a new representation in which rate or distortion are more easily quantified and controlled. In this framework, the goal of the transform is removing the statistical (Gersho & Gray, 1992) and perceptual (Epifanio, Gutiérrez, & Malo, 2003; Malo, Epifanio, Navarro, & Simoncelli, 2006) dependence between the coefficients of the new representation in order to allow an efficient scalar quantization and zero-order entropy coding of the samples. To this end, the current transform coding standards, JPEG and JPEG2000 (Wallace, 1991; Taubman & Marcellin, 2001), use fixed-basis linear transforms (2-D block discrete cosine transform [DCT] or wavelets), which are similar to adaptive linear transforms that remove second-order or higher order statistical relations of natural image samples (principal components analysis, PCA, and ICA; Hyvarinen, Karhunen, & Oja, 2001), and resemble the first linear stage in human perception models (A. Watson & Solomon, 1997). However, natural images are not that simple as a Gaussian process (fully described by its PCA components) or a linear superposition of independent patterns (the basic assumption in ICA). In fact, significant relations between the energy of the transform coefficients remain in the linear domains that are widely used for transform coding or denoising (Buccigrossi & Simoncelli, 1999; Gutiérrez, Ferri, & Malo, 2006; Malo et al., 2006). Besides this, masking experiments reveal that linear local frequency basis functions are not perceptually independent either (A. Watson & Solomon, 1997). Recent results confirm the link between human perception and statistics of natural images in this context. The statistical effect of the current cortical vision mechanisms suggests that the use of these biological image representations is highly convenient to reduce the statistical and the perceptual dependence of the image samples at the same time (Epifanio et al.; Malo et al.). These results are consistent with the literature that seeks for statistical explanations of the cortical sensors' organization (Barlow, 2001; Malo & Gutiérrez, 2006; Simoncelli, 2003).

These statistical and perceptual results suggest that achieving the desired independence necessarily requires the introduction of nonlinearities after the commonly used linear image representations *prior* to their scalar quantization. Recently, two different nonlinear approaches have been used to improve the results of image-coding schemes based on linear transforms and linear perception models. On one hand, more accurate nonlinear perception models have been applied after the linear transform for image representation (Malo et al., 2006). On the other hand, support vector machine (SVM) learning has been used for nonlinear feature selection in the linear local DCT representation domain (Gómez-Pérez, Camps-Valls, Gutiérrez, & Malo, 2005; Robinson & Kecman, 2003). Both methodologies will be jointly exploited and analyzed in this chapter.

The rationale to apply the support vector regressor (SVR) in image-coding applications is taking advantage of the sparsity property of this function approximation tools. This is carried out by using tunable ε-insensitivities to select relevant training samples, thus representing the signal with a small number of support vectors while restricting the error below the ε bounds. Therefore, an appropriate ε-insensitivity profile is useful to (a) discard statistically redundant samples, and (b) restrict the perceptual error introduced in the approximated signal. Therefore, the choice of the domain for ε-insensitivity design is a key issue in this application.

The use of SVMs for image compression was originally presented in Robinson and Kecman (2000), where the authors used the standard ε-insensitive SVR (Smola & Schölkopf, 2004) to learn the image gray levels in the spatial domain. A constant insensitivity zone per sample is reasonable in the spatial domain because of the approximate stationary behavior of the luminance samples of natural images. However, these samples are strongly coupled both from the statistical and the perceptual points of view. First, there is a strong *statistical correlation* between neighboring luminance values in the spatial domain, and second, coding errors independently introduced in this domain are *quite visible* on top of a highly correlated background. These are the basic reasons to make the promising SVR approach inefficient in this domain.

The formulation of SVRs in the local DCT domain was fundamental to achieve the first competitive results (Robinson & Kecman, 2003). In this case, Robinson and Kecman also used a constant ε-insensitivity, but according to a qualitative human-vision-based reasoning, they *a priori* discarded the high-frequency coefficients in the SVR training. This is equivalent to using a variable ε-insensitivity profile: a finite value for the low-frequency samples and an infinite value for the high-frequency samples. This heuristic makes statistical and perceptual sense since the variance of the local frequency samples is concentrated in the low-frequency coefficients and the visibility of these patterns is larger. Therefore, it is appropriate to ensure a limited error in the low-frequency region while allowing more distortion in the high-frequency region.

However, the qualitative ideal low-pass ε-insensitivity profile in Robinson and Kecman (2003) can be improved by using a rigorous formulation for the ε-insensitivity design. Specifically, the ε-insensitivity in a given image representation domain has to be constructed to restrict the maximum perceptual error (MPE) in a perceptually Euclidean domain. This MPE restriction idea is the key issue for the good subjective performance of the quantizers used in the JPEG and JPEG2000 standards (Wallace, 1991; Zeng, Daly, & Lei, 2002), as pointed out in Malo et al. (2006) and Navarro, Gutiérrez, and Malo (2005).

In Camps-Valls et al. (2006) and Gomez et al. (2005), the MPE restriction procedure was applied using different perception models to obtain the appropriate ε-insensitivity, which may be constant or variable (Camps-Valls, Soria-Olivas, Pérez-Ruixo, Artés-Rodriguez, Pérez-Cruz, & Figueiras-Vidal, 2001). However, it is worth noting that depending on the accuracy of the considered perception model, certain image representations are not suitable for SVR training.

In this chapter, we analyze the general procedure to take human vision models into account in SVR-based image-coding schemes. Specifically, we derive the condition for image representation selection and the associated ε-insensitivity profiles.

The structure of the chapter is as follows. The next section motivates the need for considering human perception in dealing with the coding noise, which poses the problem of a proper (perceptually meaningful) transformation. Then we review the computational models that account for the effects shown in the previous section. Next, the chapter formulates the problem of the design and application of suitable insensitivity profiles for SVM training that give rise to perceptually acceptable distortions. Finally, we show some experimental results on benchmark images, and then end this chapter with some conclusions and further work.

Visibility of Noise

The distortion introduced in SVM-based image coding is due to the approximation error given by the use of a limited number of support vectors. However, the qualitative nature of this distortion strongly depends on the image-representation domain and on the insensitivity profile used to select support vectors.

In this section, we show that the visibility of some distortion not only depends on the energy of the noise (mean squared error, MSE, and PSNR), but also on its frequency nature and on the background signal. Figure 1 summarizes the effects reported in the perception literature (Campbell and Robson, 1968; Heeger, 1992; A. Watson & Solomon, 1997), namely, *frequency sensitivity and masking*, that will determine the appropriate image-representation domain and insensitivity profiles for SVM training. The issue of selecting an appropriate domain of image representation is an important concern in other domains of vision computing and image processing (see Chapters XII and XIV in this book).

In this example, equal-energy random noise of different frequency bands and horizontal orientation has been added on top of three different background images: two synthetic images and one natural image. The synthetic images consist of patches of periodic functions of different frequency bands (3 cpd, 6 cpd, 12 cpd, and 24 cpd) and different orientations (horizontal, vertical, and diagonal). The two synthetic background images (first and second rows) differ in their energy (contrast or amplitude of the periodic functions). Several conclusions can be extracted from Figure 1.

1. **Mean squared error is not perceptually meaningful:** A remarkable fact is that the energy of the noise (or the MSE) does not correlate with the visibility of the noise at all (Girod, 1993; Malo, Pons, & Artigas, 1997; Pons, Malo, Artigas, & Capilla, 1999; Teo & Heeger, 1994).

Figure 1. Equal-energy noise of different-frequency content—3 cpd, 6 cpd, 12 cpd, and 24 cpd—shown on top of different backgrounds. All images have the same MSE distance with regard to the corresponding original image, but the visibility of the noise is quite different.

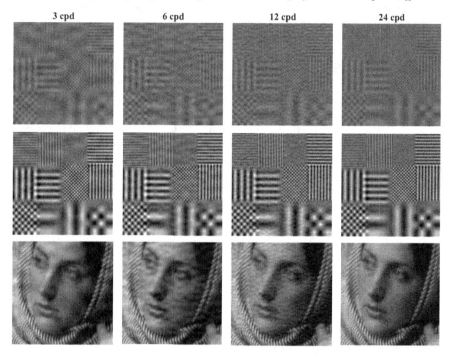

2. **Frequency selectivity:** Noise visibility strongly depends on its frequency nature: low-frequency and high-frequency noise are less visible in all cases. This is because human perception is mediated by frequency analyzers that have different sensitivity. Therefore, more noise (larger SVM insensitivity) will be perceptually acceptable in different frequency bands.

3. **Automasking:** For a given noise frequency (for a given column in Figure 1), noise visibility decreases with the energy of the background signal: The same distortion is less visible in high-contrast backgrounds. This is because the perceptual frequency analyzers are nonlinear; their slope (sensitivity) is bigger for low-contrast signals while it is smaller for high-contrast signals. This phenomenon is usually referred to as masking since a high-contrast signal masks the distortion because it saturates the response of the frequency analyzers. Therefore, more noise (larger SVM insensitivity) will be perceptually acceptable in high-contrast regions.

4. **Cross-masking:** Note however, that for the same noise frequency and background signal contrast (within every specific image in Figure 1), noise visibility depends on the similarity between signal and distortion. Low-frequency noise is more visible in high-frequency backgrounds than in low-frequency backgrounds (e.g., left figure of second row). In the same way, high-frequency noise is more visible in low-frequency

backgrounds than in high-frequency backgrounds (e.g., right image of the second row). That is, some signal of a specific frequency strongly masks the corresponding frequency analyzer, but it induces a smaller sensitivity reduction in the analyzers tuned to different frequencies. Besides that, the reduction in sensitivity of a specific analyzer is larger as the distance between the background frequency and the frequency of the analyzer is smaller. For instance, in the left image of the second row, the visibility of the low-frequency noise (sensitivity of the perceptual low-frequency analyzer) is small in the low-frequency regions (that mask this sensor) but progressively increases as the frequency of the background increases. This is because the response of each frequency analyzer not only depends on the energy of the signal for that frequency band, but also on the energy of the signal in other frequency bands (cross-masking). This implies that a different amount of noise (different SVM insensitivity) in each frequency band may be acceptable depending on the energy of that frequency band and on the energy of neighboring bands.

According to these perception properties, an input dependent ε-insensitivity in a local frequency domain is required.

Linear and Nonlinear Perception Models

The general model of early visual (cortical) processing that accounts for the previously described effects includes a linear local frequency transform, T, followed by a response transform, R (A. Watson & Solomon, 1997):

$$A \xrightarrow{\quad T \quad} y \xrightarrow{\quad R \quad} r, \tag{1}$$

where in the first stage, each spatial region A of size $N \times N$ is analyzed by a filter bank, T, for example, a set of local (block) DCT basis functions. This filter bank gives rise to a vector, $y \in \mathbb{R}^{N^2}$, whose elements y_j represent the local frequency content of the signal in that spatial region (or block). The second stage, R, accounts for the different linear (or eventually nonlinear) responses of the local frequency analyzers of the first stage.

The last image representation domain, $r \in \mathbb{R}^{N^2}$, is assumed to be perceptually Euclidean (Legge, 1981; Pons et al., 1999; Teo & Heeger, 1994; A. Watson & Solomon, 1997); that is, the distortion in any component, Δr_j, is equally relevant from the perceptual point of view. This implies that the perceptual geometry of other image representations is not Euclidean, but depends on the Jacobian of the response model ∇R (Epifanio et al., 2003; Malo et al., 2006). As it will be shown in the next section, this geometric fact is the key issue to select the representation domain and the ε-insensitivity profile for perceptually efficient SVM training.

Given the first linear filter-bank stage T, different response models have been proposed for the second stage R to account for the perception effects illustrated in Figure 2, either linear or nonlinear. In the following sections, we will first review the functional form of the model and its Jacobian. Afterward, we will show that given the shape of the responses, different amounts of noise, Δy_f, are needed to obtain the same subjective distortion, thus explaining the effects described in the previous section.

Linear, Frequency-Dependent Response

In the linear model approach, each mechanism of the filter bank has a different (but constant) gain depending on its frequency:

$$r_f = \alpha_f \cdot y_f \tag{2}$$

This linear, frequency-dependent gain is given by the contrast sensitivity function (CSF; see Figure 2; Campbell & Robson, 1968).

In this case, the Jacobian of the response is a constant diagonal matrix with the CSF values on the diagonal:

$$\nabla R_{ff'} = \alpha_f \, \delta_{ff'}. \tag{3}$$

Figure 3 shows the response of two linear mechanisms tuned to different frequencies as a function of the energy (or contrast) of the stimuli of these frequencies (Peli, 1990). This linear response model accounts for the general frequency-dependent visibility of the noise shown in Figure 1: The larger the slope of the response of a mechanism tuned to a specific

Figure 2. Frequency-dependent linear gain, α_f, of the CSF model

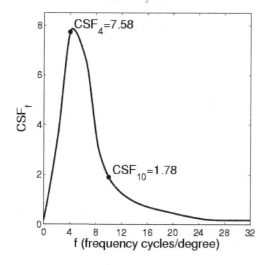

frequency, f, the smaller the distortion Δy_f needed to give rise to the same perceptual distortion $\Delta r_f = \tau$. According to the CSF, the visibility of medium frequencies is larger than the visibility of very low and high frequencies.

However, this linear model is too simple to account for masking: Note that the slope of the responses (the sensitivity of the mechanisms) is constant, so the same signal distortion on top of a signal of larger energy (or contrast) generates the same perceptual distortion. This problem can be alleviated by introducing more sophisticated (nonlinear) response models.

Nonlinear Response: Adaptive Gain Control or Divisive Normalization

The current response model for the cortical frequency analyzers is nonlinear (Heeger, 1992; A. Watson & Solomon, 1997). The outputs of the filters of the first linear stage undergo a nonlinear transform in which the energy of each linear coefficient (already weighted by a CSF-like function) is normalized by a combination of the energies of the neighboring coefficients in frequency:

$$r_f = \frac{\text{sgn}(y_f) \cdot |\alpha_f \cdot y_f|^\gamma}{\beta_f + \sum_{f'=1}^{N^2} h_{ff'} |\alpha_{f'} \cdot y_{f'}|^\gamma}, \tag{4}$$

where $h_{ff'}$ determines the interaction neighborhood in the nonlinear normalization of the energy, which is assumed to be Gaussian (A. Watson & Solomon, 1997), and

Figure 3. Responses and associated visibility thresholds of the two sensors whose slopes have been highlighted in Figure 2. The Euclidean nature of the response domain implies that two distortions, Δy_f and $\Delta y_{f'}$, induce perceptually equivalent effects if the corresponding variations in the response are the same: $\Delta r_f = \Delta r_{f'} = \tau$.

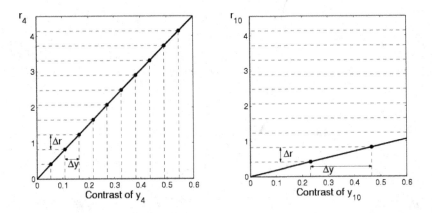

Figure 4. Parameters α and β and three frequency interaction neighborhoods (rows of h) in equation (4). The different line styles represent different frequencies: 4 cpd (solid), 10 cpd (dashed), and 18 cpd (dash-dot).

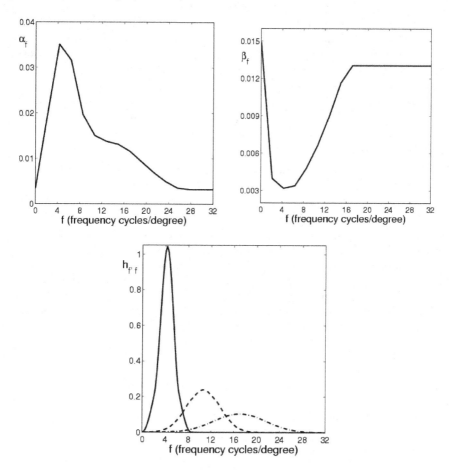

$$h_{ff'} = K_f \cdot \exp(-\|f - f'\|^2 / \sigma_{|f|}^2), \qquad\qquad (5)$$

where $\sigma_{|f|} = \frac{1}{6} |f| + 0.05$ and $|f|$ is given in cpd. See Figure 4 for the parameters in equations (4) and (5).

In this case, the Jacobian of the response is input dependent and nondiagonal:

$$\nabla R(y)_{ff'} = \mathrm{sgn}(y_f)\gamma \left(\frac{|\alpha_f \cdot y_f|^{\gamma-1}}{\beta_f + \sum_{f'=1}^{N^2} h_{ff'} |\alpha_{f'} \cdot y_{f'}|^{\gamma}} \delta_{ff'} - \frac{|\alpha_f \cdot y_f|^{\gamma}|\alpha_{f'} \cdot y_{f'}|^{\gamma-1}}{(\beta_f + \sum_{j=1}^{N^2} h_{ff'} |\alpha_{f'} \cdot y_{f'}|^{\gamma})^2} \cdot h_{ff'} \right). \qquad (6)$$

Figures 5 and 6 show examples of the response of two nonlinear mechanisms tuned to different frequencies as a function of the energy (or contrast) of stimuli of these frequencies in different masking conditions. In the first case (Figure 5), an automasking situation is considered; that is, this figure shows the response r_4 (or r_{10}) as a function of y_4 (or y_{10}) when all the other mechanisms are not stimulated, that is, $y_{f'} = 0$, $\forall f' \neq 4$ (or $\forall f' \neq 10$). In the second case (Figure 6), this automasking response is compared with the (cross-masking) response obtained when showing the optimal stimulus (y_4 or y_{10}) on top of another pattern that generates $y_6 \neq 0$.

This more elaborated response model also accounts for the frequency-dependent visibility of distortions: Note that the slope is larger for 4 cpd than for 10 cpd, thus a larger amount of distortion is required in 10 cpd to obtain the same perceived distortion. Equivalently, 4 cpd of noise is more visible than 10 cpd of noise of the same energy. This general behavior is given by the band-pass function α_f.

Moreover, it also accounts for automasking since the amount of distortion needed to obtain a constant perceptual distortion increases with the contrast of the input (see Figure 5). This is due to the fact that the response is attenuated when increasing the contrast because of the normalization term in the denominator of equation (4).

It also accounts for cross-masking since this attenuation (and the corresponding response saturation and sensitivity decrease) also occurs when other patterns $y_{f'}$ with $f' \neq f$ are present. Note how in Figure 5 the required amount of distortion increases as the contrast of the mask of different frequency is increased. Moreover, given the Gaussian shape of the interaction neighborhood, patterns of closer frequencies mask the distortion more effectively than background patterns of very different frequency. This is why the 6 cpd mask induces a larger variation of the acceptable noise in 4 cpd than in 10 cpd.

Figure 5. Responses and associated visibility thresholds of the two sensors tuned to frequencies 4 and 10 cpd in automasking (zero background) conditions. The required amount of distortion Δy_f to obtain some specific distortion in the response domain τ is shown for different contrasts of the input pattern.

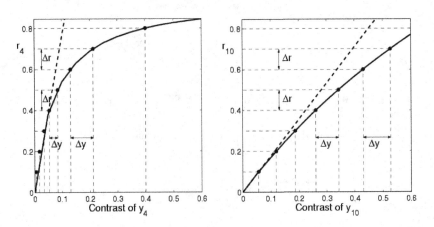

Figure 6. Responses and associated visibility thresholds of the two sensors tuned to frequencies 4 and 10 cpd when masked by a pattern of different frequency (6 cpd) at different contrast: 0 (automasking, solid line) and 0.5 (dashed line). In this case, the required amount of distortion Δy_f to obtain some specific distortion in the response domain τ at a given contrast of the stimulus increases when the contrast of the mask increases.

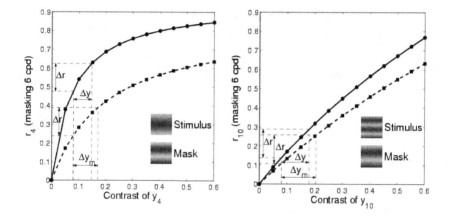

SVM ε-Insensitivity from Perceptually Acceptable Distortions

In order to obtain image approximations with a small number of support vectors, while keeping the perceptual appearance of the image good, it is necessary to derive the kind of distortions that guarantee that all the distortion coefficients in the response domain will be below a certain threshold. The appropriate domain for SVM training will be the one that makes the ε-insensitivity design feasible.

A small distortion in a spatial region of the signal ΔA induces a distortion in the perceptually meaningful response representation Δr. This distortion can be approximated by using the Jacobian of the response function:

$$\Delta r \cong \nabla R(y) \cdot \Delta y = \nabla R(T \cdot \Delta A) \cdot T \cdot \Delta A. \tag{7}$$

Then, the MPE for that spatial region, s, is given by:

$$\mathrm{MPE}_s = \| \Delta r \|_\infty = \max(\nabla R(y) \cdot \Delta y) = \max(\nabla R(T \cdot \Delta A) \cdot T \cdot \Delta A). \tag{8}$$

The global perceived distortion in an image with n spatial regions will be a particular spatial pooling (q-norm) of these n local distortions from each local (block) response representation:

$$\text{MPE} = \| (\text{MPE}_1, \cdots, \text{MPE}_n) \|_q = \left(\sum_s \text{MPE}_s^q \right)^{1/q}, \tag{9}$$

where q is the summation exponent in this spatial pooling.

Some distortion in a block ΔA, or in the local frequency domain, Δy, is perceptually acceptable if it generates a distortion in the perceptual response domain in which the distortion in every response coefficient is below a threshold τ. As stated in the introduction, the role of SVM regression in the context of image coding is reducing the size of the signal description (reducing the number of support vectors) while keeping the MPE below a threshold in every spatial region, that is, $\text{MPE}_s < \tau, \forall s$. This can be incorporated in the SVM training by using an appropriate ε-insensitivity profile, that is, given a different ε for each training sample.

The MPE restriction determines a geometric condition to derive the ε profile. In the response representation domain, this condition is quite simple, taking:

$$\varepsilon_r(f) = \tau, \tag{10}$$

it is obviously guaranteed that the distortions Δr_f will be bounded by τ, $\forall f$. This set of scalar restrictions $\varepsilon_r(f)$ is equivalent to constrain the vector distortion Δr into an n-dimensional cube of side τ.

The corresponding n-dimensional boundary region in other representation domains can be obtained operating backward from the cube in the response representation. However, depending on the complexity of the transformation from the response representation to the desired representation, the shape of the n-dimensional boundary region may be quite complicated for ε design. Let us analyze the difficulty for ε design in previously reported image-representation domains, namely, the spatial domain (Robinson & Kecman, 2000) and the block DCT domain (Gomez et al., 2005; Robinson & Kecman, 2003).

In the block DCT domain, the profile $\varepsilon_y(f)$, for a given input signal y_o, is determined by the boundaries of the n-dimensional region that fulfills the condition:

$$[\nabla R(y_o) \cdot \Delta y]_f \leq \tau \tag{11}$$

for all possible distortions Δy with $|\Delta y_f| \leq \varepsilon_y(f)$.

Analogously, in the spatial domain, the profile $\varepsilon_A(x)$ for a given input signal A_o is determined by the boundaries of the n-dimensional region that fulfills the condition:

$$[\nabla R(A_o) \cdot T \cdot \Delta A]_f \leq \tau \tag{12}$$

for all possible distortions ΔA with $|\Delta A_x| \leq \varepsilon_A(x)$.

If the matrix, ∇R or $\nabla R \cdot T$, that acts on the distortion vectors, Δy or ΔA, is not diagonal, the above conditions determine n-dimensional boxes not aligned with the axes of the representation. This implies that the distortions in different coefficients should be coupled, which is not guaranteed by the SVM regression.

This is an intrinsic problem of the spatial domain representation because T is an orthogonal filter bank that is highly nondiagonal. Therefore, the spatial domain is very unsuitable for perceptually efficient SVM regression.

The situation may be different in the DCT domain when using a simplified (linear) perception model. In this particular case, the Jacobian ∇R is diagonal (equation (3)), so the condition in equation (11) reduces to:

$$| \Delta y_f | \le \frac{\tau}{\alpha_f}, \tag{13}$$

or equivalently,

$$\varepsilon_y(f) = \frac{\tau}{\alpha_f}, \tag{14}$$

which is the frequency-dependent ε-insensitivity proposed in Gomez et al. (2005). This implies a more accurate image reproduction (smaller $\varepsilon_y(f)$) for low and medium frequencies, and it allows the introduction of substantially more distortion (larger $\varepsilon_y(f)$) in the high-frequency region. This reasoning is the justification of the ad hoc coefficient selection made in the original formulation of SVMs in the DCT domain for image coding (Robinson & Kecman, 2003). This ideal low-pass approximation of the CSF may be a too-crude approximation in some situations, leading to blocky images.

Despite the relatively good performance of the SVM coding approaches based on either rigorous (Gomez et al., 2005) or oversimplified (Robinson & Kecman, 2003) linear models, remember that linear models cannot account for automasking and cross-masking effects, and thus the introduction of nonlinear response models is highly convenient.

The current nonlinear response model (equation (4)) implies a nondiagonal Jacobian (equation (6)). Therefore, when using this perception model, it is not possible to define the ε-insensitivity in the DCT domain because of the perceptual coupling between coefficients in this domain. According to this, when using the more accurate perception models, the appropriate domain for SVM training is the perceptual response domain, hence using a constant insensitivity.

Experimental Results

In this section, we show the performance of several SVM-based image-coding schemes. First, some guidelines for model development are given, where explicit examples of the different behavior of the SVM sample selection are given depending on the image-representation domain. Then we analyze the developed coding strategies in terms of (a) the distribution of support vectors, and (b) the effect that these distributions have in the compression performance.

Model Development

In the SVR image-coding framework presented here, the whole image is first divided in blocks, and then a particular SVR is trained to learn some image representation of each domain. Afterwards, the signal description (the weights) obtained by the SVR are subsequently quantized, giving rise to the encoded block. In this section, we analyze examples of this procedure using four image representations (or ε-insensitivity design procedures): (a) the spatial representation using constant insensitivity profile (Robinson & Kecman, 2003), (b) the DCT representation using constant insensitivity in the low-frequency coefficients and discarding (infinite insensitivity) the coefficients with frequency bigger than 20 cpd, RK-i as reported in Robinson and Kecman (2005), (c) the DCT representation using CSF-based insensitivity (equation (14)), CSF-SVR as reported in Gomez et al. (2005), and (d) the proposed nonlinearly transformed DCT representation using equations (4) and (5) (NL-SVR). In this latter case, and taking into account the perceptual MPE concept, constant ε-insensitivity was used.

After training, the signal is described by the Lagrange multipliers of the support vectors needed to keep the regression error below the thresholds ε_i. Increasing the thresholds reduces the number of required support vectors, thus reducing the entropy of the encoded image and increasing the distortion. In all experiments, we used the RBF kernel, trained the SVR models without the bias term b, and modeled the absolute value of the DCT (or response) coefficients. For the sake of a fair comparison, all the free parameters (ε-insensitivity, penalization parameter C, Gaussian width of the RBF kernel σ, and weight quantization coarseness) were optimized for all the considered models. In the NL-SVM case, the parameters of the divisive normalization used in the experiments are shown in Figure 4. In every case, rather than adjusting directly the ε, we tuned iteratively the modulation parameter τ to produce a given compression ratio (target entropy). Note that high values of τ increase the width of the ε tube, which in turn produce lower numbers of support vectors and consequently yield higher compression ratios.

Figure 7 shows the performance of SVR in different image-representation domains at 0.5 bits/pix. Each panel represents the image vector (and the selected samples by the SVR learning) corresponding to the highlighted block as well as a zoom of the resulting reconstructed image. The top-left figure represents the result of the encoding and reconstruction of the image in the spatial domain. In the DCT-based cases, after transforming the 16×16 blocks using a 2-D DCT, and zigzagging its 256 coefficients, we perform support vector regression through (top-right) the RKi-1 algorithm, (bottom-left) CSF-SVR, and (bottom-right) NL-SVR. Then, the resulting support vectors (circles) are used to reconstruct the signal. These illustrative examples show that using the same SVR abilities, (a) the spatial domain representation is highly unsuitable for SVR-based image coding, and (b) SVR-CSF and the NL-SVR take into account higher frequency details by selecting support vectors in the high-frequency range when necessary, something that is not accomplished with the RKi-1 method. This second effect enhances the subjective behavior of these methods. The advantage of the nonlinear method is that it gives rise to better contrast reproduction.

Figure 7. SVR performance (selected samples) in different image-representation domains (at 0.5 bits/pix)

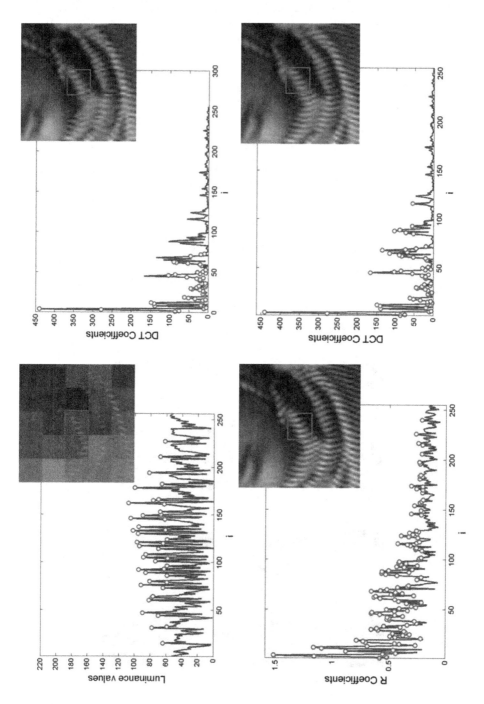

Figure 8. Analysis of the influence of the profile on SVM-based image-coding schemes in the DCT domain. The top panel shows the distribution of support vectors for each ε profile as a function of the frequency in the Lena image. The bottom panel shows (a) a zoom of the original Lena image at 8 bits/pixel (the bit rate for this example is 0.3 bpp; 27:1), (b) the ε-SVR (constant insensitivity in the DCT domain), (c) RKi-1, and (d) CSF-SVR.

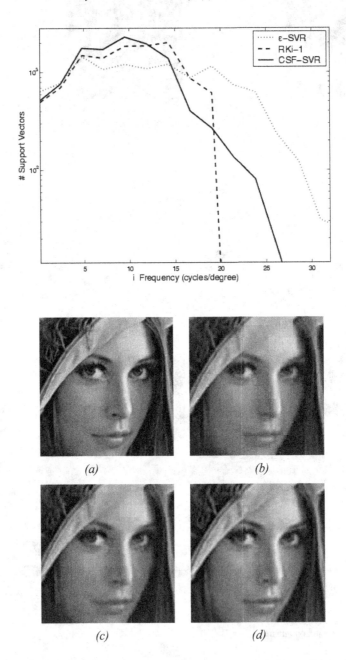

Distribution of Support Vectors in the DCT Domain

Tailoring different ε profiles produces critically different support vector distributions in the frequency domain and hence different error distributions in this domain. Therefore, different ε profiles lead to results of quite different perceptual quality. Figure 8 (left) shows a representative example of the distribution of the selected SVs by the ε-SVR (constant insensitivity in the DCT domain), the RKi-1, and the CSF-SVR models. These distributions reflect how the selection of a particular insensitivity profile modifies the learning behavior of the SVMs.

In Figure 8 (right), we illustrate the effect that the considered ε_i profile has on the encoded images. Using a straightforward constant ε for all coefficients (ε-SVR approach) concentrates more support vectors in the low-frequency region because the variance of these DCT coefficients in natural images is higher (Clarke, 1981; Malo, Ferri, Albert, Soret, & Artigas, 2000). However, it still yields a relatively high number of support vectors in the high-frequency region. This is inefficient because of the low subjective relevance of that region (see Figure 2). Considering these vectors will not significantly reduce the (perceptual) reconstruction error while it increases the entropy of the encoded signal. The RKi-1 approach (Robinson & Kecman, 2003) uses a constant ε, but the authors solve the above problem by neglecting the high-frequency coefficients in training the SVM for each block. This is equivalent to the use of an arbitrarily large insensitivity for the high-frequency region. As a result, this approach relatively allocates more support vectors in the low- and medium-frequency regions. This modification of the straightforward uniform approach is qualitatively based on the basic low-pass behavior of human vision. However, such a crude approximation (that implies no control of the distortion in the high-frequency region) can introduce annoying errors in blocks with sharp edges. The CSF-SVR approach uses a variable ε according to the CSF, and thus takes into account the perception facts reviewed previously, giving rise to a (natural) concentration of support vectors in the low- and medium-frequency region. Note that this concentration is even bigger than in the RKi-1 approach. However, the proposed algorithm does not neglect any coefficient in the learning process. This strategy naturally reduces the number of allocated support vectors in the high-frequency region with regard to the straightforward uniform approach, but it does not prevent selecting some of them when it is necessary to keep the error below the selected threshold, which may be relevant in edge blocks.

The visual effect of the different distribution of the support vectors due to the different insensitivity profiles is clear in Figure 8 (right). First, it is obvious that the perceptually based training leads to better overall subjective results: The annoying blocking artifacts of the ε-SVR and RKi-1 algorithms are highly reduced in the CSF-SVR, giving rise to smoother and perceptually more acceptable images. Second, the blocking artifacts in the ε-SVR and RKi-1 approaches may come from different reasons. On the one hand, the uniform ε-SVR wastes (relatively) too many support vectors (and bits) in the high-frequency region in such a way that noticeable errors in the low-frequency components (related to the average luminance in each block) are produced. However, note that due to the allocation of more vectors in the high-frequency region, it is the method that better reproduces details. On the other hand, neglecting the high-frequency coefficients in the training (RKi-1 approach) does reduce the blocking a little bit, but it cannot cope with high-contrast edges that also produce a lot of energy in the high-frequency region (for instance, Lena's cheek on the dark hair background).

Compression Performance

In this section, we analyze the performance of the algorithms through rate-distortion curves (Figure 9) and explicit examples for visual comparison (Figure 10). In order to assess the quality of the coded images, three different measures were used: the standard (Euclidean) RMSE, the MPE (Gomez et al., 2005; Malo et al., 2006; Malo et al., 2000), and the (also

Figure 9. Average rate-distortion curves over four standard images (Lena, Barbara, Boats, Einstein) using objective and subjective measures for the considered SVM approaches (RKi-1 is dotted, CSF-SVR is dashed, and NL-SVR is solid). JPEG (dotted squares) has also been included for reference purposes. (a) RMSE distortion (top left), (b) MPE (Gomez et al., 2005; Malo et al., 2006; Malo et al., 2000) (top right), and (c) SSIM (Wang et al., 2004) (bottom).

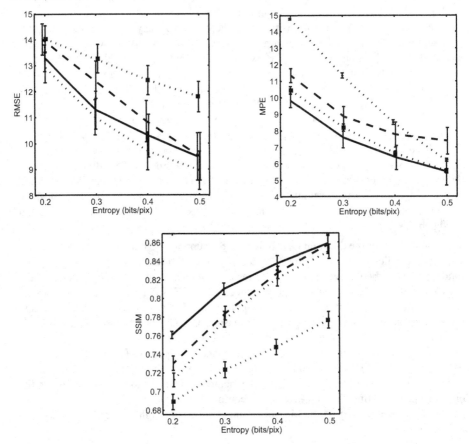

Figure 10. Examples of decoded Lena (a-d) and Barbara (e-h) images at 0.3 bits/pix, encoded by using JPEG (a, e), RKi-1 (b, f), CSF-SVR (c, g), and NL-SVR (d, h)

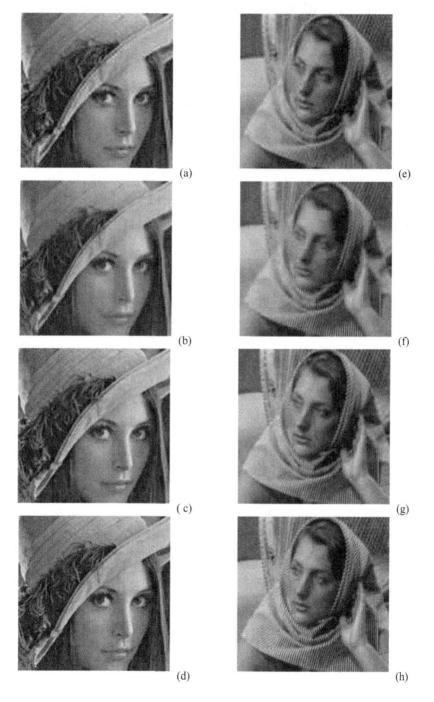

(a)

(e)

(b)

(f)

(c)

(g)

(d)

(h)

perceptually meaningful) structural similarity (SSIM) index (Wang, Bovik, Sheikh, & Simoncelli, 2004).

According to the standard Euclidean MSE point of view, the performance of the SVM algorithms is basically the same (note the overlapped big deviations in Figure 9a). However, it is widely known that the MSE results are not useful to represent the subjective quality of images, as extensively reported elsewhere (Girod, 1993; Teo & Heeger, 1994; A. B. Watson & Malo, 2002). When using more appropriate (perceptually meaningful) quality measures (Figures 9b-9c), the NL-SVR outperforms previously reported SVM methods.

Figure 10 shows representative results of the considered SVM strategies on standard images (Lena and Barbara) at the same bit rate (0.3 bits/pix). The visual inspection confirms that the numerical gain in MPE and SSIM shown in Figure 9 is also perceptually significant. Some conclusions can be extracted from this figure. First, as previously reported in Gomez et al. (2005), RKi-1 leads to poorer (blocky) results because of the too-crude approximation of the CSF (as an ideal low-pass filter) and the equal relevance applied to the low-frequency DCT coefficients. Second, despite the good performance yielded by the CSF-SVR approach to avoid blocking effects, it is worth noting that high-frequency details are smoothed (e.g., see Barbara's scarf). These effects are highly alleviated by introducing SVR in the nonlinear domain. See, for instance, Lena's eyes, her hat's feathers, or the better reproduction of the high-frequency pattern in Barbara's clothes.

Conclusion, Discussion, and Further Work

In this chapter, we have analyzed the use and performance of SVR models in image compression. A thorough revision of perception and statistics facts became strictly necessary to improve the standard application of SVR in this application field. First, the selection of a suitable (and perceptually meaningful) working domain requires one to map the input data first with a linear transformation and then with an (optional) nonlinear second transformation. Second, working in a given domain also imposes certain constraints on the definition of the most suitable insensitivity zone for training the SVR. As a consequence, the joint consideration of domain and insensitivity in the proposed scheme widely facilitates the task of function approximation, and enables a proper selection of support vectors rather than a reduced amount of them.

Several examples have illustrated the capabilities of using SVR in transform coding schemes, and revealed it to be very efficient in terms of perceptually meaningful rate-distortion measurements and visual inspection. However, further studies should be developed in the immediate future, which could lead to some refinements and improved compression, for example, by performing sparse learning regression in more sophisticated nonlinear perceptual domains, or by replacing the DCT with wavelet transforms. Finally, further research should be addressed to analyze the statistical effects of SVM feature extraction and its relation to more general nonlinear ICA techniques (Hyvarinen et al., 2001; Murray & Kreutz-Delgado, 2004).

References

Barlow, H. B. (2001). Redundancy reduction revisited. *Network: Comp. Neur. Sys., 12*, 241-253.

Buccigrossi, R., & Simoncelli, E. (1999). Image compression via joint statistical characterization in the wavelet domain. *IEEE Transactions on Image Processing, 8*(12), 1688-1701.

Campbell, F., & Robson, J. (1968). Application of Fourier analysis to the visibility of gratings. *Journal of Physiology, 197*(3), 551-566.

Camps-Valls, G., Soria-Olivas, E., Pérez-Ruixo, J., Artés-Rodriguez, A., Pérez-Cruz, F., & Figueiras-Vidal, A. (2001). A profile-dependent kernel-based regression for cyclosporine concentration prediction. *Neural Information Processing Systems (NIPS): Workshop on New Directions in Kernel-Based Learning Methods.* Available at http://www.uv.es/~gcamps

Clarke, R. (1981). Relation between the Karhunen-Loeve transform and cosine transforms. In *Proceedings IEE, Pt. F, 128*(6), 359-360.

Epifanio, I., Gutiérrez, J., & Malo, J. (2003). Linear transform for simultaneous diagonalization of covariance and perceptual metric matrix in image coding. *Pattern Recognition, 36*(8), 1799-1811.

Gersho, A., & Gray, R. (1992). *Vector quantization and signal compression.* Boston: Kluwer Academic Press.

Girod, B. (1993). What's wrong with mean-squared error. In A. B. Watson (Ed.), *Digital images and human vision* (pp. 207-220). MIT Press.

Gómez-Pérez, G., Camps-Valls, G., Gutierrez, J., & Malo, J. (2005). Perceptual adaptive insensitivity for support vector machine image coding. *IEEE Transactions on Neural Networks, 16*(6), 1574-1581.

Gutierrez, J., Ferri, F., & Malo, J. (2006). Regularization operators for natural images based on non-linear perception models. *IEEE Trans. Im. Proc., 15*(1), 189-200.

Heeger, D. J. (1992). Normalization of cell responses in cat striate cortex. *Visual Neuroscience, 9*, 181-198.

Hyvarinen, A., Karhunen, J., & Oja, E. (2001). *Independent component analysis.* New York: John Wiley & Sons.

Legge, G. (1981). A power law for contrast discrimination. *Vision Research, 18*, 68-91.

Malo, J., Epifanio, I., Navarro, R., & Simoncelli, E. (2006). Non-linear image representation for efficient perceptual coding. *IEEE Trans. Im. Proc., 15*(1), 68-80.

Malo, J., Ferri, F., Albert, J., Soret, J., & Artigas, J. M. (2000). The role of perceptual contrast non-linearities in image transform coding. *Image & Vision Computing, 18*(3), 233-246.

Malo, J., & Gutiérrez, J. (2006). V1 non-linearities emerge from local-to-global non-linear ICA. *Network: Comp. Neural Syst., 17*(1), 85-102.

Malo, J., Pons, A., & Artigas, J. (1997). Subjective image fidelity metric based on bit allocation of the human visual system in the DCT domain. *Image & Vision Computing, 15*(7), 535-548.

Murray, J. F., & Kreutz-Delgado, K. (2004). Sparse image coding using learned overcomplete dictionaries. *IEEE International Workshop on Machine Learning for Signal Processing (MLSP 2004)*.

Navarro, Y., Gutiérrez, J., & Malo, J. (2005). Gain control for the chromatic channels in JPEG2000. In *Proceedings of 10t^h International Conference of AIC, 1*(1), 539-542.

Peli, E. (1990). Contrast in complex images. *JOSA A, 7*, 2032-2040.

Pons, A. M., Malo, J., Artigas, J. M., & Capilla, P. (1999). Image quality metric based on multidimensional contrast perception models. *Displays, 20*, 93-110.

Robinson, J., & Kecman, V. (2000). The use of support vector machines in image compression. In *Proceedings of the International Conference on Engineering Intelligence Systems, EIS2000, 36* (pp. 93-96).

Robinson, J., & Kecman, V. (2003). Combining support vector machine learning with the discrete cosine transform in image compression. *IEEE Transactions on Neural Networks, 14*(4), 950-958.

Simoncelli, E. (2003). Vision and the statistics of the visual environment. *Current Opinion in Neurobiology, 13*, 144-149.

Smola, A. J., & Schölkopf, B. (2004). A tutorial on support vector regression. *Statistics and Computing, 14*, 199-222.

Taubman, D., & Marcellin, M. (2001). *JPEG2000: Image compression fundamentals, standards and practice*. Boston: Kluwer Academic Publishers.

Teo, P., & Heeger, D. (1994). Perceptual image distortion. *Proceedings of the SPIE Conference: Human Vision, Visual Processing, and Digital Display V, 2179* (pp. 127-141).

Wallace, G. (1991). The JPEG still picture compression standard. *Communications of the ACM, 34*(4), 31-43.

Wang, Z., Bovik, A. C., Sheikh, H. R., & Simoncelli, E. P. (2004). Image quality assessment: From error visibility to structural similarity. *IEEE Trans. Im. Proc., 13*(4), 600-612.

Watson, A., & Solomon, J. (1997). A model of visual contrast gain control and pattern masking. *Journal of the Optical Society of America A, 14*(9), 2379-2391.

Watson, A. B., & Malo, J. (2002). Video quality measures based on the standard spatial observer. In *Proceedings of the IEEE International Conference on Image Proceedings* (Vol. 3, pp. 41-44).

Zeng, W., Daly, S., & Lei, S. (2002). An overview of the visual optimization tools in JPEG2000. *Sig.Proc.Im.Comm., 17*(1), 85-104.

Chapter XIV

Image Classification and Retrieval with Kernel Methods

Francesca Odone, Università degli Studi di Genova, Italy

Alessandro Verri, Università degli Studi di Genova, Italy

Abstract

In this chapter we review some kernel methods useful for image classification and retrieval applications. Starting from the problem of constructing appropriate image representations, we describe in depth and comment on the main properties of various kernel engineering approaches that have been recently proposed in the computer vision and machine learning literature for solving a number of image classification problems. We distinguish between kernel functions applied to images as a whole and kernel functions looking at image features. We conclude by presenting some current work and discussing open issues.

Introduction

The problem of *content-based image classification* loosely refers to associating a given image to one of a predefined set of classes using the visual information contained in the image. Despite decades of research, the solutions proposed so far to this multifaceted problem, even if confined to some restricted application domains, do not seem to reach the required levels of effectiveness and efficiency. This is not surprising if one realizes that this deceivingly simple problem is intertwined with the understanding of how human intelligence works.

In more prosaic terms, content-based image classification can be seen as a core element of many engineering applications, including video surveillance (where image classification is used to detect dangerous objects or situations, or automatically identify objects or people), data mining (for automatic image annotation or to support image search engines), automatic guidance (here, image classification is useful for view-based automatic localization), or other robotics applications that require object recognition.

Recent advances in kernel methods made it possible the development of a number of promising techniques for addressing particular applications and enabled a better understanding of the subtleties of the general problem from the viewpoint of statistical learning. For an introduction to kernel methods, see Chapter I.

The aim of this chapter is to describe some of these advances, discuss their strengths and weaknesses, and relate them to an application domain whenever it is possible. In particular, we will stress the importance of designing appropriate *kernel functions* (also referred to as *kernels* in the reminder of the chapter) for a given data type or a data representation.

Before moving on, we introduce the terminology we adopted in this chapter and list the main computer vision problems that can be viewed as instances of *image classification*. A first image classification problem is *object detection*: the aim is finding one or more instances of an object in an image. From the classification viewpoint, it often boils down to classifying image subregions. A second problem is *view-based object recognition* (the difference from object detection is mostly semantic): objects to be detected are instances of a certain category (e.g., faces or cars), while objects to be recognized are instances of the same object viewed under different conditions (e.g., my face or my car). A third class is *visual categorization*. It refers to associating an image to two (binary classification) or more (multiclass classification) image categories (e.g., indoor or outdoor, or other higher level image descriptions).

The rest of the chapter is organized in five sections. First, we comment on the specific properties of images that should be taken into account in the design of a kernel method. Second, we discuss kernel methods that were proposed in image classification and retrieval problems with emphasis on the selected image representation. Third, we describe kernel functions that are applied to image global structures. Fourth, we discuss kernel functions of local nature that have been receiving increasing attention in the last few years. Finally, we present and comment on some current work and open issues in the field.

Image Specificity

An important issue of statistical learning approaches, like support vector machines (SVMs) or other kernel methods, is which kernel function to use for which problem. A number of general-purpose kernel functions are available, but the use of an appropriate kernel function for the problem at hand is likely to lead to a substantial increase in the generalization ability of the learning system. The challenge of building kernel functions is to satisfy certain mathematical requirements while incorporating the prior knowledge of the application domain.

In the image context, one has to deal with specific issues giving rise to extremely difficult problems, the solution of which is still beyond reach. A first common issue all image classification problems are facing is the large variability of the inputs. Images depend on various parameters controlling format, size, resolution, and compression quality, which make it difficult to compare image visual content, or simply to recognize the same visual content in an image saved with different parameters. This is in sharp contrast to other application domains like, for example, text categorization and bioinformatics.

Raw images are rich in content and they lead to large feature vectors. The information they carry is often redundant, thus feature selection or image subsampling is always advisable. One of the main targets of computer vision is extracting useful information from images, including interest points (such as corners), geometric shapes (like lines or circles), and signal variations (for instance, edges or ridges; Trucco & Verri, 1998). It is common practice to use these simple but well-established techniques to find more compact representations for image classification. This gives rise to a second issue in engineering kernel functions for images: the difficulty of extracting image descriptors, or feature vectors, of equal size in different images. Kernel methods are typically designed to be applied to descriptions of equal length. Visual cues in images, instead, are often more naturally described in terms of feature vectors of varying size, in accordance to the image content. Further feature selection or normalization could be used to obtain equal-length vectors, but the expressiveness of the description could be flawed. Appropriate kernel functions for dealing with this problem can be a more convincing answer.

A third peculiar aspect of images is the coexistence of short-range and long-range spatial correlation in the signal. Short-range correlation is hard to characterize due to the unknown scale at which one is analyzing the information content, while long-range correlation is difficult to capture due to both the changing geometry of 3-D objects viewed in 2-D images and the segmentation problem (i.e., telling which part of the image is part of which object).

A fourth characteristic of image classification problems (common to other application domains) is the large number of classes. The number of object classes or image categories to be recognized in practical scenarios reaches easily the order of at least hundreds or thousands (e.g., recognizing who is who from a picture or classifying dynamic events from image sequences).

No general approach has been developed for dealing with these specific problems, though all the approaches we describe in the following, either implicitly or explicitly, provide partial solutions that, in some cases, appear to be sufficient for a particular application.

Searching for the Appropriate Representation

A specific kernel function can be regarded as a particular feature mapping. In this section, we review some of the first methods proposed after interest rose by the introduction of support vector machines (Vapnik, 1995) as the core of trainable systems. A common trait of these methods is the emphasis on the relevance of the choice of which representation to use for which problem. In retrospective, this choice can be viewed as an explicit version of kernel function selection.

An application for which SVMs since their early days proved particularly effective is *object detection*. Usually they are applied to searching common objects with a relatively low interclass variability, such as faces, pedestrians, and cars. These categories are interesting to video surveillance and traffic-monitoring systems.

The structure of these methods is usually as follows. In the training phase, the system takes a set of possibly aligned and normalized images of the class of interest (the positive examples) and a set of images that do not represent the class (the negative examples). In the test phase, the system slides a fixed-size window over the input image and uses the trained classifier to decide whether the observed pattern contains the object of interest. To deal with multiple scales, the image is iteratively resized and the search is repeated across scales.

One of the first works proposing this approach was Osuna, Freund, and Girosi (1997), in which a face-detection system was proposed. The data description was very simple—a vectorization of 19×19 pixel patches—and it relied on the high repeatability of the human face structure at low resolution. Care was taken in selecting the training set and accurately processing it. (The data set used, the Center for Biological and Computational Learning [CBCL] database, publicly available,[1] contains perfectly correlated frontal faces cropped to exclude all background and hair.)

Also, they described a procedure to select useful negative data among the false positives obtained on running the system over a data set that did not contain faces. Selecting appropriate negative examples for a task is extremely important as the class of negatives is usually richer and more variable. Often at run time, as in the case of faces, positive examples are a minority. Figure 1 shows a common picture of a group of people. At fixed scale, it contains

Figure 1. A test image of the MIT-CMU frontal faces test set[2]

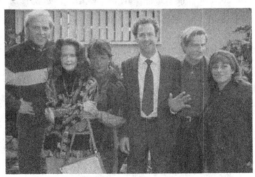

six positive patches and about 190,000 negative patches since the image is 610×395 pixels and each face is about 50×50 pixels. If a multiscale search is performed, the number of negatives grows accordingly.

Faces are an interesting object class because they show a very peculiar common structure, especially when observed at low resolution, and include much symmetry. Other object classes (pedestrians and, even more, cars) present a much higher interclass variability and often require more care in the representation.

Papageorgiou and Poggio (2000) presented a face-, pedestrian-, and car-detection method based on SVMs. The method used Haar wavelets to represent images, and an architecture similar to the one described above. The images are transformed to the space of wavelet coefficients, providing a multiresolution representation that captures different levels of detail. Also, Haar wavelets can be computed efficiently. The authors presented results that are still considered a reference for the field.

The global approach proved to work well for detecting objects under fixed viewing conditions. However, problems occur when the viewpoint and pose vary. One possible solution is to try and include samples of all possible situations in the training set, but this is not always feasible (for instance, if the training set is given and fixed) and can be impractical if object variability is too high. The *component-based approach* (Heisele, Ho, & Poggio, 2001) tackles this problem for the case of face detection, arguing that when relative position changes, small components vary less than the pattern describing the whole object. In the component-based approach, a face is decomposed into semantically meaningful components (eyes, mouth, and nose). Each component is represented by a set of examples and modeled by training a linear SVM. The main issue is how to include geometric relationships between components. Mohan, Papageorgiou, and Poggio (2001) provide a two-level strategy based on first testing for the presence of components and then checking if the geometrical configuration of detected components corresponds to a learned geometrical model of a face.

Another issue of interest in the component-based approach is how to automatically choose components. Heisele, Verri, and Poggio (2002) suggest an approach based on the availability of a data set of 3-D synthetic face models. First the user manually selects points of interest on one model—the selection can be automatically expanded to the other models—and finally a learning procedure selects the best rectangular shaped components around the selected points. Alternative approaches, completely automatic, have been later proposed in the literature (Franceschi, Odone, Smeraldi, & Verri, 2005; Ullman, Vidal-Naquet, & Sali, 2002; Viola & Jones, 2004).

Another application that has been extensively studied as an interesting learning problem is *object recognition*, in which a specific object has to be identified against a number of other objects. This problem may be specialized for a number of applications, including automatic guidance and localization. In the special case where the objects are human faces, it opens to *face recognition*, an extremely lively research field, with applications to video surveillance and security.[3] The main difficulty of this problem is finding methods able to recognize the same object in different poses and under varying illumination conditions and yet discriminate between similar objects.

Pontil and Verri (1998) show the performances of SVMs with standard polynomial kernel functions on identifying objects belonging to a collection from the COIL database.[4] The database includes 72 views of each object. The objects are acquired in a controlled environment on a dark background. For the experiments, the images were reduced to 32×32 pixels. Each object was represented with 36 images evenly selected among the 72 views. The remaining 36 images were used as tests. Given the relatively small number of examples and the large number of classes, they used a one-vs.-one approach to multiclass classification. The filtering effect of the averaging preprocessing step was enough to induce very high recognition rates even in the presence of a large amount of noise added to the test set. A limitation of the system was due to the global approach of the classifier, ill suited to deal with occlusions and clutter. A way to circumvent this problem is to use components, as described above, or local features (see the section on kernel functions for local features). Another way is to engineer classifiers that are more tolerant to local changes than the linear and polynomial kernel functions (see the Hausdorff kernel of the next section).

Kernel Functions for the Whole Image

The computer vision literature on techniques for evaluating the similarity between images or image patches is vast. Some methods are based on comparing dense low-level information, others on (a) extracting features, (b) building sparse image representations, and then (c) comparing them. The two different approaches that inspired two different families of kernel functions for images are typically based on fixed-length or on variable-length representations respectively.[5] In this section, we discuss the former approach, describing kernel functions that exploit dense and redundant image descriptions derived from the whole image. The next section is dedicated to the latter method and deals with image representations of variable length, based on the combination of sparse local information.

Low-level image descriptions are either based directly on pixels, or on building dense histogram-based representations. In the first case, it is advisable to exploit spatial correlation, whilst the second case uses information about relative frequencies.

In this section, we first discuss kernel functions for template matching that can be used on raw pixel descriptions, and then describe state-of-the-art kernel functions for histograms.

Kernel Functions for Template Matching

If the input data are raw pixels, kernel functions can be derived from correlation measures. In particular, cross-correlation is exactly the linear kernel applied to the pixel grey level, while the sum of squared differences (SSD) has been proved a conditionally positive definite function that can be used as a kernel for binary SVMs even without being a Mercer's kernel (Poggio, Mukherjee, Rifkin, Rakhlin, & Verri, 2001). If these correlation measures are applied directly to the whole image, they do not take into account spatial image correlation.

Raw pixels have been successfully compared with Gaussian radial basis function (RBF), where the choice of σ tunes the degree of correlation between neighbouring pixels that one wants to consider. One of the first attempts to use explicitly the prior knowledge on images for designing appropriate kernel functions can be found in Schölkopf, Simrad, Smola, and Vapnik (1998), in which a variant of polynomial kernels of degree d taking into account short-range spatial correlations is described. Another way of dealing with short-range correlations in images is provided by *compactly supported (CS) kernels*.

Definition of Compactly Supported Kernels

A kernel K_r is compactly supported if it vanishes from a certain distance r between $\mathbf{x}$ and $\mathbf{y}$:

$$K_r(\mathbf{x},\mathbf{y}) = \begin{cases} K(\mathbf{x},\mathbf{y}) & if \|\mathbf{x}-\mathbf{y}\| < r \\ 0 & otherwise \end{cases} \tag{1}$$

From the algorithmic viewpoint, the most interesting property of CS kernels is that they lead to sparse Gram matrices and thus to a reduction of the algorithmic complexity. Unfortunately, the most common examples of CS kernels—triangular, circular, and spherical kernels (Genton, 2001)—are not positive definite in higher dimensions. Furthermore, truncating a positive definite kernel does not lead in general to a positive definite kernel (Boughorbel et al., 2005b).

In Boughorbel, Tarel, Fleuret, & Boujemaa (2005), an extension to triangular and circular kernels to high dimensions is proposed called geometric compactly supported (GCS) kernels. These kernels are based on the intersection of two *n*-dimensional balls of equal radius, proved to be positive definite. The work includes a recursive implementation of the kernel computation. The GCS kernel could be used directly on pixel patterns, but the authors apply it to color histograms and present experiments on an image-categorization task (3,200 images of six classes). By tuning the parameter (the radius), they obtain results comparable to the Laplacian kernel.

Definition of Hausdorff Kernel

Well-known weaknesses of template matching are illumination and pose variations and occlusions. In Odone, Barla, and Verri (2005), it was proposed a kernel for images explicitly derived from a similarity measure designed to be tolerant to small variations and occlusion (Odone, Trucco, & Verri, 2001). The similarity measure, loosely inspired by the Hausdorff distance, aimed at compensating for small illumination changes and small local transformations by comparing each pixel of one image with a neighbourhood in space and grey levels of the other image. In the 1-D case, if A and B are grey-level images, this can be written as:

$$h_A(B) = \sum_{i=1}^{N} U(\varepsilon - |A[i] - B[s(i)]|), \tag{2}$$

where U is the unit step function, and $s(i)$ is the pixel of B most similar to the grey value of pixel i of A. Symmetry was restored by taking the average:

$$H(A,B) = \frac{1}{2}(h_A(B) + h_B(A)). \tag{3}$$

In Odone et al. (2005), a variation of H was proposed, leading to a Mercer's kernel K_S. The variation is based on rewriting the similarity measure using binary representations of images. The idea is to compute the inner product between A and B^S, the convolution of B with a suitable stencil (or pattern of weights) S. A kernel is obtained by restoring symmetry:

$$K_S(A,B) = \frac{1}{2}(A \cdot B^S + B \cdot A^S). \tag{4}$$

Positive definiteness is ensured if and only if the sum of the off-centered entries in the stencil does not exceed the central entry (Odone et al., 2005). Experimental evidence is given that K_S can be used to build effective methods for view-based 3-D object recognition.

Kernels for Histograms

As pointed out in Chapelle, Haffner, & Vapnik (1999), the discrete nature of histograms suggests that more suitable kernels than the standard ones may be used.

A common trick to use distance measures for histograms as kernels is to place them on the exponential part of RBF Gaussian kernels instead of the L^2 norm. See, for instance, Jing, Li, Zhang, and Zhang (2003), where an RBF kernel is engineered in order to use the earth mover's distance (EMD) as a dissimilarity measure (more details in the next section), or Belongie, Fowlkes, Chung, and Malik (2002), where an RBF kernel based on χ^2 has been shown to be of Mercer's type.

Chapelle et al. (1999) propose a family of kernels, the generalized RBF kernels, that seem to be better suited than the Gaussian for dealing with image histograms. These kernels, in essence, ensure heavier tails than the Gaussian kernels in the attempt to contrast the well-known phenomenon of diagonally dominant kernel matrices in high-dimensional inputs.

Definition of Generalized RBF Kernels

Let A and B be the histograms of images I and J, respectively. Each of them has M bins A_i and B_i $i=1,...,M$. The generalized RBF kernel is defined as:

$$K_{HT}(A,B) = \exp\left(-\frac{1}{2\sigma^2}\sum_i \left|A_i^a - B_i^a\right|^b\right). \tag{5}$$

If $b = 1$, the kernels are usually referred to as Laplacian kernels, while if $b = 0.5$, they are called *sublinear kernels*. K_{HT} satisfies the Mercer's condition if $0 \le b \le 2$, while the choice of *a* does not impact the function's positive definiteness.

Histogram intersection (Swain & Ballard, 1991) is one of the few examples of similarity measures for histograms that have been used directly as a kernel function. This similarity measure is very effective for color indexing, being well suited to deal with color and scale changes, and quite tolerant to clutter. Furthermore, histogram intersection can be computed efficiently and adapted to search for partially occluded objects in images. The effectiveness of histogram intersection as a similarity measure for color indexing raised the question of whether or not this measure can be adopted in kernel-based methods.

Definition of Histogram Intersection

Let *A* and *B* be the histograms of images I and J respectively. The *histogram-intersection* kernel is defined as:

$$K_{HI}(A,B) = \sum_{i=1}^{M} \min\{A_i, B_i\}. \tag{6}$$

In Odone et al. (2005), K_{HI} is shown to be a Mercer's kernel by finding an explicit feature mapping after which histogram intersection is an inner product. Let us first assume that I and J have both *N* pixels. Histogram *A* is represented with a *P*-dimensional binary vector **A** *(P=M*N)*:

$$\mathbf{A} = \left(\underbrace{\overbrace{1,\cdots,1}^{A_1},\overbrace{0,\cdots,0}^{N-A_1}}_{1st-bin}, \underbrace{\overbrace{1,\cdots,1}^{A_2},\overbrace{0,\cdots,0}^{N-A_2}}_{2nd-bin}, \cdots, \underbrace{\overbrace{1,\cdots,1}^{A_M},\overbrace{0,\cdots,0}^{N-A_M}}_{Mth-bin} \right). \tag{7}$$

In this representation, each bin A_i is transformed in a binary vector of length *N*, with a number of *1*s proportional to the value of A_i, and zeros elsewhere. Similarly, *B* is represented with a binary vector **B**. It can be readily seen that $K_H(A,B)$ is equal to the standard inner product between corresponding vectors **A** and **B**. Thus, K_{HI} is a Mercer's kernel and the binary vector described above represents the result of the explicit mapping between input and feature space. It is possible to deal with arbitrary-sized images by first normalizing the histograms. In Odone et al, (2005) can be found more details and comments on the proof.

Boughorbel, Tarel, and Boujemaa (2005a) propose a generalized version of the histogram-intersection kernel that can be used without histogram normalization and applied to a more general class of features.

Definition of Generalized Histogram Intersection

Let *A* and *B* be the histograms of images I and J respectively. The generalized histogram-intersection kernel is defined as:

$$K_{GHI}(A,B) = \sum_{i=1}^{M} \min\left\{ \mid A_i \mid^{\beta}, \mid B_i \mid^{\beta} \right\}. \qquad (8)$$

The authors show that K_{GHI} is positive definite for all $\beta \geqslant 0$. See Boughorbel et al. (2005c) for details.

The histogram-intersection kernel was applied in Odone et al. (2005) to two binary image classification problems: indoor-outdoor and cityscape-noncityscape classifications. In the first case, it was shown as being comparable, and in the second case it was superior to heavy-tails kernels. An interesting advantage of histogram intersection is that it does not need parameter tuning. In Boughorbel, Tarel, and Boujemaa (2005a), the generalized histogram intersection is applied to a six-class image-categorization problem. With a suitable choice of parameter β, this kernel outperformed both Laplacian and histogram intersection kernels.

Kernel Functions for Local Features

The global approach to image classification is sensitive to changes due to perspective distortion, occlusions, illumination variations, and clutter. In the previous section, we have mentioned the Hausdorff kernel, which was an attempt to embed tolerance to local variations in a correlation measure. Another drawback of global approaches is that the descriptions obtained are redundant, and may contain misleading information, such as flat areas or background. While for background elimination an appropriate preprocessing (segmentation) is needed, redundancy can be better addressed with local descriptions. Local features (Lowe, 2004; Mikolajczyk & Schmid, 2003; Schmid & Mohr, 1997) are powerful image descriptors to tackle image classification. The local approach suggests that keeping only important point sets leads to a more compact description and makes it easier to control occlusions and illumination changes.

The main problem in combining kernel methods with local image features is that local approaches produce feature vectors of different size. This is due to the fact that there is no guarantee that applying the same point-detector algorithm to different images will produce the same number of points. On the other hand, kernel methods are based on computing inner products between feature vectors in appropriate feature spaces and thus assume that all feature vectors have the same size (i.e., they belong to the same space). Obviously, as pointed out in Wallraven, Caputo, and Graf (2003), simple heuristics such as zero-padding to make all vectors uniform in size are not applicable here.

Another property of local feature descriptions, and in general of all set descriptions, is that there is no obvious structuring, for example, no ordering, among the vector elements. Thus, no assumption of the correlation of vectors can be used. Lacking internal structure in the feature sets, the construction of local kernels is often computationally challenging.

This section provides a brief review on kernels for image local key points, showing how they deal with variable-length feature vectors. Other interesting pointers can be found in the section on sequence classification in Chapter III; the literature on kernel engineering for genomic sequences provides useful insights on how to build kernels for variable-size descriptions.

The reminder of the section is organized as follows. We first briefly review past work on kernels for sets. We then describe in some detail the *matching kernel* (Wallraven et al., 2003), one the first attempts of using local image descriptors in kernel methods; here we will also discuss a modification of the local kernel that has been recently proposed (Boughorbel, 2005). We then describe a very recent work on designing kernels for *pyramid local descriptions* (Grauman & Darrell, 2005). We conclude the section with a kernel for regions, discussing the links with the local feature case.

Kernels for Sets

Among the kernels for structured data proposed (that include strings, DNA, and trees), kernels for sets have been extensively studied for their peculiarity of dealing with unordered data.

A common approach to define a global similarity between feature sets $X = \{x_1, ..., x_m\}$ and $Y = \{y_1, ..., y_n\}$ of different sizes is to combine the local similarities between (possibly all) pairs of vector elements:

$$K(X,Y) = \Im(K_l(x_i, y_j)). \tag{9}$$

The simplest way of comparing sets is the summation kernel:

$$K_S(X,Y) = \sum_{i=1}^{m} \sum_{j=1}^{n} k(\mathbf{x}_i, \mathbf{y}_j). \tag{10}$$

K_S has been proved to be a Mercer kernel, provided that k is a Mercer kernel (Haussler, 1999). In practical applications, this kernel is not of great interest. Together with being computationally heavy, it mixed good and bad correspondences in the same result.

Wolf and Shashua (2003) propose a Mercer kernel for sets of vectors based on the concept of principal angles between two linear subspaces. To guarantee that the kernel is positive definite, there is an underlying assumption that sets must have the same size. This assumption makes the kernel impractical if one wants to use it to match image features.

An alternative approach to design kernels for sets of variable sizes is to fit a distribution to the set and define the kernel on such distributions. Kernel construction amounts at measuring the similarity between distributions. The main drawbacks of such an approach are that an assumption on the distribution needs to be made and also, in many practical cases, the feature set is not sufficiently large to give a good fit. It is worth mentioning in this context the work presented in Kondor and Jebara (2003). The authors base their work on the intuition that in many practical cases, and certainly in the case of images, it would be useful to design kernels that are relatively insensitive to transformations $x_i \longrightarrow x_i + \delta$, especially when δ is a smooth function of x. They call this property "soft invariance," and they achieve it by fitting Gaussian models to the feature sets. They define a kernel for distributions based on the Bhattacharyya's affinity:

$$K_B(X,Y) = K_B(p,p') = \int \sqrt{p(x)} \sqrt{p'(x)} dx. \tag{11}$$

From the computational viewpoint, this kernel is quite expensive as the Bhattacharyya kernel is cubic in the number of interest points.

The Matching Kernel

Wallraven et al. (2003) propose one of the first applications of a kernel for sets to local image features. They introduce a kernel function that they call local or matching kernel and apply it to object recognition. Let us first recall the definition of matching kernel both with and without position information.

Definition of Matching Kernel

Let $X = \{x_1, ..., x_m\}$ and $Y = \{y_1, ..., y_n\}$, $x_i, y_j \in \mathbb{R}^d$, $i = 1, ..., m$, $i = 1, ..., n$, be two sets of features. We may think they are some representations of point of interest extracted from two different images. Then the matching kernel, K_L, is defined as:

$$K_L(X,Y) = \frac{1}{2}(\hat{K}(X,Y) + \hat{K}(Y,X)), \tag{12}$$

where $\hat{K}(X,Y) = \frac{1}{m} \sum_{i=1}^{m} \max_{j=1,...,n} \{K_l(x_i, y_j)\}$.

In case one wants to include the features' positions in the matching procedure, the above kernel can be modified as follows. Let $P_X = \{px_1, ..., px_m\}$ and $P_Y = \{py_1, ..., py_n\}$ be the coordinates associated to feature sets X and Y. Then the local kernel K_L can be modified as:

$$\hat{K}(X,Y) = \frac{1}{m} \sum_{i=1}^{m} \max_{j=1,...,n} \{K_l(x_i, y_j)\} \exp(-(px_i - py_j)^2 / 2\sigma^2). \tag{13}$$

According to the authors, if K_l is a Mercer kernel, then also K_L (with or without geometric information) is a Mercer kernel. K_l can be chosen among the standard kernels or among the Mercer's functions for images proposed in the literature (see previous section). Unfortunately, the proof presented in Wallraven et al. (2003) is not correct, as shown in Boughorbel, Tarel, and Fleuret (2004) with a counterexample. The tricky point leading to the erroneous conclusion is that the max operator applied to Mercer kernels does not give a Mercer kernel.

The results presented there show that the proposed similarity measure is good for the problem at hand and the image representation chosen. Unfortunately, without the Mercer property, uniqueness of the solution and convergence cannot be guaranteed.

More recently, a modification of the local kernel that has the Mercer property has been proposed (Boughorbel, Tarel, & Boujemaa, 2005a). The new kernel, called *intermediate matching kernel* and designed to be positive definite, is based on using a set of virtual features.

Definition of Intermediate Matching Kernel

Let $X = \{x_1, ..., x_m\}$ and $Y = \{y_1, ..., y_n\}$, $x_i, y_j \in \mathbb{R}^d$, $i = 1, ..., m$, $i = 1, ..., n$, be two sets of features. Assuming we have built a set V of virtual features, $V = \{v_1, ..., v_p\}$, the intermediate matching kernel K_v is defined as:

$$K_V(X,Y) = \sum_{v_i \in V} K_{v_i}(X,Y),$$ (14)

with

$$K_{v_i}(X,Y) = \exp(-\|x^* - y^*\|^2 / 2\sigma^2),$$ (15)

where x^* and y^* are the elements of X and Y respectively closer to the virtual feature v_i.

The virtual features can be selected with a preprocessing procedure applied to the training set. Once all the local features are extracted from the training set, they are clustered, and the cluster centers are used as virtual features. The authors use a simple fuzzy K-means clustering algorithm, for which the number of clusters needs to be set. According to the authors, though, the choice of the number of clusters is not so crucial as it may be expected: With a higher number of clusters, the recognition becomes more accurate, but the performances rapidly saturate. Experimental evidence shows that the best results are obtained by computing virtual features on homogeneous training images belonging to one class. Each class is then implicitly represented by a set of virtual features; once the virtual features are selected, they are all joined together to form a vocabulary of features for the problem at hand. This approach appears to be related with the bag-of-features approach discussed in the next section.

In Boughorbel (2005) are presented experiments on object recognition with two different data sets. They include an interesting comparison among two different versions of the original matching kernel, the compactly supported kernel applied locally, and the intermediate matching kernel. The experiments highlight the superiority of the intermediate matching kernel, both in performance and generalization ability.

The Pyramid Kernel

Grauman and Darrell (2005) propose a rather complex representation based on mapping a feature set to a multiresolution histogram. The kernel is basically a multiresolution extension of the histogram-intersection kernel described before.

According to the authors, this approach is more efficient in terms of computational complexity than the other local methods presented here. From the point of view of the algorithm, the more interesting aspect of this approach is that it is not based on building a global similarity by combining local similarities. Instead, it compares directly an overall representation of local features, capturing implicitly possible feature co-occurrences and features' joint statistics.

Definition of Pyramid Kernel

Let $X = \{x_1, ..., x_m\}$ and $Y = \{y_1, ..., y_n\}$, $x_i, y_j \in \Re^d$, $X, Y \in \mathcal{X}$. $\mathcal{X}$ is the input space of set vectors. Let us assume that all features are bounded by a d-dimensional hypersphere of diameter D.

We first map each feature vector in a multiresolution histogram according to the following function:

$$\Psi(X) = [H_{-1}(X), H_0(X), ..., H_L(X)], \quad L = \lceil \log_2 D \rceil. \tag{16}$$

$H_i(X)$ is a histogram of X with d-dimensional bins of side length 2^i. The presence of i=-1 will be clear when the kernel is introduced.

The pyramid match kernel, K_Δ, is defined as follows:

$$\tilde{K}_\Delta(\Psi(X), \Psi(Y)) = \sum_{i=0}^{L} \frac{1}{2^i} (K_{HI}(H_i(X), H_i(Y)) - K_{HI}(H_{i-1}(X), H_{i-1}(Y))). \tag{17}$$

The normalization term with the bin size tells us that matches found at finer resolutions are weighted more. The difference means that if the same match appears at different resolutions, only the match found at the finer resolution is kept. To avoid favoring larger input sets, a final normalization step is added:

$$K_\Delta(\Psi(X), \Psi(Y)) = 1/\sqrt{C}\tilde{K}_\Delta(\Psi(X), \Psi(Y)), \tag{18}$$

where

$$C = \tilde{K}(\Psi(X), \Psi(X))\tilde{K}(\Psi(Y), \Psi(Y)). \tag{19}$$

For the proof that K_Δ is a Mercer kernel, see Grauman and Darrell (2005). The results presented compare favorably to previous approaches on the database ETH-80.[6] Preliminary results on the complex Caltech[7] database are also reported.

Dealing with Regions

A popular approach to image categorization is to first perform image segmentation, and then represent the global image content with descriptions of the segmented regions. This approach is usually referred to as region-based approach. Similar to descriptions based on local features, region-based descriptions have variable lengths.

Jing et al. (2003) use SVMs with a region-based representation in the relevance feedback approach to image retrieval. Images are first segmented, then all regions bigger than a threshold are used to compose the image representation. The authors tackle the problem of variable-length vectors by embedding a similarity measure popular for image retrieval, the EMD (Rubner et al., 1998), in a Gaussian kernel.

Definition of EMD Kernel

Let $X = \{x_1, \ldots, x_m\}$ and $Y = \{y_1, \ldots, y_n\}$, $x_i, y_j \in \mathbb{R}^d$. (20)

$$K_{EMD}(X, Y) = \exp(-EMD(X, Y) / 2\sigma^2),$$ (21)

where $x_i, y_j \in \mathbb{R}^d$ describe possible regions representations; the authors suggest color moments or autocorrelograms.

Current Work

The main drawbacks of current local approaches are that their attempts to exploit spatial correlation are very limited and thus the feature vectors obtained lack any internal structure. This increases the algorithmic complexity and also limits the description power of the data available. Without any prior information on mutual positions, in principle, all features of one vector should be combined with all features of the other vector. A possible approach to overcome this problem is to combine similar features in order to reduce their number, similar to what stemming does for text processing. One possible approach is to cluster similar features and possibly find *representative* features that describe the cluster. Boughorbel, Tarel, and Boujemaa (2005b) adopt this approach to engineer the intermediate matching kernel described in the previous section. The representative features are the centroids of the computed clusters and they are used as virtual features to compare indirectly the real features extracted from the images. Csurka, Dance, Fan, Willamowsky, and Bray (2004) use a similar approach to define their *bag of key points*, which will be briefly described later in this section. Very effective representatives can be found if the training data are linked by a coherent structure, that is, they depict different views of the same scene, or even better, they belong to an image sequence and have temporal coherence. This will be briefly described at the end of the section.

Bag of Key Points

The idea of a bag of key points was proposed in the context of visual categorization (Csurka et al., 2004). The bag-of-key-points approach can be sketched as follows: (a) Extract and represent interesting points for all images of the training set (mixing all the classes), (b) identify the key-point "bags" with a clustering technique, (c) represent all images as bags of features using a histogram-like approach—for each feature of the image belonging to a given cluster, the bin corresponding to the cluster is increased by one element, and (d) train a learning system on such representations; the authors show that the best performances are obtained with linear SVM classifiers organized in a one-against-all tournament system.

The idea of bags of key points is inspired by the bags of words successfully used in text categorization (Joachims, 1998), where all the bags (clusters of features) identified in the second stage represent the *vocabulary* of features for the problem at hand.

The authors present results on visual categorization using two different object data sets of seven and five classes respectively, showing good recognition rates. The histogram-based representation is perhaps too simple as it discards not only any information on the geometry of the features, but also information on how well each feature fits the corresponding bin. In a more recent work, the authors proposed a preliminary study on using geometric information to improve visual categorization (Csurka, Willamowsky, Dance, & Perronnin, 2005).

Trains of Key Points

The bags-of-key-points approach is very attractive as it models in a simple way all characterizing features of the objects one wants to describe. The weakest part of it is clustering, where the number of feature classes needs to be fixed or estimated with some heuristics; if the number of clusters is not estimated correctly, the whole modeling would be flawed. Depending on the application domain, the bag-of-features structure can be kept while substituting the clustering with more reliable ways of finding feature classes and their representatives. One example of such domains is view-based 3-D object identification in case the training data are represented by image sequences of the objects of interest (Barla, Odone, & Verri, 2002; Pontil & Verri, 1998). In this case, one can exploit the temporal coherence between adjacent images and use a tracking algorithm, such as Kalman, to find groups of similar features over the sequence. If one wants to exploit additional information about features scale and orientation during the tracking phase, nonlinear tracking algorithms (Julier & Uhlmann, 1997) are advisable. The results of robust tracking will be trains of features that follow the interesting points over time. Similar to using clusters centers, each train of

Figure 2. Sample frames taken from the training sets of three different objects

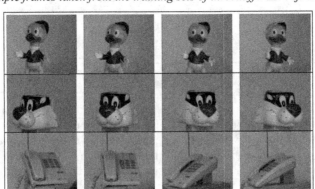

features may be represented, for instance, by virtual features made of the average feature and its standard deviation.

We are currently working on such feature-based representations of 3-D objects. Figure 2 shows sample frames of the images belonging to three objects of our data set, and Figure 3 shows examples of the local distinctive points detected in SIFT (Lowe, 2004).

Finally, Figure 4 shows the results of some experiments illustrating the appropriateness of our representations on test images that do not belong to the sequence. The images on top contain patches around the points where the features have been located on the test image. The images on the bottom represent the test images as a combination of the virtual features that matched features of the test data. These results indicate that trains of key points are good candidates for building feature vectors for view-based 3-D object recognition.

Discussion

Despite the growing number of contributions in this area in the last few years, much more work remains to be done. We think that three areas in particular deserve more attention. First,

Figure 3. Local distinctive features located on sample images

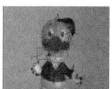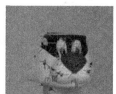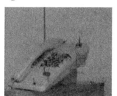

Figure 4. Features on test images and a visualization of the virtual features that represent them

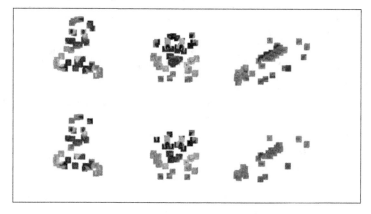

most of the methods developed so far have been fine-tuned on certain training and test sets. As a result, the role played by the prior knowledge implicitly embedded in the developed system is likely to undermine the generalization ability of the proposed methods applied to fresh data. This problem can presumably be overcome by promoting data exchanges and third-party assessment of the described techniques.

Second, the importance of long-range correlation, or geometry, is still underestimated. While it is conceivable that not much 3-D geometry structure information is needed to tackle most (though not all) image classification problems, the relative position of visual features of the same object is known to be both perceptually relevant and crucial to obtain results robust to occlusions.

Finally, we argue that segmentation should be brought back into the picture. The complexity of image classification tasks requires that the various problems should be addressed making use of all the relevant and available information. Perfect segmentation is presumably impossible to obtain, but the current state of the art of image segmentation could be taken as an interesting starting point for developing more sophisticated (and perhaps computationally intensive) image classifiers. An example of kernel-based image segmentation is kernel PCA segmentation. The interested reader is referred to Chapter XIV.

Acknowledgments

The authors would like to thank S. Boughorbel and J. P. Tarel for useful comments to the manuscript, A. Barla for all the joint work on kernels for global representations, and E. Arnaud and E. Delponte for their work and their expertise on particle filtering and local key points.

References

Barla, A., Odone, F., & Verri, A. (2002). Hausdorff kernel for 3D object acquisition and detection. In *Proceedings of the European Conference on Computer Vision* (Vol. 4, pp. 20-33).

Belongie, S., Fowlkes, C., Chung, F., & Malik, J. (2002). Spectral partitioning with indefinite kernels using the Nyström extension. In *Proceedings of the European Conference on Computer Vision* (Vol. 3, pp. 531-542).

Bishof, H., Wildenauer, H., & Leonardis, A. (2001). Illumination insensitive eigenspaces. In *Proceedings of the IEEE International Conference on Computer Vision* (pp. 233-238).

Boughorbel, S. (2005). *Kernels for image classification with support vector machines.* Unpublished doctoral dissertation, Université Paris.

Boughorbel, S., Tarel, J. P., & Boujemaa, N. (2005a). Generalized histogram intersection kernel for image recognition. *International Conference on Image Processing* (Vol. 3, pp. 161-164).

Boughorbel, S., Tarel, J. P., & Boujemaa, N. (2005b). The intermediate matching kernel for image local features. *International Joint Conference on Neural Networks* (pp. 889-894).

Boughorbel, S., Tarel, J. P., & Fleuret, F. (2004). Non-Mercer kernels for SVM object recognition. In *Proceedings of British Machine Vision Conference* (pp. 137-146).

Boughorbel, S., Tarel, J. P., Fleuret, F., & Boujemaa, N. (2005). The GCS kernel for SVM-based image recognition. *International Conference on Artificial Neural Networks* (Vol. 2, pp. 595-600).

Chapelle, O., Haffner, P., & Vapnik, V. (1999). SVMs for histogram based image classification. *IEEE Transactions on Neural Networks, 9*, 1-11.

Csurka, G., Dance, C., Fan, L., Willamowsky, J., & Bray, C. (2004). Visual categorization with bags of keypoints. *Proceedings of the ECCV International Workshop on Statistical Learning in Computer Vision.*

Csurka, G., Willamowsky, J., Dance, C., & Perronnin, F. (2005). Incorporating geometry information with weak classifiers for improved generic visual categorization. In *Proceedings of the International Conference on Image Analysis and Processing* (pp. 612-620).

Franceschi, E., Odone, F., Smeraldi, F., & Verri, A. (2005). *Feature selection with non-parametric statistics.* Proceedings of the IEEE International Conference on Image Processing, Genova, Italy.

Genton, M. (2001). Classes of kernels for machine learning: A statistics perspective. *Journal of Machine Learning Research, 2*, 299-312.

Grauman, K., & Darrell, T. (2005). *The pyramid match kernel: Discriminative classification with sets of image features.* In Proceedings of the IEEE International Conference on Computer Vision, Beijing, China.

Haussler, D. (1999). *Convolution kernels on discrete structures* (Tech. Rep. No. UCS-CRL-99-10). Santa Cruz, CA: UC Santa Cruz.

Heisele, B., Ho, P., & Poggio, T. (2001). Face recognition with support vector machines: Global versus component based approach. In *Proceedings of the International Conference on Computer Vision* (pp. 688-694).

Heisele, B., Verri, A., & Poggio, T. (2002). Learning and vision machines. In *Proceedings of the IEEE, 90*(7), 1164-1177.

Jing, F., Li, M., Zhang, H., & Zhang, B. (2003). Support vector machines for region-based image retrieval. In *Proceedings of the IEEE International Conference on Multimedia & Expo* (Vol. 2, pp, 4-22).

Joachims, T. (1998). Text categorization with support vector machines: Learning with many relevant features. *European Conference on Machine Learning* (pp. 137-142).

Jonsson, K., Matas, J., Kittler, J., & Li, Y. (2000). Learning support vectors for face verification and recognition. *Proceedings of the IEEE International Conference on Automatic Face and Gesture Recognition* (pp. 28-30).

Julier, S., & Uhlmann, J. (1997). A new extension of the Kalman filter to nonlinear systems. In *International Symposium Aerospace/Defense Sensing, Simulations, and Controls* (pp. 34-46).

Kondor, R., & Jebara, T. (2003). A kernel between sets of vectors. Presented at the *International Conference on Machine Learning (ICML)* (pp. 361-368).

Lowe, D. G. (2004). Distinctive image features from scale invariant keypoints. *International Journal of Computer Vision, 60*(2), 91-110.

Mikolajczyk, K., & Schmid, C. (2003). A performance evaluation of local descriptors. In *Proceedings of the Conference on Computer Vision and Pattern Recognition* (Vol. 2, pp. 257-263).

Mohan, A., Papageorgiou, C., & Poggio, T. (2001). Example-based object detection in images by components. *IEEE Transactions on Pattern Analysis and Machine Intelligence, 23*(4), 349-361.

Odone, F., Barla, A., & Verri, A. (2005). Building kernels from binary strings for image matching. *IEEE Transactions on Image Processing, 14*(2), 169-180.

Odone, F., Trucco, E., & Verri, A. (2001). General purpose matching of grey-level arbitrary images. In *Proceedings of the 4th International Workshop on Visual Forms* (pp. 573-582).

Osuna, E., Freund, R., & Girosi, F. (1997). Training support vector machines: An application to face detection. In *Proceedings of the IEEE Conference on Computer Vision and Pattern Recognition* (pp. 17-19).

Papageorgiou, C., & Poggio, T. (2000). A trainable system for object detection. *International Journal of Computer Vision, 38*(1), 15-33.

Poggio, T., Mukherjee, S., Rifkin, R., Rakhlin, A., & Verri, A. (2001). In *Proceedings of the Conference on Uncertainty in Geometric Computation* (pp. 22-28).

Pontil, M., & Verri, A. (1998). Support vector machines for 3D object recognition. *IEEE Transactions on Pattern Analysis and Machine Intelligence, 6*, 637-646.

Roobaert, D., Zillich, M., & Eklundh, J. O. (2001). A pure learning approach to background invariant object recognition using pedagogical support vector learning. In *Proceedings of the IEEE Conference on Computer Vision and Pattern Recognition* (Vol. 2, pp. 351-357).

Rubner, Y., Tomasi, C., & Guibas, L. J. (1998). A metric for distributions with applications to image databases. In *Proceedings of the IEEE International Conference on Computer Vision,* Bombay, India (pp. 59-66).

Schmid, C., & Mohr, R. (1997). Local greyvalue invariants for image retrieval. *IEEE Transactions on Pattern Analysis and Machine Intelligence, 19*(5), 530-535.

Schölkopf, B., Simard, P., Smola, A., & Vapnik V. (1998). Prior knowledge in support vector kernels. In *Proceedings on the Advances in Neural Information Processing Systems (NIPS)* (Vol. 10, pp. 640-646).

Swain, M. J., & Ballard, D. H. (1991). Color indexing. *Journal of Computer Vision, 7*(1), 11-32.

Trucco, E., & Verri, A. (1998). *Introductory techniques for 3-D computer vision.* Prentice-Hall.

Ullman, S., Vidal-Naquet, M., & Sali, E. (2002). Visual features of intermediate complexity and their use in classification. *Nature Neuroscience, 5*(7), 1-6.

Vapnik, V. V. (1995). *The nature of statistical learning theory.* Berlin, Germany: Springer-Verlag.

Viola, P., & Jones, M. (2004). Robust real-time object detection. *International Journal of Computer Vision, 57*(2), 137-154.

Wallraven, C., Caputo, B., & Graf, A. (2003). *Recognition with local features: The kernel recipe.* In Proceedings of the IEEE International Conference on Computer Vision, Nice, France.

Wolf, L., & Shashua, A. (2003). Learning over sets using kernel principal angles. *Journal of Machine Learning Research, 4*(10), 913-931.

Endnotes

[1]   The CBCL database http://cbcl.mit.edu/projects/cbcl/software-datasets/ includes faces, pedestrian, and cars.

[2]   The image of Figure 1 belongs to the MIT/CMU test set. The Combined MIT/CMU Test Set of Frontal Faces is currently available for download at http://www.ri.cmu.edu/projects/project_419.html

[3]   The reader interested in face recognition is referred to the *Face Recognition Home Page* at http://www.face-rec.org/

[4]   The COIL database of 100 objects is available for download at http://www1.cs.columbia.edu/CAVE/

[5]   On this respect, image classification shares some similarities with genomic sequence classification, see Chapter III of this book (Vert, 2006).

[6]   Available for download at http://www.vision.ethz.ch/projects/categorization/

[7]   A dataset of 101 objects available for download at http://www.vision.caltech.edu/Image_Datasets/Caltech101/

Chapter XV

Probabilistic Kernel PCA and its Application to Statistical Modeling and Inference

Daniel Cremers, University of Bonn, Germany

Timo Kohlberger, Siemens Corporate Research, USA

Abstract

We present a method of density estimation that is based on an extension of kernel PCA to a probabilistic framework. Given a set of sample data, we assume that this data forms a Gaussian distribution, not in the input space but upon a nonlinear mapping to an appropriate feature space. As with most kernel methods, this mapping can be carried out implicitly. Due to the strong nonlinearity, the corresponding density estimate in the input space is highly non-Gaussian. Numerical applications on 2-D data sets indicate that it is capable of approximating essentially arbitrary distributions. Beyond demonstrating applications on 2-D data sets, we apply our method to high-dimensional data given by various silhouettes of a 3-D object. The shape density estimated by our method is subsequently applied as a statistical shape prior to variational image segmentation. Experiments demonstrate that the resulting segmentation process can incorporate highly accurate knowledge on a large variety of complex real-world shapes. It makes the segmentation process robust to misleading information due to noise, clutter and occlusion.

Introduction

One of the challenges in the field of image segmentation is the incorporation of prior knowledge on the shape of the segmenting contour. A common approach is to learn the shape of an object statistically from a set of training shapes, and to then restrict the segmenting contour to a submanifold of familiar shapes during the segmentation process. For the problem of segmenting a specific known object, this approach was shown to drastically improve segmentation results (cf. Cremers, 2001; Leventon, Grimson, & Faugeras, 2000; Tsai et al., 2001).

Although the shape prior can be quite powerful in compensating for misleading information due to noise, clutter, and occlusion in the input image, most approaches are limited in their applicability to more complicated shape variations of real-world objects. Commonly, the permissible shapes are assumed to form a multivariate Gaussian distribution, which essentially means that all possible shape deformations correspond to linear combinations of a set of eigenmodes, such as those given by principal component analysis (PCA; cf. Cootes, 1999; Cremers, 2002; Kervrann & Heitz, 1998; Klassen, Srivastava, Mio, & Joshi, 2004; Leventon et al., 2000; Staib & Duncan, 1992). In particular, this means that for any two permissible shapes, the entire sequence of shapes obtained by a linear morphing of the two shapes is permissible as well. Such Gaussian shape models have recently been proposed for implicitly represented shapes as well (cf. Leventon et al., 2000; Rousson, Paragios, & Deriche, 2004; Tsai et al., 2001).[1] Once the set of training shapes exhibits highly nonlinear shape deformations, such as different 2-D views of a 3-D object, one finds distinct clusters in shape space corresponding to the stable views of an object. Moreover, each of the clusters may by itself be quite non-Gaussian. The Gaussian hypothesis will then result in a mixing of the different views, and the space of accepted shapes will be far too large for the prior to sensibly restrict the contour deformation.

A number of models have been proposed to deal with nonlinear shape variation. However, they often suffer from certain drawbacks. Some involve a complicated model construction procedure (Chalmond & Girard, 1999). Some are supervised in the sense that they assume prior knowledge on the structure of the nonlinearity (Heap & Hogg, 1996). Others require prior classification with the number of classes to be estimated or specified beforehand, and each class being assumed Gaussian (Cootes, 1999; Hogg, 1998). Some cannot be easily extended to shape spaces of higher dimension (Hastie & Stuetzle, 1989).

In this chapter, we present a density-estimation approach that is based on Mercer kernels (Courant & Hilbert, 1953; Mercer, 1909) and that does not suffer from any of the mentioned drawbacks. The proposed model can be interpreted as an extension of kernel PCA (Schölkopf, 1998) to the problem of density estimation. We refer to it as probabilistic kernel PCA. This chapter comprises and extends results that were published from two conferences (Cremers, 2001; Cremers, 2002) and in a journal paper (Cremers, 2003). Then, we review the variational integration of a linear shape prior into Mumford-Shah-based segmentation. Next, we give an intuitive example for the limitations of the linear shape model. Afterward, we present the nonlinear density estimate based on probabilistic kernel PCA. We compare it to related approaches and give estimates of the involved parameters. In the next section, we illustrate its application to artificial 2-D data and to silhouettes of real objects. Then this nonlinear shape prior is integrated into segmentation. We propose a variational integration of similarity invariance. We give numerous examples of segmentation with and without shape prior on static images and tracking sequences that finally confirm the properties of the nonlinear shape prior: It can encode very different shapes and generalizes to novel views without blurring or mixing different views. Furthermore, it improves segmentation by reducing the dimension of the search space by stabilizing with respect to clutter and noise and by reconstructing the contour in areas of occlusion.

Bayesian Approach to Image Segmentation

The goal of image segmentation is to partition the image $I : \Omega \subset \mathbb{R}^r \rightarrow \mathbb{R}^d$ into meaningful regions, where meaningful typically refers to a separation of regions that can be ascribed to different objects or to the background.[2] In this sense, the problem of image segmentation is closely related to higher level image-analysis problems such as image parsing, object boundary detection, and object recognition. As will become apparent in the subsequent pages, this connection is even more pronounced once prior knowledge about specific objects of interest is introduced into the segmentation process.

Within a generative Bayesian framework, a segmentation can be obtained by determining the boundary $\hat{C}$ that maximizes the conditional probability:

$$P(C|I) = \frac{P(I|C)\,P(C)}{P(I)}. \tag{1}$$

For the optimization, the denominator is a constant and can therefore be neglected. The first factor in the numerator requires a model of the image-formation process to specify the probability of a measurement I given a boundary C. The second factor in equation (1) allows one to impose a prior $P(C)$ on the space of contours specifying which contours are a priori more or less likely. Note that the interpretation of densities $P(C)$ on infinite-dimensional spaces requires the definition of appropriate measures and addressing the issue of integrability. A thorough treatment of density estimation on infinite-dimensional spaces is, however, beyond the scope of this work.

The inversion of the image-formation process is the central goal of all image analysis, yet it is generally an ill-posed problem: Important information about the world may be lost due to the projection of the scene onto two dimensions, due to partial occlusions of the objects of interest, or due to complicated interaction of light and objects. Many of these effects (light variations due to interreflections and scattering, camera sensor noise, etc.) can be approximated by appropriate statistical models. The Bayesian formula in equation (1) can thus be interpreted as an inversion of the image-formation process in a stochastic setting.

In the following, we shall consider one of the simplest intensity models for image segmentation, namely, we will assume that the intensities of objects and background are random samples drawn from respective Gaussian distributions. This model is one of the most popular image-formation models; different variations of it can be traced back to the works of Ising (1925) on ferromagnetism, and the Mumford-Shah functional (Mumford & Shah,

1989) and its statistical interpretation by Zhu and Yuille (1996). There exist a number of practical implementations via partial differential equations (Chan & Vese, 2001; Cremers, 2002; Cremers, Schnörr, Weickert, & Schellewald, 2000; Figueiredo, Leitao, & Jain, 2000; Ronfard, 1994; Tsai, Yezzi, & Willsky, 2001), and extensions of this intensity model to texture (Rousson, Brox, & Deriche, 2003), motion (Cremers & Soatto, 2005), and dynamic texture segmentation (Doretto, Cremers, Favaro, & Soatto, 2003).

Assume the image plane Ω is made up of k regions $\{\Omega_i\}_{i=1,...,k}$, each of which corresponds to an object or to the background. The intensity $I(x)$ of each pixel of region Ω_i is assumed to be distributed according to a Gaussian of the form:

$$P_i(I(x)) = \frac{1}{\sqrt{2\pi}\sigma} \exp\left(-\frac{(I(x) - u_i)^2}{2\sigma^2}\right). \tag{2}$$

For simplicity, we shall assume that all Gaussians have the same variance σ. The extension to allow separate variances σ_i for each region Ω_i is straightforward. More sophisticated intensity models, such as mixture models, kernel density estimators, and spatially varying intensity models, are conceivable. But these are not the focus of the present work.

Assuming the intensity of all pixels to be independent, the probability of measuring an intensity image I given a partition by a boundary C into regions $\{\Omega_1, ..., \Omega_k\}$ is given by:

$$P(I|C) = P(I|\{\Omega_1, ..., \Omega_k\}) = \prod_{i=1}^{k} \prod_{x \in \Omega_i} (P_i(I(x)))^{dx}. \tag{3}$$

The exponent dx denotes the bin size of the discretization and guarantees a consistent continuum limit. If, for example, we discretize the image plane with twice as many pixels of half the size, then we obtain the same expression.

Given this image-formation model, the maximization of the a posteriori probability in equation (1) can be implemented by minimizing its negative logarithm, which is given by a functional of the form:

$$E(C) = E_{image}(C) + E_{shape}(C) = \frac{1}{2\sigma^2} \sum_i \int_{\Omega_i} (I(x) - u_i)^2 \, dx - \log P(C). \tag{4}$$

Minimizing this functional leads to a piecewise constant approximation of the intensity image I. The most common generic prior on the segmentation C is one which favors boundaries C of minimal length $L(C)$:

$$P(C) \propto \exp(-\nu\, L(C)), \quad E_{shape}(C) = \nu\, L(C), \text{ with } \nu > 0. \tag{5}$$

Generic shape priors of the form in equation (5) are common to most established segmentation methods, such as the snakes (Kass, Witkin, & Terzopoulos, 1988) or the Mumford-Shah functional (Mumford & Shah, 1989). While they provide good performance in general-purpose segmentation schemes, coping with noise, and guaranteeing smooth segmentation boundaries, they also induce a tendency of the segmentation scheme to suppress small-scale details.

It is not clear a priori why a shorter contour length should be favored over a longer one. However, if we are given some prior knowledge about the shape of objects of interest. for example, in terms of a set of training silhouettes, then it is possible to introduce this information into the segmentation process.

Statistical Shape Priors in Variational Image Segmentation

The idea to introduce object-specific shape knowledge into segmentation methods was pioneered by Grenander, Chow, and Keenan (1991). Statistical shape models were developed among others by Cootes, Taylor, Cooper, and Graham (1995). The probabilistic integration in the above variational framework was developed in Cremers (2002). The construction of more sophisticated statistical shape priors $P(C)$ by means of a probabilistic extension of kernel PCA is the focus of this book chapter.

One of the central questions when modeling statistical shape priors is how to represent shape. We proposed an implementation of the functional of equation (4) with a parameterized spline curve:

$$C_z : [0,1] \to \mathbb{R}^2, \qquad C_z(s) = \sum_{n=1}^{N} \begin{pmatrix} x_n \\ y_n \end{pmatrix} B_n(s), \tag{6}$$

where B_n are quadratic, uniform, and periodic B-spline basis functions (Farin, 1997), and $z = (x_1, y_1, ..., x_N, y_N)^\top$ denotes the vector of control points. In particular, we proposed to measure the length of the contour by the squared L_2-norm:

$$L(C) = \int_0^1 \left(\frac{dC}{ds} \right)^2 ds, \tag{7}$$

rather than the usual L_1-norm. As a consequence, the subsequent energy minimization simultaneously enforces an equidistant spacing of control points. This length constraint induces a rubber-band-like behavior of the contour and thereby prevents the formation of cusps during the contour evolution. Since it is the same length constraint that is used for the classical snakes (Kass et al., 1988), we obtain a hybrid model that combines the external energy of the Mumford-Shah functional with the internal (shape) energy of the snakes. For this reason, the functional of equation (4) with length constraint in equation (7) is called a *diffusion snake*.

As discussed above, one can replace the simple length constraint by a more sophisticated statistical shape energy $E_{shape}(C)$, which measures the dissimilarity of the given contour

Figure 1. Segmentation with linear shape prior on an image of a partially occluded hand: Initial contour (left), segmentation without shape prior (center), and segmentation with shape prior (right) are shown. The statistical shape prior compensates for misleading information due to noise, clutter, and occlusion. Integration into the variational framework effectively reduces the dimension of the search space and enlarges the region of convergence.

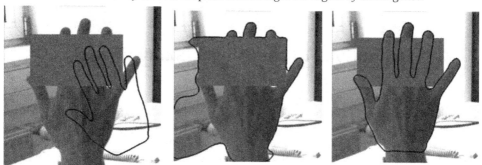

with respect to a set of training contours. Minimizing the total energy given by equation (4) will enforce a segmentation that is based on both the input image I and the similarity to a set of training shapes. Given the spline representation in equation (6) of the contour, shape statistics can then be obtained by estimating the distribution of the control point vectors corresponding to a set of contours that were extracted from binary training images.

In order to study the interaction between statistical shape knowledge and image gray-value information, we restricted the shape statistics in Cremers (2002) to a commonly employed model by assuming the training shapes to form a multivariate Gaussian distribution in shape space. This corresponds to a quadratic energy on the spline control point vector z:

$$E_c(C_z) = \frac{1}{2}(z - z_0)'C^{-1}(z - z_0),$$

(8)

where z_0 denotes the mean control point vector and C the covariance matrix after appropriate regularization (Cremers, 2002). The effect of this shape energy[3] in dealing with clutter and

Figure 2. Left: Projection of the training shapes and the estimated energy onto the first two principal components for a set containing right (+) and left (■) hands. Right: Sampling along the first principal component shows the mixing of different classes in the Gaussian model. Note that according to the Gaussian model, the mean shape (central shape) is the most probable shape.

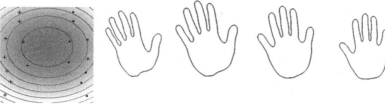

occlusion is exemplified in Figure 1. For the input image f of a partially occluded hand, we performed a gradient descent to minimize the total energy of equation (4) without ($\alpha = 0$) and with ($\alpha > 0$) shape prior. Incorporating the shape prior draws the evolving contour to a submanifold of familiar shapes. Thus the resulting segmentation process becomes insensitive to misleading information due to clutter and occlusion.

Limitations of the Linear Shape Model

Unfortunately, the linear shape statistics in equation (8) are limited in their applicability to more complicated shape deformations. As soon as the training shapes form distinct clusters in shape space, such as those corresponding to the stable views of a 3-D object, or if the shapes of a given cluster are no longer distributed according to a hyper-ellipsoid, the Gaussian shape prior tends to mix classes and blur details of the shape information in such a way that the resulting shape prior is no longer able to effectively restrict the contour evolution to the space of familiar shapes.

A standard way to numerically verify the validity of the Gaussian hypothesis is to perform statistical tests such as the χ^2-test. In the following, we will demonstrate the "non-Gaussianity" of a set of sample shapes in a different way because it gives a better intuitive understanding of the limitations of the Gaussian hypothesis in the context of shape statistics.

Figure 2, left side, shows the training shapes corresponding to nine views of a right hand and nine views of a left hand projected onto the first two principal components and the level lines of constant energy for the Gaussian model in equation (8). Note that if the training set were Gaussian distributed, then all projections should be Gaussian distributed as well. Yet in the projection in Figure 2, left side, one can clearly distinguish two separate clusters containing the right hands (+) and the left hands (■).

As suggested by the level lines of constant energy, the first principal component, that is. the mayor axis of the ellipsoid, corresponds to the deformation between right and left hands. This morphing from a left hand to a right hand is visualized in more detail in the right images of Figure 2. Sampling along the first principal component around the mean shape shows a mixing of shapes belonging to different classes. Obviously, the Gaussian model does not accurately represent the distribution of training shapes. In fact, according to the Gaussian model, the most probable shape is the mean shape given by the central shape in Figure 2. In this way, sampling along the different eigenmodes around the mean shape can give an intuitive feeling for the quality of the Gaussian assumption.

Density Estimation in Feature Space

In the following, we present an extension of the above method that incorporates a strong nonlinearity at almost no additional effort. Essentially, we propose to perform a density estimation not in the original space but in the feature space of nonlinearly transformed data.[4]

The nonlinearity enters in terms of Mercer kernels (Courant & Hilbert, 1953), which have been extensively used in pattern recognition and machine learning (cf. Aizerman, Braverman, & Rozonoer, 1964; Boser, Guyon, & Vapnik, 1992). In the present section, we will introduce the method of density estimation, discuss its relation to kernel principal component analysis (kernel PCA; Schölkopf, 1998), and propose estimates of the involved parameters. Finally, we will illustrate the density estimate in applications to artificial 2-D data and to 200-dimensional data corresponding to silhouettes of real-world training shapes. In order not to break the flow of the argument, further remarks on the relation of distances in feature space to classical methods of density estimation are postponed to Appendix A.

Gaussian Density in Kernel Space

Let $z_1, ..., z_m \in \mathbb{R}^n$ be a given set of training data. Let ϕ be a nonlinear mapping from the input space to a potentially higher dimensional space Y. The mean and the sample covariance matrix of the mapped training data are given by:

$$\phi_0 = \frac{1}{m} \sum_{i=1}^{m} \phi(z_i), \quad \tilde{C}_\phi = \frac{1}{m} \sum_{i=1}^{m} (\phi(z_i) - \phi_0)(\phi(z_i) - \phi_0)'. \tag{9}$$

Denote the corresponding scalar product in Y by the Mercer kernel (Courant & Hilbert, 1953):

$$k(x, y) := \langle \phi(x), \phi(y) \rangle, \quad \text{for } x, y \in \mathbb{R}^n. \tag{10}$$

Denote a mapped point after centering with respect to the mapped training points by:

$$\tilde{\phi}(z) := \phi(z) - \phi_0, \tag{11}$$

and the centered kernel function by

$$\tilde{k}(x, y) := \langle \tilde{\phi}(x), \tilde{\phi}(y) \rangle$$

$$= k(x, y) - \frac{1}{m} \sum_{k=1}^{m} \left(k(x, z_k) + k(y, z_k) \right) + \frac{1}{m^2} \sum_{k,l=1}^{m} k(z_k, z_l). \tag{12}$$

We estimate the distribution of the mapped training data by a Gaussian probability density in the space Y (see Figure 3). The corresponding energy, given by the negative logarithm of the probability, is a Mahalanobis type distance in the space Y:

$$E_\phi(z) = \tilde{\phi}(z)' C_\phi^{-1} \tilde{\phi}(z). \tag{13}$$

It can be considered a nonlinear measure of the dissimilarity between a point z and the training data. The regularized covariance matrix C_ϕ is obtained by replacing all zero eigenvalues of the sample covariance matrix $\tilde{C}_\phi$ by a constant $\lambda_\perp$:

$$C_\phi = V \Lambda V' + \lambda_\perp (I - VV'), \tag{14}$$

where Λ denotes the diagonal matrix of nonzero eigenvalues $\lambda_1 \le ... \le \lambda_r$ of $\tilde{C}$, and V is the matrix of the corresponding eigenvectors $V_1, ..., V_r$. By definition of $\tilde{C}_\phi$, these eigenvectors lie in the span of the mapped training data:

$$V_k = \sum_{i=1}^{m} \alpha_i^k \tilde{\phi}(z_i), \qquad 1 \le k \le r. \tag{15}$$

Schölkopf et al. (1998) showed that the eigenvalues λ_k of the covariance matrix and the expansion coefficients $\{\alpha_i^k\}_{i=1,...,m}$ in equation (15) can be obtained in terms of the eigenvalues and eigenvectors of the centered kernel matrix as follows. Let K be the $m \times m$ kernel matrix with entries $K_{ij} = k(z_i, z_j)$. Moreover, let $\tilde{K}$ be the centered kernel matrix with entries $\tilde{K}_{ij} = \tilde{k}(z_i, z_j)$. With equation (12), one can express the centered kernel matrix as a function of the uncentered one:

$$\tilde{K} = K - KE - EK + EKE, \qquad \text{where } E_{ij} = \frac{1}{m} \ \forall \ i, j = 1, ..., m. \tag{16}$$

With these definitions, the eigenvalues $\lambda_1, ..., \lambda_r$ of the sample covariance matrix are given by $\lambda_k = \frac{1}{m} \tilde{\lambda}_k$, where $\tilde{\lambda}_k$ are the eigenvalues of $\tilde{K}$, and the expansion coefficients $\{\alpha_i^k\}_{i=1,...,m}$ in equation (15) form the components of the eigenvector of $\tilde{K}$ associated with the eigenvalue $\tilde{\lambda}_k$.

Inserting equation (14) splits energy (equation (13)) into two terms:

$$E_\phi(z) = \sum_{k=1}^{r} \lambda_k^{-1} (V_k, \tilde{\phi}(z))^2 \ + \ \lambda_\perp^{-1} (|\tilde{\phi}(z)|^2 - \sum_{k=1}^{r} (V_k, \tilde{\phi}(z))^2). \tag{17}$$

With expansion equation (15), we obtain the final expression of our energy:

$$E_\phi(z) = \sum_{k=1}^{r} \left(\sum_{i=1}^{m} \alpha_i^k \tilde{k}(z_i, z) \right)^2 \cdot \left(\lambda_k^{-1} - \lambda_\perp^{-1} \right) + \lambda_\perp^{-1} \cdot \tilde{k}(z, z). \tag{18}$$

As in the case of kernel PCA, the nonlinearity ϕ only appears in terms of the kernel function. This allows one to specify an entire family of possible nonlinearities by the choice of the associated kernel. For all our experiments, we used the Gaussian kernel:

Figure 3. Nonlinear mapping into $Y = F \oplus \overline{F}$ *and the distances DIFS and DFFS*

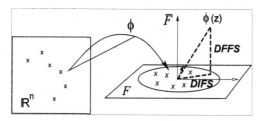

$$k(x, y) = \frac{1}{(2\pi\sigma^2)^{\frac{n}{2}}} \exp\left(-\frac{\|x - y\|^2}{2\sigma^2}\right). \tag{19}$$

For a justification of this choice, we refer to Appendix A, where we show the relation of the proposed energy with the classical Parzen estimator.

Relation to Kernel PCA

Just as in the linear case (cf. Moghaddam & Pentland, 1995), the regularization of equation (14) of the covariance matrix causes a splitting of the energy into two terms (equation (17)), which can be considered as a *distance in feature space* (DIFS) and a *distance from feature space* (DFFS; see Figure 3). For the purpose of pattern reconstruction in the framework of kernel PCA, it was suggested to minimize a reconstruction error (Schölkopf, 1998) that is identical with the DFFS. This procedure is based on the assumption that the entire plane spanned by the mapped training data corresponds to acceptable patterns. However, this is not a valid assumption: Already in the linear case, moving too far along an eigenmode will produce patterns that have almost no similarity to the training data, although they are still accepted by the hypothesis. Moreover, the distance DFFS is not based on a probabilistic model. In contrast, energy (equation (18)) is derived from a Gaussian probability distribution. It minimizes both the DFFS and the DIFS.

The kernel PCA approach has been studied in the framework of statistical shape models (Romdhani, Gong, & Psarrou, 1999; Twining & Taylor, 2001). Our approach differs from these two in three ways. First, our model is based on a probabilistic formulation of kernel PCA (as discussed above). Second, we derive a *similarity invariant* nonlinear shape model, as will be detailed later. Third, we introduce the nonlinear shape dissimilarity measure as a shape prior in variational segmentation.

On the Regularization of the Covariance Matrix

A regularization of the covariance matrix in the case of kernel PCA, as done in equation (14), was first proposed in Cremers (2001) and has also been suggested more recently in [45]. The choice of the parameter $\lambda_\perp$ is not a trivial issue. For the linear case, such regularizations of the covariance matrix have also been proposed (Cremers, 2001; Moghaddam & Pentland, 1995; Roweis, 1998; Tipping, 2001). There, the constant $\lambda_\perp$ is estimated as the mean of the replaced eigenvalues by minimizing the Kullback-Leibler distance of the corresponding densities. However, we believe that in our context, this is not an appropriate regularization of the covariance matrix. The Kullback-Leibler distance is supposed to measure the error with respect to the correct density, which means that the covariance matrix calculated from the training data is assumed to be the correct one. But this is not the case because the number of training points is limited. For essentially the same reason this approach does not extend to the nonlinear case considered here: Depending on the type of nonlinearity ϕ, the covariance matrix is potentially infinite-dimensional such that the mean over all replaced eigenvalues will be zero. As in the linear case (Cremers, 2002), we therefore propose to choose:

$$0 < \lambda_\perp < \lambda_r, \tag{20}$$

which means that unfamiliar variations from the mean are less probable than the smallest variation observed on the training set. In practice, we fix $\lambda_\perp = \lambda_r/2$.

On the Choice of the Hyperparameter σ

The last parameter to be fixed in the proposed density estimate is the hyperparameter σ in equation (19). Let μ be the average distance between two neighboring data points:

$$\mu^2 := \frac{1}{m} \sum_{i=1}^{m} \min_{j \neq i} |z_i - z_j|^2 . \tag{21}$$

In order to get a smooth energy landscape, we propose to choose σ in the order of μ. In practice, we used:

$$\sigma = 1.5 \, \mu \tag{22}$$

for most of our experiments. We chose this somewhat heuristic measure μ for the following favorable properties.

- μ is insensitive to the distance of clusters as long as each cluster has more than one data point.
- μ scales linearly with the data points.
- μ is robust with respect to the individual data points.

Density Estimate for Silhouettes of 2-D and 3-D Objects

Although energy (equation (13)) is quadratic in the space Y of mapped points, it is generally not convex in the original space, showing several minima and level lines of essentially arbitrary shape. Figure 4 shows artificial 2-D data and the corresponding lines of constant energy $E_\phi(z)$ in the original space. The modes of the associated density are located around the clusters of the input data.

For a set of binarized views of objects, we automatically fit a closed quadratic spline curve around each object. All spline curves have $N = 100$ control points, set equidistantly.

The polygons of control points $z = (x_1, y_1, x_2, y_2, ..., x_N, y_N)$ are aligned with respect to translation, rotation, scaling, and cyclic permutation (Cremers, 2002). This data was used to determine the density estimate $E_\phi(z)$ in equation (18).

For the visualization of the density estimate and the training shapes, all data were projected onto two of the principal components of a linear PCA. Note that due to the projection, this

Figure 4. Density estimate (equation (13)) for artificial 2-D data. Distributions of variable shape are well estimated by the Gaussian hypothesis in the feature space. We used the kernel (equation 19) with $\sigma = 1.5\ \mu$.

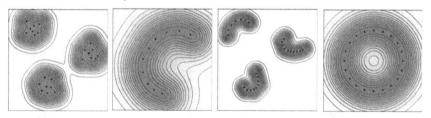

Figure 5. Model comparison. Density estimates for a set of left (■) and right (+) hands, projected onto the first two principal components. From left to right: Aligned contours, simple Gaussian, mixture of Gaussians, Gaussian in feature space (equation 13). Both the mixture model and the Gaussian in the feature space capture the two-class structure of the data. However, the estimate in the feature space is unsupervised and produces level lines that are not necessarily ellipses.

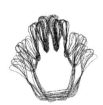 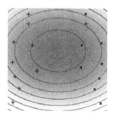 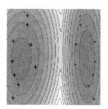 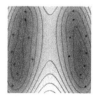

Figure 6. Density estimate for views of two 3-D objects. The training shapes of the duck (white +) and the rabbit (■) form distinct clusters in shape space, which are well captured by the energy level lines shown in appropriate 2-D projections.

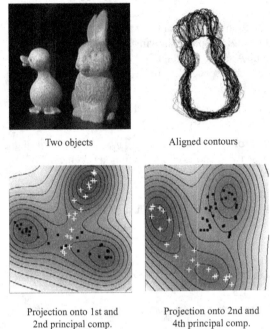

Two objects   Aligned contours

Projection onto 1st and   Projection onto 2nd and
2nd principal comp.   4th principal comp.

visualization only gives a very rough sketch of the true distribution in the 200-dimensional shape space.

Figure 5 shows density estimates for a set of right hands and left hands. The estimates correspond to the hypotheses of a simple Gaussian in the original space, a mixture of Gaussians, and a Gaussian in feature space. Although both the mixture model and our estimate in feature space capture the two distinct clusters, there are several differences. First the mixture model is supervised: The number of classes and the class membership must be known. Second, it only allows level lines of elliptical shape, corresponding to the hypothesis that each cluster by itself is a Gaussian distribution. The model of a Gaussian density in feature space does not assume any prior knowledge and produces level lines that capture the true distribution of the data even if individual classes do not correspond to hyper-ellipsoids.

This is demonstrated on a set of training shapes that correspond to different views of two 3-D objects. Figure 6 shows the two objects, their contours after alignment, and the level lines corresponding to the estimated energy density (equation (13)) in appropriate 2-D projections.

Nonlinear Shape Statistics in
Variational Image Segmentation

Minimization by Gradient Descent

Energy (equation (13)) measures the similarity of a shape C_z parameterized by a control point vector z with respect to a set of training shapes. For the purpose of segmentation, we introduce this energy as a shape energy E_{shape} in the functional equation (4).

The total energy must be simultaneously minimized with respect to the control points defining the contour and with respect to the segmenting gray values $\{u_i\}$. Minimizing the total energy including the length constraint (equation (7)) with respect to the contour C_z (for fixed $\{u_i\}$) results in the evolution equation:

$$\frac{\partial C_z(s,t)}{\partial t} = -\frac{dE_{image}}{dC_z} = (e_s^+ - e_s^-) \cdot n_s + \nu \frac{d^2 C_z}{ds^2}, \tag{23}$$

where the terms e_s^+ and e_s^- denote the energy density $e = (f - u_i)^2$, inside and outside the contour $C_z(s)$, respectively, and n_s denotes the normal vector on the contour. The constants $\{u_i\}$ are updated in alternation with the contour evolution to be the mean gray value of the adjoining regions $\{\Omega_i\}$. The contour evolution equation (23) is transformed into an evolution equation for the control points z by introducing equation (6) of the contour as a spline curve. By discretizing on a set of nodes s_j along the contour, we obtain a set of coupled linear differential equations. Solving for the coordinates of the ith control point and including the term induced by the shape energy we obtain:

$$\frac{dx_i(t)}{dt} = \sum_{j=1}^{N} \left(\mathbf{B}^{-1} \right)_{ij} [\left(e_j^+ - e_j^- \right) n_x(s_j,t) + \nu \, (x_{j-1} - 2x_j + x_{j+1})] - \alpha \left[\frac{dE_{shape}(z)}{dz} \right]_{2i-1},$$

$$\frac{dy_i(t)}{dt} = \sum_{j=1}^{N} \left(\mathbf{B}^{-1} \right)_{ij} [\left(e_j^+ - e_j^- \right) n_y(s_j,t) + \nu \, (y_{j-1} - 2y_j + y_{j+1})] - \alpha \left[\frac{dE_{shape}(z)}{dz} \right]_{2i}. \tag{24}$$

The cyclic tridiagonal matrix $\mathbf{B}$ contains the spline basis functions evaluated at these nodes.

The three terms in the evolution equation (24) can be interpreted as follows:

- The first term forces the contour toward the object boundaries by maximizing a homogeneity criterion in the adjoining regions, which compete in terms of their energy densities e^+ and e^-.

- The second term enforces an equidistant spacing of control points, thus minimizing the contour length. This prevents the formation of cusps during the contour evolution.

- The last term pulls the control point vector toward the domains of familiar shapes, thereby maximizing the similarity of the evolving contour with respect to the training shapes. It will be detailed in the next section.

Invariance in the Variational Framework

By construction, the density estimate (equation (13)) is not invariant with respect to translation, scaling, and rotation of the shape C_z. We therefore propose to eliminate these degrees of freedom in the following way: Since the training shapes were aligned to their mean shape z_0 with respect to translation, rotation, and scaling and then normalized to unit size, we shall do the same to the argument z of the shape energy before applying our density estimate E_ϕ.

We therefore define the shape energy by:

$$E_{shape}(z) = E_\phi(\tilde{z}), \quad \text{with } \tilde{z} = \frac{R_\theta \, z_c}{|R_\theta \, z_c|}, \tag{25}$$

where z_c denotes the control point vector after centering,

$$z_c = \left(I_n - \frac{1}{n} A \right) z, \quad \text{with } A = \begin{pmatrix} 1 & 0 & 1 & 0 & \cdots \\ 0 & 1 & 0 & 1 & \cdots \\ 1 & 0 & 1 & 0 & \cdots \\ \vdots & \vdots & \vdots & \vdots & \ddots \end{pmatrix}, \tag{26}$$

and R_θ denotes the optimal rotation of the control point polygon z_c with respect to the mean shape z_0. We will not go into detail about the derivation of R_θ. Similar derivations can be found in [50,18]. The final result is given by the formula:

$$\tilde{z} = \frac{M \, z_c}{|M \, z_c|}, \quad \text{with } M = I_n \otimes \begin{pmatrix} z'_0 \, z_c & -z_0 \times z_c \\ z_0 \times z_c & z'_0 \, z_c \end{pmatrix}, \tag{27}$$

where $\otimes$ denotes the Kronecker product and $z_0 \times z_c := z'_0 \, R_{\pi/2} z_c$.

The last term in the contour evolution equation (24) is now calculated by applying the chain rule:

$$\frac{dE_{shape}(z)}{dz} = \frac{dE_\phi(\tilde{z})}{d\tilde{z}} \cdot \frac{d\tilde{z}}{dz} = \frac{dE_\phi(\tilde{z})}{d\tilde{z}} \cdot \frac{d\tilde{z}}{dz_c} \cdot \frac{dz_c}{dz}. \tag{28}$$

Since this derivative can be calculated analytically, no additional parameters enter the above evolution equation to account for scale, rotation, and translation.

Other authors (cf. Chen, Thiruvenkadam, Tagare, Huang, Wilson, & Geiser, 2001) propose to explicitly model a translation, an angle, and a scale, and minimize with respect to these quantities (e.g., by gradient descent). In our opinion, this has several drawbacks. First, it introduces four additional parameters, which makes numerical minimization more complicated; parameters to balance the gradient descent must be chosen. Second, this approach mixes the degrees of freedom corresponding to scale, rotation, and shape deformation. Third, potential local minima may be introduced by the additional parameters. On several segmentation tasks, we were able to confirm these effects by comparing the two approaches.

Since there exists a similar closed-form solution for the optimal alignment of two polygons with respect to the more general affine group (Wermann & Weinshall, 1995), the above approach could be extended to define a shape prior that is invariant with respect to affine transformations. However, we do not elaborate this for the time being.

Numerical Results

In the following, we will present a number of numerical results obtained by introducing the similarity invariant nonlinear shape prior from equations (25) and (18) into the Mum-

Figure 7. Segmenting partially occluded images of several objects. While the linear prior draws the segmenting contour towards the mean shape, the nonlinear one permits the segmentation process to distinguish between the three training shapes. Introduction of the shape prior upon stationarity of the contour (top right) causes the contour to evolve normal to the level lines of constant energy into the nearest local minimum, as indicated by the white curves in the projected density estimate (bottom right).

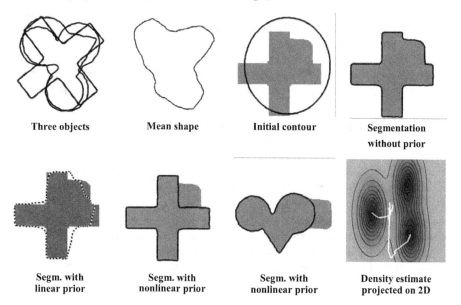

| Three objects | Mean shape | Initial contour | Segmentation without prior |

| Segm. with linear prior | Segm. with nonlinear prior | Segm. with nonlinear prior | Density estimate projected on 2D |

ford-Shah-based segmentation process as discussed above. The results are ordered so as to demonstrate different properties of the proposed shape prior.

Linear vs. Nonlinear Shape Prior

Compared to the linear case of equation (8), the nonlinear shape energy is no longer convex. Depending on the input data, it permits the formation of several minima corresponding to different clusters of familiar contours. Minimization by gradient descent will end up in the nearest local minimum. In order to obtain a certain independence of the shape prior from the initial contour, we propose to first minimize the image energy E_{shape} by itself until stationarity, and to then include the shape prior E_{shape}. This approach guarantees that we will extract as much information as possible from the image before deciding on which of the different clusters of accepted shapes the obtained contour resembles most.

Figure 7 shows a simple example of three artificial objects. The shape prior (equation (25)) was constructed on the three aligned silhouettes shown on the top left. The mean of the three shapes (second image) indicates that the linear Gaussian is not a reliable model for this training set. The next images show the initial contour for the segmentation of a partially occluded image of the first object, the final segmentation without prior knowledge, the final segmentation after introducing the linear prior, and the final segmentation upon introduction of the nonlinear prior. Rather than drawing the contour toward the mean shape (as does the linear prior), the nonlinear one draws the evolving contour toward one of the encoded shapes. Moreover, the same nonlinear prior permits a segmentation of an occluded version of the other encoded objects.

The bottom right image in Figure 7 shows the training shapes and the density estimate in a projection on the first two axes of a (linear) PCA. The white curves correspond to the path of the segmenting contour from its initialization to its converged state for the two segmentation processes respectively. Note that upon introducing the shape prior, the corresponding contour descends the energy landscape in the direction of the negative gradient to end up in one of the minima. The example shows that, in contrast to the linear shape prior, the nonlinear one can well separate different objects without mixing them. Since each cluster in this example contains only one view for the purpose of illustration, the estimate of equation (22) for the kernel width σ does not apply; instead, we chose a smaller granularity of $\sigma = \mu/4$.

Simultaneous Encoding of Several Training Objects

The following example is an application of our method that shows how the nonlinear shape prior can encode a number of different alphabetical letters and thus improve the segmentation of these letters in a given image.

We want to point out that there exists a vast number of different methods for optical character recognition. We do not claim that the present method is optimally suited for this task, and we do not claim that it outperforms existing methods. The following results only show that our rather general segmentation approach with the nonlinear shape prior can be applied to

Figure 8. (a) Original image region of 200×200 pixels. (b) Subsampled to 16×16 pixels (used as input data). (c) Upsampled low-resolution image using bilinear interpolation.

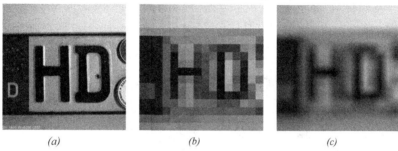

(a)   (b)   (c)

Figure 9. (a) Aligned training shapes, (b) projection onto the first and third (linear) principal component, (c) mean shape

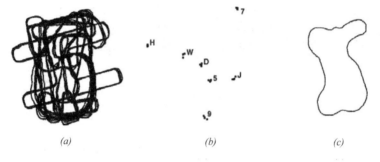

(a)   (b)   (c)

a large variety of tasks and that it permits to simultaneously encode the shape of several objects.

A set of seven letters and digits were segmented (several times) without any shape prior in an input image as the one shown in Figure 8a. The obtained contours were used as a training set to construct the shape prior. Figure 9 shows the set of aligned contours and their projection into the plane spanned by the first and third principal component (of a linear PCA). The clusters are labeled with the corresponding letters and digits. Again, the mean shape, shown in Figure 8c, indicates that the linear model is not an adequate model for the distribution of the training shapes.

In order to generate realistic input data, we subsampled the input image to a resolution of 16×16 pixels, as shown in Figure 8b. Such low-resolution input data are typical in this context. As a first step, we upsampled this input data using bilinear interpolation, as shown in Figure 8c.

Given such an input image, we initialized the contour, iterated the segmentation process without prior until stationarity, and then introduced either the linear or the nonlinear shape

Figure 10. (a) Segmentation without prior, (b) segmentation upon introduction of the linear prior, (c) final segmentation with the nonlinear prior, and (d) appropriate projections of the contour evolution with nonlinear prior into the space of contours show the convergence of the contour toward one of the learnt letters.

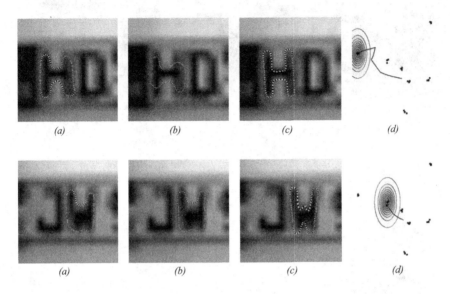

prior. Figure 10 shows segmentation results without prior, with the linear prior, and with the nonlinear prior. Again, the convergence of the segmenting contour toward one of the learnt letters is visualized by appropriate projections onto the first two linear principal components of the training contours.[5]

Figure 11 shows results of the segmentation approach with the same nonlinear shape prior applied to two more shapes. Again, the nonlinear shape prior improves the segmentation results. This demonstrates that one can encode information on a set of fairly different shapes into a single shape prior.

Generalization to Novel Views

In all of the above examples, the nonlinear shape prior merely permitted a reconstruction of the training shapes (up to similarity transformations). The power of the proposed shape prior lies in the fact that it not only can encode several very different shapes, but also that the prior is a *statistical* prior: It has the capacity to generalize and abstract from the fixed set of training shapes. As a consequence, the respective segmentation process with the nonlinear prior is able to segment novel views of an object that were not present in the training set. This aspect of the nonlinear statistical shape prior will be demonstrated in the following examples.

Figure 11. (a) Initial contour, (b) final segmentation without prior, and (c) final segmentation upon introduction of the nonlinear prior. With a single nonlinear prior, a number of fairly different shapes can be reconstructed from the subsampled and smoothed input image.

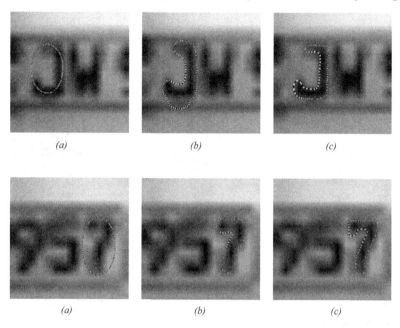

(a)   (b)   (c)

(a)   (b)   (c)

The training set consists of nine right and nine left hands, shown together with the estimated energy density in a projection onto the first two principal components in Figure 12 (right side). Rather than mixing the two classes of right and left hands, the shape prior clearly separates several clusters in shape space. The final segmentations without (left) and with (center) prior shape knowledge show that the shape prior compensates for occlusion by filling up information where it is missing. Moreover, the statistical nature of the prior is demonstrated by the fact that the hand in the image is not part of the training set. This can be seen in the projection (Figure 12, right side), where the final segmentation (white box) does not correspond to any of the training contours (black crosses).

Tracking 3-D Objects with Changing Viewpoint

In the following, we present results of applying the nonlinear shape statistics for an example of tracking an object in 3-D with a prior constructed from a large set of 2-D views. For this purpose, we binarized 100 views of a rabbit; two of them and the respective binarizations are shown in Figure 13. For each of the 100 views, we automatically extracted the contours and aligned them with respect to translation, rotation, scaling, and cyclic permutation of the control points. We calculated the density estimate (equation (13)) and the corresponding shape energy (equation (25)).

Figure 12. Segmentation with a nonlinear shape prior containing right (×) and left (■) hands, shown in the projected energy plot on the right. The input image is a right hand with an occlusion. After the Mumford-Shah segmentation becomes stationary (left image), the nonlinear shape prior is introduced, and the contour converges toward the final segmentation (center image). The contour evolution in its projection is visualized by the white curve in the energy density plot (right). Note that the final segmentation (white box) does not correspond to any of the training silhouettes, nor to the minimum (i.e., the most probable shape) of the respective cluster.

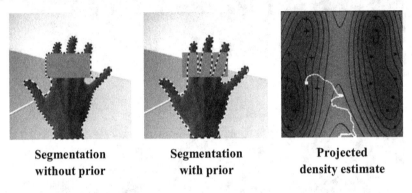

| **Segmentation without prior** | **Segmentation with prior** | **Projected density estimate** |

Figure 13. Example views and binarization used for estimating the shape density.

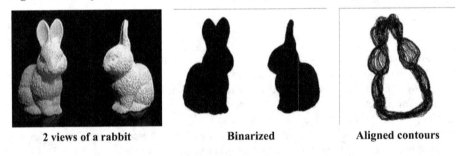

| **2 views of a rabbit** | **Binarized** | **Aligned contours** |

In a film sequence, we moved and rotated the rabbit in front of a cluttered background. Moreover, we artificially introduced an occlusion afterward. We segmented the first image by the modified Mumford-Shah model until convergence before the shape prior was introduced. The initial contour and the segmentations without and with prior are shown in Figure 14. Afterward, we iterated 15 steps in the gradient descent on full energy for each frame in the sequence.[6] Some sample screen shots of the sequence are shown in Figure 15. Note that the viewpoint changes continuously.

The training silhouettes are shown in 2-D projections with the estimated shape energy in Figure 16. The path of the changing contour during the entire sequence corresponds to the white curve. The curve follows the distribution of training data well, interpolating in areas

Figure 14. Beginning of the tracking sequence: initial contour, segmentation without prior, segmentation upon introducing the nonlinear prior on the contour

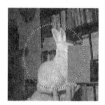
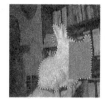
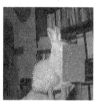

Initial contour   No prior   With prior

Figure 15. Sample screen shots from the tracking sequence

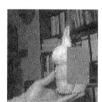
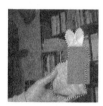
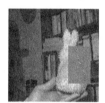

Figure 16. Tracking sequence visualized. Training data (▮), estimated energy density, and the contour evolution (white curve) in appropriate 2-D projections are shown. The contour evolution is restricted to the valleys of low energy induced by the training data.

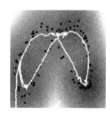
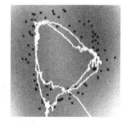

Projection onto 1st and 2nd
principal component

Projection onto 2nd and 4th
principal component

where there are no training silhouettes. Note that the intersections of the curve and of the training data in the center (Figure 16, left side) are only due to the projection on 2-D. The results show that, given sufficient training data, the shape prior is able to capture fine details such as the ear positions of the rabbit in the various views. Moreover, it generalizes well to novel views not included in the training set and permits a reconstruction of the occluded section throughout the entire sequence.

Conclusion

We presented a variational integration of nonlinear shape statistics into a Mumford-Shah-based segmentation process. The statistics are derived from a novel method of density estimation that can be considered as an extension of the kernel PCA approach to a probabilistic framework. The original training data are nonlinearly transformed to a feature space. In this higher dimensional space, the distribution of the mapped data is estimated by a Gaussian density. Due to the strong nonlinearity, the corresponding density estimate in the original space is highly non-Gaussian, allowing several shape clusters and banana- or ring-shaped data distributions.

We integrated the nonlinear statistics as a shape prior in a variational approach to segmentation. We gave details on appropriate estimations of the involved parameters. Based on the explicit representation of the contour, we proposed a closed-form, parameter-free solution for the integration of invariance with respect to similarity transformations in the variational framework.

Applications to the segmentation of static images and image sequences show several favorable properties of the nonlinear prior.

- Due to the possible multimodality in the original space, the nonlinear prior can encode a number of fairly different training objects.

- It can capture even small details of shape variation without mixing different views.

- It copes for misleading information due to noise and clutter, and enables the reconstruction of occluded parts of the object silhouette.

- Due to the statistical nature of the prior, a generalization to novel views not included in the training set is possible.

Finally, we showed examples where the 3-D structure of an object is encoded through a training set of 2-D projections.

By projecting onto the first principal components of the data, we managed to visualize the training data and the estimated shape density. The evolution of the contour during the segmentation of static images and image sequences can be visualized by a projection into this density plot. In this way, we verified that the shape prior effectively restricts the contour evolution to the submanifold of familiar shapes.

Acknowledgments

We thank Christoph Schnörr for support and many fruitful discussions.

References

Aizerman, M. A., Braverman, E. M., & Rozonoer, L. I. (1964). Theoretical foundations of the potential function method in pattern recognition learning. *Automation and Remote Control, 25*, 821-837.

Boser, B. E., Guyon, I. M., & Vapnik, V. N. (1992). A training algorithm for optimal margin classifiers. *Proceedings of the 5th Annual ACM Workshop on Computer Learning Theory* (pp. 144-152).

Chalmond, B., & Girard, S. C. (1999). Nonlinear modeling of scattered multivariate data and its application to shape change. *IEEE Transactions on Patter Analysis and Machine Intelligence, 21*(5), 422-432.

Chan, T. F., & Vese, L. A. (2001). A level set algorithm for minimizing the Mumford-Shah functional in image processing. *IEEE Workshop on Variational and Level Set Methods* (pp. 161-168).

Chen, Y., Thiruvenkadam, S., Tagare, H., Huang, F., Wilson, D., & Geiser, E. (2001). On the incorporation of shape priors into geometric active contours. *IEEE Workshop on Variational and Level Set Methods* (pp. 145-152).

Cootes, T. F., Breston, C., Edwards, G., & Taylor, C. J. (1999). A unified framework for atlas matching using active appearance models. In Lecture notes in computer science: Vol. 1613. In *Proceedings of International Conference on Inf. Proc. in Med. Imaging* (pp. 322-333). Springer.

Cootes, T. F., & Taylor, C. J. (1999). A mixture model for representing shape variation. *Image and Vision Computing, 17*(8), 567-574.

Cootes, T. F., Taylor, C. J., Cooper, D. M., & Graham, J. (1995). Active shape models: Their training and application. *Comp. Vision Image Underst., 61*(1), 38-59.

Courant, R., & Hilbert, D. (1953). *Methods of mathematical physics* (Vol. 1). New York: Interscience Publishers.

Cremers, D. (2002, May). Reprinted from Publication title: Nonlinear shape statistics in Mumford–Shah based segmentation. In A. Heyden et al. (Eds.), *Europ. Conference on Comp. Vis.* (Vol. 2351, pp. 93-108), Copenhagen. Copyright (2002), with permission from Springer.

Cremers, D. (2003). Reprinted from Publication title: Shape statistics in kernel space for variational image segmentation. *Pattern Recognition*, 36(9), 1929-1943. Copyright (2003), with permission from Elsevier.

Cremers, D., Kohlberger, T., & Schnörr, C. (2001). Reprinted from publication title: Nonlinear shape statistics via kernel spaces. In B. Radig & S. Florczyk (Eds.), *Pattern recognition* (Vol. 2191, pp. 269-276). Munich, Germany. Copyright (2001), with permission from Springer.

Cremers, D., Schnörr, C., & Weickert, J. (2001). Diffusion snakes: Combining statistical shape knowledge and image information in a variational framework. *IEEE First International Workshop on Variational and Level Set Methods* (pp. 137-144).

Cremers, D., Schnörr, C., Weickert, J., & Schellewald, C. (2000). Diffusion snakes using statistical shape knowledge. In G. Sommer & Y. Y. Zeevi (Eds.), *Lecture notes in computer science: Vol 1888. Algebraic frames for the perception-action cycle* (pp. 164-174). Kiel, Germany: Springer.

Cremers, D., & Soatto, S. (2005). Motion competition: A variational framework for piecewise parametric motion segmentation. *International Journal of Computer Vision, 62*(3), 249-265.

Cremers, D., Tischhäuser, F., Weickert, J., & Schnörr, C. (2002). Diffusion snakes: Introducing statistical shape knowledge into the Mumford-Shah functional. *International Journal of Computer Vision, 50*(3), 295-313.

Doretto, G., Cremers, D., Favaro, P., & Soatto, S. (2003). Dynamic texture segmentation. *IEEE International Conference on Computer Vision, 2*, 1236-1242.

Dryden, I. L., & Mardia, K. V. (1998). *Statistical shape analysis.* Chichester, UK: Wiley.

Farin, G. (1997). *Curves and surfaces for computer-aided geometric design.* San Diego, CA: Academic Press.

Figueiredo, M., Leitao, J., & Jain, A. K. (2000). Unsupervised contour representation and estimation using B-splines and a minimum description length criterion. *IEEE Transactions on Image Processing, 9*(6), 1075-1087.

Girolami, M., & He, C. (2003). Probability density estimation from optimally condensed data samples. *IEEE Transactions on Pattern Analysis and Machine Intelligence, 25*(10), 1253-1264.

Grenander, C., Chow, Y., & Keenan, D. M. (1991). *Hands: A pattern theoretic study of biological shapes.* New York: Springer.

Hastie, D., & Stuetzle, W. (1989). Principal curves. *Journal of the American Statistical Association, 84*, 502-516.

Heap, T. (1998). Wormholes in shape space: Tracking through discontinuous changes in shape. *International Conference on Computer Vision* (pp. 97-106).

Heap, T., & Hogg, D. (1996). Automated pivot location for the Cartesian-polar hybrid point distribution model. In *British Machine Vision Conference* (pp. 97-106).

Ising, E. (1925). Beitrag zur theorie des ferromagnetismus. *Zeitschrift für Physik, 23*, 253-258.

Kass, M., Witkin, A., & Terzopoulos, D. (1988). Snakes: Active contour models. *International Journal of Computer Vision, 1*(4), 321-331.

Kervrann, C., & Heitz, F. (1998). A hierarchical Markov modeling approach for the segmentation and tracking of deformable shapes. *Graphical Models and Image Processing, 60*, 173-195.

Klassen, E., Srivastava, A., Mio, W., & Joshi, S. H. (2004). Analysis of planar shapes using geodesic paths on shape spaces. *IEEE Transactions on Pattern Analysis and Machine Intelligence, 26*(3), 372-383.

Leventon, M., Grimson, W., & Faugeras, O. (2000). Statistical shape influence in geodesic active contours. *CVPR, 1*, 316-323.

Mercer, J. (1909). Functions of positive and negative type and their connection with the theory of integral equations. *Philos. Trans. Roy. Soc. London, A, 209*, 415-446.

Moghaddam, B., & Pentland, A. (1995). Probabilistic visual learning for object detection. *IEEE International Conference on Computer Vision* (pp. 786-793).

Mumford, D., & Shah, J. (1989). Optimal approximations by piecewise smooth functions and associated variational problems. *Comm. Pure Appl. Math., 42*, 577-685.

Osher, S. J., & Sethian, J. A. (1988). Fronts propagation with curvature dependent speed: Algorithms based on Hamilton–Jacobi formulations. *Journal of Comp. Phys., 79*, 12-49.

Parzen, E. (1962). On the estimation of a probability density function and the mode. *Annals of Mathematical Statistics, 33*, 1065-1076.

Romdhani, S., Gong, S., & Psarrou, A. (1999). A multi-view non-linear active shape model using kernel PCA. In *Proceedings of the British Machine Vision Conference* (Vol. 2, pp. 483-492).

Ronfard, R. (1994). Region-based strategies for active contour models. *International Journal of Computer Vision, 13*(2), 229-251.

Rosenblatt, F. (1956). Remarks on some nonparametric estimates of a density function. *Annals of Mathematical Statistics, 27*, 832-837.

Rousson, M., Brox, T., & Deriche, R. (2003). Active unsupervised texture segmentation on a diffusion based feature space. In *Proceedings of IEEE Conference on Computer Vision Pattern Recognition* (pp. 699-704).

Rousson, M., Paragios, N., & Deriche, R. (2004). Implicit active shape models for 3D segmentation in MRI imaging. In *Lecture notes in computer science: (Vol. 2217). International Conference on Medical Image Computing and Computer Assisted Intervention (MICCAI)* (pp. 209-216). Springer.

Roweis, S. (1998). EM algorithms for PCA and SPCA. *Advances in Neural Information Processing Systems, 10*, 626-632.

Schölkopf, B., Mika, S., Smola, A., Rätsch, G., & Müller, K.-R. (1998). Kernel PCA pattern reconstruction via approximate pre-images. *International Conference on Artificial Neural Networks (ICANN)*, 147-152.

Schölkopf, B., Smola, A., & Müller, K.-R. (1998). Nonlinear component analysis as a kernel eigenvalue problem. *Neural Computation, 10*, 1299-1319.

Staib, L. H., & Duncan, J. S. (1992). Boundary finding with parametrically deformable models. *IEEE Transactions on Pattern Analysis and Machine Intelligence, 14*(11), 1061-1075.

Tipping, M. E. (2001). Sparse kernel principal component analysis. *Advances in Neural Information Processing Systems, NIPS 13*.

Tipping, M. E., & Bishop, C. M. (1997). *Probabilistic principal component analysis* (Tech. Rep. No. Woe-19). UK: Neural Computing Research Group, Aston University.

Tsai, A., Yezzi, A., Wells, W., Tempany, C., Tucker, D., Fan, A., et al. (2001). Model-based curve evolution technique for image segmentation. *Computer Vision Pattern Recognition*, 463-468.

Tsai, A., Yezzi, A. J., & Willsky, A. S. (2001). Curve evolution implementation of the Mumford-Shah functional for image segmentation, denoising, interpolation, and magnification. *IEEE Transactions on Image Processing, 10*(8), 1169-1186.

Twining, C. J., & Taylor, C. J. (2001). Kernel principal component analysis and the construction of non-linear active shape models. In *Proceedings of the British Machine Vision Conference* (pp. 23-32).

Werman, M., & Weinshall, D. (1995). Similarity and affine invariant distances between 2D point sets. *IEEE Transactions on Pattern Analysis and Machine Intelligence, 17*(8), 810-814.

Zhu, S. C., & Yuille, A. (1996). Region competition: Unifying snakes, region growing, and Bayes/MDL for multiband image segmentation. *IEEE Transactions on Pattern Analysis and Machine Intelligence, 18*(9), 884-900.

Endnotes

[1] Implicit shape representations and level set methods (Osher, 1988) have become increasingly popular as they allow to cope with shapes of varying topology. This chapter is focused on explicit shape representations. A more detailed comparison of advantages and drawbacks of both representations is beyond the scope of this work.

[1] In this chapter, we consider 2D gray value images, such that $r = 2$ and $d = 1$.

Appendix A.

From Feature-Space Distance to the Parzen Estimator

In this section, we will link the feature-space distances that induce our shape dissimilarity measure to classical methods of density estimation. The derivation of the energy (equation (18)) was based on the assumption that the training data after a nonlinear mapping corresponding to the kernel (equation (19)) are distributed according to a Gaussian density in the space Y. The final expression (equation (18)) resembles the well-known Parzen estimator (Parzen, 1962; Rosenblatt, 1956), which estimates the density of a distribution of training

Figure A.1. Sample vectors randomly distributed on two spirals (left), corresponding estimates of Parzen (middle), and generalized Parzen (right) for appropriate values of the kernel width σ.

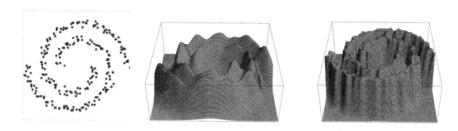

data by summing up the data points after convolution with a Gaussian (or some other kernel function).

In fact, the energy associated with an isotropic (spherical) Gaussian distribution in feature space is (up to normalization) equivalent to a Parzen estimator in the original space. With the definitions of equations (11) and (12), this energy is given by the Euclidean feature space distance

$$E_{sphere}(z) = |\tilde{\phi}(z)|^2 = \tilde{k}(z,z) = -\frac{2}{m}\sum_{i=1}^{m} k(z,z_i) + \text{const.} \tag{A.1}$$

Up to scaling and a constant, this is the Parzen estimator.

The proposed energy (equation (13)) can therefore be interpreted as a generalization of the Parzen estimator obtained by moving from a spherical distribution in feature space to an ellipsoidal one. Due to the regularization of the covariance matrix in equation (14), equation (13) contains a (dominant) isotropic component given by the last term in equation (18). We believe that this connection to the Parzen estimator justifies the assumption of a Gaussian in feature space and the choice of localized (stationary) kernels such as equation (19).

Numerical simulations show that the remaining anisotropic component in equation (18) has an important influence. Figure A.1 shows the example of a set of 2-D points thath were randomly sampled along two spirals (left). The middle and right images show the Parzen and the generalized Parzen for appropriate values of the kernel width σ. Note that the spiral structures are more pronounced by the generalized Parzen. However, a more detailed theoretical study of the difference between the Euclidean distance in feature space (equation (A.1)) and the Mahalanobis distance in feature space (equation (13)) is beyond the scope of this work.

Chapter XVI

Hyperspectral Image Classification with Kernels

Lorenzo Bruzzone, University of Trento, Italy

Luis Gomez-Chova, Universitat de València, Spain

Mattia Marconcini, University of Trento, Italy

Gustavo Camps-Valls, Universitat de València, Spain

Abstract

The information contained in hyperspectral images allows the characterization, identification, and classification of land covers with improved accuracy and robustness. However, several critical problems should be considered in the classification of hyperspectral images, among which are (a) the high number of spectral channels, (b) the spatial variability of the spectral signature, (c) the high cost of true sample labeling, and (d) the quality of data. Recently, kernel methods have offered excellent results in this context. This chapter reviews the state-of-the-art hyperspectral image classifiers, presents two recently proposed kernel-based approaches, and systematically discusses the specific needs and demands of this field.

Introduction to Remote Sensing

Materials in a scene reflect, absorb, and emit electromagnetic radiation in different ways depending on their molecular composition and shape. Remote sensing exploits this physical fact and deals with the acquisition of information about a scene (or specific object) at a short, medium, or long distance. The radiation acquired by an (airborne or satellite) sensor is measured at different wavelengths, and the resulting spectral signature (or *spectrum*) is used to identify a given material. The field of *spectroscopy* is concerned with the measurement, analysis, and interpretation of such spectra (Richards & Jia, 1999; Shaw & Manolakis, 2002). Figure 1 shows the application of imaging spectroscopy to perform satellite remote sensing.

Hyperspectral sensors are a class of imaging spectroscopy sensors acquiring hundreds of contiguous narrow bands or channels. Hyperspectral sensors sample the reflective portion of the electromagnetic spectrum ranging from the visible region (0.4-0.7 μm) through the near infrared (about 2.4 μm) in hundreds of narrow contiguous bands about 10 nm wide.[1] Hyperspectral sensors represent an evolution in technology from earlier multispectral sensors, which typically collect spectral information in only a few discrete, noncontiguous bands.

The high spectral resolution characteristic of hyperspectral sensors preserves important aspects of the spectrum (e.g., shape of narrow absorption bands), and makes the differentiation of different materials on the ground possible. The spatially and spectrally sampled information can be described as a data cube (colloquially referred to as "the hypercube"), which includes

Figure 1. Principle of imaging spectroscopy

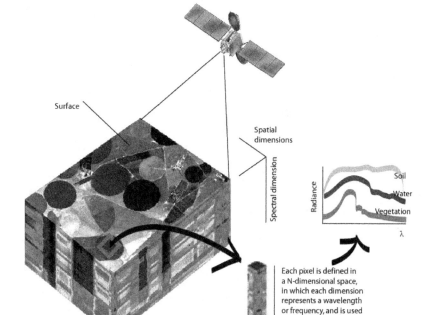

two spatial coordinates and the spectral one (or wavelength). As a consequence, each image pixel is defined in a high-dimensional space where each dimension corresponds to a given wavelength interval in the spectrum, $\mathbf{x}_i \in \mathbb{R}^N$, where N is the number of spectral channels or bands.

Remote sensing images acquired by previous-generation multispectral sensors (such as the widely used Landsat thematic mapper sensor) have shown their usefulness in numerous Earth-observation (EO) applications. In general, the relatively small number of acquisition channels that characterizes multispectral sensors may be sufficient to discriminate among different land-cover classes (e.g., forestry, water, crops, urban areas, etc.). However, their discrimination capability is very limited when different types (or conditions) of the same species (e.g., different types of forest) are to be recognized. Hyperspectral sensors can be used to deal with this problem and represents a further step ahead in achieving the main general goals of remote sensing, which are the following:

1.   Monitoring and modeling the processes on the Earth's surface and their interaction with the atmosphere.

2.   Obtaining quantitative measurements and estimations of geo, bio, and physical variables.

3.   Identifying materials on the land cover and analyzing the acquired spectral signatures by satellite or airborne sensors.

To attain such objectives, the remote sensing community has evolved to a multidisciplinary field of science that embraces physics, chemistry, signal theory, computer science, electronics, and communications. From a *machine learning* and *signal and image processing* point of view, all these problems and applications are tackled under specific formalisms (see Table 1), and among all of them, the classification of hyperspectral images has become an important field of remote sensing, where kernel methods have shown excellent capabilities.

Kernel Methods in
Hyperspectral Image Classification

The information contained in hyperspectral images allows more accurate and robust characterization, identification, and classification of the land covers (Swain, 1978). Nevertheless, unlike multispectral data, hyperspectral images cannot be analyzed by manual photo interpretation as the hundreds of available spectral channels (images) do not make it possible to accomplish this task. Consequently, many researchers have turned to techniques for addressing hyperdimensional classification problems from the fields of statistics and machine learning in order to automatically generate reliable supervised and unsupervised classifiers. Unsupervised methods are not sensitive to the ratio between the number of labeled samples and number of features since they work on the whole image, but the correspondence between clusters and classes is not ensured. Consequently, supervised methods are preferable when the desired input-output mapping is well defined and a data set of true labels is available. However, several critical problems arise when dealing with the supervised classification of hyperspectral images.

Table 1. A taxonomy for remote sensing methods and applications

Topic	Fields & Tools	Objectives & Problems	Examples	Methods & Techniques
Classification and Clustering	Pattern recognition	Monitoring the evolution and changes of the Earth's cover	Urban monitoring, crop fields, mineral detection, change detection	k-NN (k-nearest neighbors), linear discriminant, neural networks, SVM and kernel methods, etc.
Biophysical Parameter Estimation	Regression and function approximation	Monitoring the Earth's cover at a local and global scale	Water quality, desertification, vegetation indexes, temperature, biomass, ozone, chlorophyll	Linear regression, statistical approaches, neural networks, SVR (support vector regression), inverse techniques using nonlinear forward models coupled with constrained optimization
Physical Model Development	Probability density function (PDF) estimation and feature selection	Atmospherical models, improved classification, unmixing, etc.	Estimating the spectral signature density, spectral libraries, subpixel vegetation density, land covers	Parzen, Gaussian mixtures, support vectors, etc.
Image Coding	Transform coding and vision computing	Compress the huge amount of acquired data	Transmission of airborne or satellite sensor to Earth station, avoid redundancy and errors, realistic quick-looks	PCA (principal components analysis), discrete cosine transform (DCT), wavelets, SPIHT, etc.
Spectral Channel Selection	Filtering and wrapping	Ranking and channel selection	Efficient transmission, model development, compression	PCA, sequential floating search selection (SFFS), etc.
Browsing and Cataloging	Databases and warehousing	Managing, sorting, browsing, and retrieving in huge image databases	Users seek for specific features in images(w/wnclouds,temperature, day, sensor, etc.)	Spectral libraries, preclassification, correlation, kernel methods
Spectral Unmixing	Signal processing and machine learning	Making independent the mixture of spectra present in a pixel, restoration, classification with pure pixels, etc.	Unmixing and subpixel techniques	Constrained or unconstrained independent component analysis (ICA), linear or nonlinear unmixing, kernels and pre-images, etc.
Image Rectification and Restoration	Image and signal processing	Correct distorted or degraded images	Raw data contain rotated, distorted, non-ideally-square pixels, compare images at different acquisition times	Geometrical transformations, image-correction techniques, ortho-rectification, etc.
Image Enhancement	Image and signal processing, de-noising, de-blurring	Efficient display of images, extract relevant features	Eliminate noise in the data due to acquisition, transmission, thermal noise	Wiener, wavelets, advanced de-noising
Data Fusion	Image and signal processing, databases	Different sensors, temporal acquisitions, resolutions	Multitemporal analysis, change detection	Multiresolution and fusion methods

1.   The high number of spectral channels in hyperspectral images and the relatively low number of available labeled samples (due to the high cost of ground-truth collection process, see Figure 2a) poses the problem of the *curse of dimensionality* or Hughes phenomenon (Hughes, 1968).

2.   The spatial variability of the spectral signature of each land-cover class (which is not stationary in the spatial domain) results in a critical variability of the values of feature-vector components of each class (see Figure 2b).

3.   Uncertainty and variability on class definition (see Figure 2c).

4.   Temporal evolution of the Earth's cover (see Figure 2d).

5.   Atmospheric correction to obtain intrinsic properties of surface materials independent of intervening atmosphere, solar irradiance, and view angle.

6.   The presence of different noise sources and uncertainties in the acquired image, for example, in the measurement, instrumental and observational noise, and uncertainty in the acquisition time.

In this context, robust and accurate classifiers are needed. In the remote sensing literature, many supervised methods have been developed to tackle the multispectral image-classification problem. A successful approach to multispectral image classification is based on the use of artificial neural networks (Bischof & Leona, 1998; Bruzzone & Cossu, 2002; Giacinto, Roli, & Bruzzone, 2000; Yang, Meer, Bakker, & Tan, 1999). However, these approaches are not effective when dealing with a high number of spectral bands (Hughes phenomenon; Hughes, 1968), or when working with a low number of training samples.

Much work has been carried out in the literature to overcome the aforementioned problem. Four main approaches can be identified: (a) regularization of the sample covariance matrix in statistical classifiers, (b) adaptive statistics estimation by the exploitation of the classified (semilabeled) samples (c) preprocessing techniques based on feature selection and extraction,

Figure 2. Illustrative examples of encountered problems in hyperspectral image classification: (a) A terrestrial campaign is necessary to accurately obtain a labeled training set, (b) different sensors provide different spectral and spatial resolutions from the same scene, (c) defining a class is sometimes difficult, and (d) images from the same scene acquired at different time instants contain different spectral and spatial characteristics.

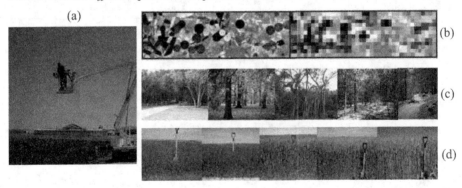

aimed at reducing and transforming the original feature space into another space of a lower dimensionality, and (d) analysis of the behaviour of the spectral signatures to model the classes

An elegant alternative approach to the analysis of hyperspectral data consists of kernel methods (Boser, Guyon, & Vapnik, 1992; Cortes & Vapnik, 1995; Cristianini & Shawe-Taylor, 2000; Schölkopf & Smola, 2002; Vapnik, 1998). A good overview of statistical learning theory can be found in Vapnik (1999). Many works have been presented in the last decade developing hyperspectral kernel classifiers. Support vector machines (SVMs) were first applied to hyperspectral image classification in Gualtieri, Chettri, Cromp, & Johnson (1999) and Gualtieri and Cromp (1998), and their capabilities were further analyzed in (Bruzzone & Melgani, 2003; Camps-Valls et al., 2004; Camps-Valls, Gómez-Chova, Calpe, Soria, Martín, & Moreno, 2003; Foody & Mathur, 2004; Huang, Davis, & Townshend, 2002; Melgani & Bruzzone, 2004) terms of stability, robustness to noise, and accuracy. Some other kernel methods have been recently presented to improve classification, such as kernel PCA (Camps-Valls et al., 2003), the kernel Fisher discriminant (KFD) analysis (Dundar & Langrebe, 2004), the regularized AdaBoosting (Reg-AB; Camps-Valls et al., 2004), or support vector clustering (SVC; Song, Cherian, & Fan, 2005; Srivastava & Stroeve, 2003). Lately, some kernel formulations have appeared in the context of target and anomaly detection (Kwon & Nasrabadi, 2004a, 2004b), which basically consists of using the spectral information of different materials to discriminate between the target and background signatures.

Finally, in Camps-Valls and Bruzzone (2005), an extensive comparison of kernel-based classifiers (RBF [radial basis function] neural networks, SVM, KFD, and regularized AdaBoosting) was conducted by taking into account the peculiarities of hyperspectral images, that is, assessment was conducted in terms of the accuracy of methods when working in noisy environments, high input dimension, and limited training sets. The next section reviews the most important results attained in this work.

Kernel Methods in Hyperspectral Image Classification: Experimental Comparisons

In this section, we perform an extensive comparison among kernel methods for hyperspectral image classification. The results are partially extracted from Camps-Valls and Bruzzone (2005).

Data Collection

Experiments are carried out using a hyperspectral image acquired by the Airborne Visible/ Infrared Imaging Spectrometer (AVIRIS), which had taken over NW Indiana's Indian Pine test site[2] in June 1992 (Landgrebe, 1992). Two different data sets are considered in the following experiments.

1. **Subset scene.** From the 16 different land-cover classes available in the original ground truth, 7 were discarded since an insufficient number of training samples were available,

and thus this fact would dismiss the planned experimental analysis. The remaining 9 classes were used to generate a set of 4,757 training samples (for the learning phase of the classifiers) and 4,588 test samples (for validating their performance). See Table 2 for details.

2.   **Whole scene.** We used the whole scene, consisting of the full 145×145 pixels, which contains 16 classes, ranging in size from 20 pixels to 2,468 pixels. See Gualtieri et al. (1999) for full details.

In both data sets, we removed 20 noisy bands covering the region of water absorption, and finally worked with 200 spectral bands.

Benchmarking Kernel-Based Classifiers

The first experimental analysis considers SVMs, KFD, Reg-RBFNN (regularized RBF neural network), and Reg-AB. In addition, we include the linear discriminant analysis (LDA) as baseline method for comparison purposes. Note that LDA corresponds to the solution of KFD if a linear kernel is adopted and no regularization is used ($C = 0$). These experiments only considered the subset scene and results were obtained using the libSVM implementation (*A Library for Support Vector Machines*).[3]

In the case of Reg-RBFNN, the number of Gaussian neurons was tuned between 2 and 50, and λ was varied exponentially in the range $\lambda = 10^{-2}, ..., 10^2$. The width and centers of the Gaussians are computed iteratively in the algorithm. In the case of SVMs and KFD, we used the Gaussian kernel (RBF) and thus, only the Gaussian width (standard deviation), σ, along with the regularization parameter(s) $C^{(*)}$, should be tuned. We tried exponentially increased sequences of σ ($\sigma = 1, ..., 50$) and C ($C = 10^{-2}, ..., 10^6$). For the case of the Reg-AB algorithm, the regularization term was varied in the range $C = [10^0, ..., 10^3]$, and the number of iterations was tuned to $T = 10$. The width and centers of the Gaussians are also computed iteratively in the algorithm. We developed one-against-all (OAA) schemes to deal with the multiclass problem for all considered classifiers. The usual procedure of cross-validation was followed to choose the best combination of free parameters.

Table 2. Number of training and test samples used in the subset scene

CLASS	TRAINING	TEST
C1 - Corn-no till	742	692
C2 - Corn-min till	442	392
C3 - Grass/Pasture	260	237
C4 - Grass/Trees	389	358
C5 - Hay-windrowed	236	253
C6 - Soybean-no till	487	481
C7 - Soybean-min till	1,245	1,223
C8 - Soybean-clean till	305	309
C9 - Woods	651	643
TOTAL	4,757	4,588

Table 3 shows the results obtained for each method in terms of overall accuracy (OA[%]) and Kappa statistic, which incorporates the diagonal (observations classified correctly) as well as the off-diagonal observations of the confusion matrix (misclassified observations) to give a more robust assessment of accuracy than overall accuracy measure. The best overall accuracy and Kappa statistic values are provided by the SVM-Poly, closely followed by the SVM-RBF and Reg-AB, yielding an overall accuracy equal to 94.44%, 94.31%, and 93.50%, respectively. KFD and Reg-RBFNN showed overall accuracies around 91%. All methods are quite correlated (correlation coefficient among outputs greater than 0.85), and the Wilcoxon rank sum test revealed that only LDA was statistically different ($p<0.0001$). Reg-RBFNN ($p = 0.67$), KFD ($p = 0.39$), and Reg-AB ($p = 0.33$) did not reject the null hypothesis at a 95% level of significance. When looking at producers' and users' accuracies, it is noteworthy that kernel-based methods obtain higher scores on classes C3, C4, C5, and C9, and that the most troublesome classes are C1, C6, C7, and C8. This has been also observed in Melgani and Bruzzone (2004), and can be explained because grass, pasture, trees, and woods are homogeneous areas that are clearly defined and labeled. Contrarily, corn and soybean classes can be particularly misrecognized because they have specific subclasses (no till, min till, clean till).

Additionally, different simulated experiments are conducted to assess the performance of kernel machines in different situations encountered in remote sensing, such as the presence of different nature (Gaussian or impulsive) and amount of noise, and training with reduced training labels.

Robustness to the Presence of Gaussian Noise

Figure 3a shows the evolution through different signal-to-noise ratios (SNRs) of the overall accuracy of the models in the test set when Gaussian noise is added to the spectral channels. We varied the SNR between 16 and 40 dB, and 100 realizations were averaged for each value, which constitutes a reasonable confidence margin for the least measured OA[%]. We can observe that SVM-Poly yields the best performance through the whole signal-to-noise domain. It is also noticeable that, when moderate noise (SNR>25dB) is introduced, SVM-RBF also shows higher overall accuracy than KFD. However, as complex situations (SNR<25dB) are simulated, KFD exhibits better accuracy than SVM-RBF, but is inferior to SVM-Poly. The superiority of the polynomial kernel to the RBF kernel was previously noticed in Camps-Valls et al. (2004) with different hyperspectral data sets and amounts of noise.

Robustness to the Presence of Impulsive Noise

Figure 3b shows the evolution of the overall accuracy in the test set when spikes of high impulsive noise ($P_o = -5$dB) are added in different number of bands (1, 5, 10, 25, 50, 100, and 150). Once again, the experiment was repeated 100 times and the averaged results are shown for each model. A similar effect to that observed in the previous experiments is obtained. SVM-Poly shows the best accuracy in the whole domain. As we increase the number of outlying bands, the accuracies of SVM-RBF and Reg-AB become slightly more

Table 3. Results after a coarse feature selection (200 input bands). Several accuracy measures are included: users, producers, overall accuracy (OA[%]), and Kappa statistic in the test set for different kernel classifiers—LDA, Reg-RBFNN, SVMs with RBF kernel (SVM-RBF) and with polynomial kernel (SVM-Poly), and KFD Analysis (with RBF kernel). The column "Parameters" gives some information about the final models. The best scores for each class are highlighted in bold-face font. The OA[%] being statistically different (at 95% confidence level) from the best model are underlined, as tested through paired Wilcoxon rank sum test. Table adapted from Camps-Valls and Bruzzone (2005).

METHOD	PARAMETERS	PRODUCERS / USERS									OA[%]	Kappa
		C1	C2	C3	C4	C5	C6	C7	C8	C9		
LDA	-	78.27	68.05	88.53	88.28	**100.00**	65.30	84.78	73.24	100.00	82.08	0.79
		84.83	75.51	81.43	98.88	**100.00**	82.95	66.07	80.58	97.51		
Reg-RBFNN	nodes: 48, $\lambda = 1e-7$	**87.43**	80.61	94.94	**99.72**	**100.00**	83.78	90.92	91.91	99.22	91.39	0.90
		91.11	92.67	96.57	95.20	99.61	84.13	86.88	88.47	**99.53**		
SVM-RBF	$\gamma = 379.27$, $C = 46.42$	**92.82**	94.95	**95.78**	96.74	**100.00**	88.80	92.67	92.74	**99.53**	94.31	0.93
		91.47	91.07	95.78	99.44	99.60	90.64	92.97	**95.15**	98.76		
SVM-Poly	$d = 7$, $C = 63.10$	**92.82**	94.95	95.78	96.84	**100.00**	**88.89**	92.76	91.35	99.43	**94.44**	**0.93**
		91.47	91.16	95.88	**99.55**	99.60	**90.74**	**93.06**	94.88	97.93		
KFD	$\gamma = 144$, $C = 15$	89.78	**95.50**	95.73	96.22	99.60	84.91	86.34	91.40	99.37	91.54	0.90
		88.87	81.12	94.51	99.44	99.60	81.91	91.50	92.88	98.76		
Reg-AB	$\lambda = 1e-6$, $T = 10$, nodes: 8, $\phi = 1/2$	91.47	86.98	94.09	99.16	**100.00**	88.56	90.67	**94.17**	99.22	93.50	0.92
		100.00	**94.19**	**96.95**	97.79	**100.00**	85.71	89.87	90.93	**99.53**		

Figure 3. Behaviour of the overall accuracy in the test set vs. different amounts of (top left) Gaussian noise added to input features, (top right) when spikes of $P_o = -5dB$ are added in different number of bands, and (bottom) vs. different rates of samples used for training. Figures adapted from Camps-Valls and Bruzzone (2005).

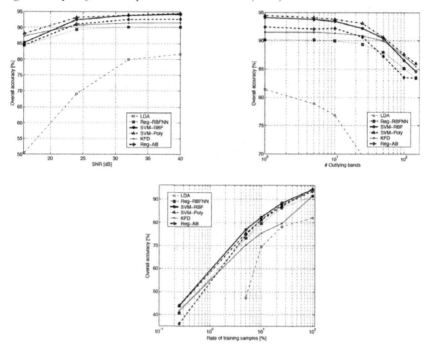

degraded than those exhibited by KFD. However, situations with too many outlying bands are uncommon. Both SVMs and KFD show better performance than Reg-RBFNN or LDA, but statistical differences were only observed with respect to LDA ($p<0.001$) in all cases.

Working with Reduced Training Sets

In the last experiment, we test models regarding their ability to deal with a limited number of labeled training samples. This is an important problem in hyperspectral remote sensing applications, given the economical cost of true labeling and the high dimension of the input feature space. Five different situations are analyzed in this setup: 0.25%, 5%, 10%, 25%, and 100% of the original training samples were randomly selected to train the models and to evaluate their accuracy on the total test set. These situations correspond to training sets containing 12, 229, 459, 1147, and 4588 samples, respectively. The experiment was repeated 100 times to avoid biased estimations.

Figure 3c shows the evolution of the overall accuracy as a function of the percentage of training samples used. The first case (12 samples) constitutes an example of a strongly ill-posed problem, in which LDA cannot be developed since the input dimension is higher than the number of available training samples. In this limit situation, SVMs (both kernels) shows a better performance than the other methods, although these results are in a very low range of accuracy (OA<50%). As the rate of training samples is increased, and more common situations are tested, nonlinear kernel methods follow a similar trend, but SVMs and Reg-AB always keep a clear advantage of 3 to 8% with respect KFD and Reg-RBFNN. Moreover, KFD shows a poor performance in the major part of situations and requires an expensive computational cost as more samples become available, which, for some practical applications, is certainly a critical constraint.

Recent Kernel Developments

So far, in the context of hyperspectral image classification, kernel classifiers have followed an inductive pixel-based approach for pattern recognition. Despite the good performance observed in such limited situations (mainly due to the use of richer oversampled spectra and homogeneous land covers), kernel machines can be adapted to the special characteristics of the classification of hyperspectral images. In the following, we present two recent kernel developments for this purpose: (a) a transductive SVM approach, which can deal with unlabeled samples to improve recognition performance (Bruzzone, Chi, & Marconcini, 2005; Chi & Bruzzone, 2005), and (b) a full family of composite kernels for efficient combination of spatial and spectral information in the scene (Camps-Valls, Gómez-Chova, Muñoz-Marí, Vila-Francés, & Calpe-Maravilla, 2006).

Transductive SVMs for Semisupervised Classification

Given the high economical and practical cost of true sample labeling, many different semisupervised classification algorithms have been presented in the literature. Semisupervised methods jointly exploit labeled and unlabeled patterns in the phase of the estimation of classifier parameters, and thus, they require a reformulation of a basic inductive algorithm such as the standard SVM.

Formulation

In this section, we present a transductive SVM (T-SVM) recently presented in the literature (Bruzzone et al., 2005; Bruzzone, Chi, & Marconcini, in press; Chi & Bruzzone, 2005), which is specifically designed to tackle the problem of multispectral and hyperspectral image classification. T-SVMs gradually search the optimal classification hyperplane in the feature space with a transductive process that incorporates unlabeled samples in the training phase.

Let the given training set $S = \{\mathbf{x}_l\}_{l=1}^{\ell}$ made up of ℓ labeled samples, and the associated labels $Y = \{y_l\}_{l=1}^{\ell}$. The unlabeled set:

$$S^* = \left\{\mathbf{x}_u^*\right\}_{u=1}^{m}$$

consists of m unlabeled samples, and the corresponding predicted labels:

$$Y^* = \left\{ y_u^* \right\}_{u=1}^m$$

are obtained according to the classification model after learning with the training set: $\mathbf{x}_l, \mathbf{x}_u^* \in \mathbb{R}^N$ and $y_l, y_u^* \in \{-1, +1\}$. Like in the inductive case, let us define a nonlinear mapping $\phi(\bullet)$, usually to a higher (possibly infinite) dimensional (Hilbert) feature space, $\phi : \mathbb{R}^N \longrightarrow F$. The T-SVM technique is based on an iterative algorithm. At the initial iteration, a standard inductive SVM (I-SVM) is used to obtain an initial separating hyperplane based on training data alone $\{\mathbf{x}_l\}_{l=1}^\ell$. Then pseudo labels $\left\{ y_u^* \right\}_{u=1}^m$ are given to the unlabeled samples $\left\{ \mathbf{x}_u^* \right\}_{u=1}^m$, which are thus called semilabeled patterns. After that, a subset of the semilabeled samples selected according to a given criterion (i.e., transductive samples) is used to define a hybrid training set made up of these samples and the original training patterns in S. The resulting hybrid training set is used at the following iterations to find a more reliable discriminant hyperplane with respect to the distribution of all patterns of the image. This hyperplane separates (S, Y), (S^*, Y^*) with maximal margin in a nonlinear nonseparable case as follows:

$$\min_{\mathbf{w}, \xi_l, \xi_u^*, b} \left\{ \frac{1}{2} \| \mathbf{w} \|^2 + C \sum_{l=1}^\ell \xi_l + C^* \sum_{u=1}^d \xi_u^* \right\} \tag{1}$$

constrained to

$$y_l (\langle \phi(\mathbf{x}_l), \mathbf{w} \rangle + b) \geq 1 - \xi_l \qquad \forall l = 1, \dots, \ell, \tag{2}$$

$$y_u^* (\langle \phi(\mathbf{x}_u^*), \mathbf{w} \rangle + b) \geq 1 - \xi_u^* \qquad \forall u = 1, \dots, d, \tag{3}$$

$$\xi_l \geq 0 \qquad \forall l = 1, \dots, \ell, \tag{4}$$

$$\xi_u^* \geq 0 \qquad \forall u = 1, \dots, d, \tag{5}$$

where $\mathbf{w}$ and b define a linear classifier in the kernel space. In order to handle nonseparable training and transductive data, similar to I-SVMs, the slack variables ξ_l, ξ_u^* and the associated penalty values C, C^* of both training and transductive samples are introduced. d ($d \leq m$) denotes the number of selected unlabeled samples in the transductive process. Note that, with this notation, if $d = m$, all the unlabeled samples are used for transductive learning, like in Chen, Wang, and Dong (2003) and Joachims (1999). For ease of computation on the quadratic optimization problem, the Lagrange theory is employed. The resulting quadratic programming problem leads to formalize the following decision function implemented by the classifier for any test vector $\mathbf{x}$:

$$f(\mathbf{x}) = \mathrm{sgn} \left(\sum_{l=1}^\ell y_l \cdot \alpha_l \cdot \kappa(\mathbf{x}_l, \mathbf{x}) + \sum_{u=1}^d y_u^* \cdot \alpha_u^* \cdot \kappa(\mathbf{x}_u^*, \mathbf{x}) + b \right), \tag{6}$$

where b can be easily computed from the Lagrange multipliers α_l, α_u^* that are neither 0 nor C, as commonly conducted in the standard I-SVM algorithm (Schölkopf & Smola, 2002). Five interesting issues should be addressed.

- **Selection of transductive samples.** Due to the fact that support vectors bear the richest information (i.e., they are the only patterns that affect the position of the separating hyperplane), among the informative samples (i.e., the ones in the margin band), unlabeled samples closest to the margin bounds have the highest probability to be correctly classified. Therefore, in the algorithm, at each iteration from both the upper (positive) and the lower (negative) side of the margin, the $P \geq 1$ (P is a user-defined parameter) transductive samples closest to the margin bounds assigned to the label +1 and –1, respectively, are taken. If the number of unlabeled samples in one side of the margin is lower than P, the labeling is done anyway. The procedure is iterated until convergence (see the following). A dynamical adjustment is necessary for taking into account that the position of the hyperplane changes at each iteration. If the label of a transductive pattern at iteration $(i + 1)$ is different from the one at iteration (i) (label inconsistency), such a label is erased and the pattern is reset to the unlabeled state. In this way, it is possible to reconsider this pattern at the following iterations of the transductive learning procedure.

- **Regularization parameter of transductive samples.** In the learning process of T-SVMs, a proper choice for the regularization parameters C and C^* is very important. The purpose of C and C^* is to control the number of misclassified samples that belong to the original training set and the unlabeled set, respectively. On increasing their values, the penalty associated with errors on the training and transductive samples increases. In other words, the larger the regularization parameter, the higher the influence of the associated samples on the selection of the discriminant hyperplane. As regards the transductive procedure, it has to be taken into account that the statistical distribution of transductive patterns could be rather different compared to that of the original training data (i.e., in ill-posed problems, the available labeled samples are often not representative enough of the test data distribution). Thus, they should be considered gradually in the transductive process so as to avoid instabilities in the learning process. For this reason, we adopted a weighting strategy based on a temporal criterion. For each binary subproblem, we propose to increase the regularization parameter for the transductive patterns C^* in a quadratic way, depending on the number of iterations, as follows:

$$C^{*(i)} = \frac{C^{*\max} - C^{*(0)}}{G^2} i^2 + C^{*(0)}, \quad G, i \in \mathbb{N}, \; C^* \in \mathbb{R}^+, \tag{7}$$

where i is the ith iteration of the transductive learning process, $C^{*(0)}$ is the initial regularization value for transductive samples (this is a user-defined parameter), $C^{*\max}$ is the maximal cost value of transductive samples and is related to that of training patterns (i.e., $C^{*\max} = \lambda \cdot C$, $\lambda \leq 1$ being a constant), and G (another user-defined value) is the growth rate, which, together with the maximum regularization value, controls the asymptotic convergence of the algorithm. Based on equation (7), we can define an indexing table so as to identify regularization values of transductive samples easily according to the number of iterations included in the training set.

- **Convergence criterion.** From a theoretical viewpoint, it can be assumed that the convergence is reached if any of the originally unlabeled samples lies into the margin band. Nevertheless, such a choice might result in a high computational load. More-over, it may happen that even if the margin band is empty, the number of inconsistent patterns at the current iteration is not negligible. For these reasons, we empirically defined that the convergence is reached if both the number of mislabeled samples at the previous iteration and the number of remaining unlabeled samples in the margin at the current iteration are lower than or equal to $a \cdot l$, where l is the number of origi-nally labeled samples and a is a constant fixed a priori that tunes the sensitivity of the learning process. A reasonable empirical choice is $a = 0.02$.

It is worth noting that as in all semisupervised methods, also for the proposed T-SVM, it is not possible to guarantee an increase of accuracy in all cases at convergence. If the initial accuracy is particularly low (i.e., most of the semilabeled samples are incorrectly classified), it is not possible to obtain good performances. The correct convergence of the learning, in fact, depends on the definition of the transductive samples considered and, implicitly, on the similarity between the problems represented by the training patterns and the unlabeled samples. Nevertheless, this effect is common to all semisu-pervised classification approaches and it is not peculiar of the proposed method (see, for example, Shahshahani & Landgrebe, 1994).

- **Multiclass problem.** As in standard I-SVMs, T-SVMs inherit the multiclass problem. Therefore, the transductive process too has to be based on a structured architecture made up of binary classifiers. However, there is an important difference between I-SVMs and T-SVMs that leads to a fundamental constraint when considering multiclass architectures. A requirement of the learning procedure of binary T-SVMs is that it must be possible to give a proper classification label to all unlabeled samples. Therefore, the choice of adopting a one-against-all strategy is mandatory (see Shahshahani & Langrebe, 1994). At each iteration, in fact, all the transductive patterns should be labeled. Hence, we cannot employ a one-against-one (OAO) strategy because it is not possible to consider only samples that are supposed to belong to two specific information classes without labeling all the others.

- **Model selection.** Concerning the selection of the T-SVM parameters (i.e., the kernel parameters, the regularization parameter, and the growth rate), in general we suggest three main strategies depending on the number of originally available labeled pat-terns.

(i)   From a theoretical viewpoint, a very reliable strategy involves the extension of the k-fold cross-validation to the transductive framework. $k+1$ disjoints labeled sets must be defined: k sets, $T_1, .., T_k$, of (approximately) equal size, and a validation set, V. For any given set of parameters, the T-SVM must be trained k times. Each time $k-1$ subsets are put together to form the training set $S = \{T_1 \cup T_2 \cup \dots \cup T_k\} - T_i$, $i = 1, \dots, k$, whereas the remaining set T_i and the validation set V, both considered without their labels, are put together to form the unlabeled set $S^* = T_i \cup V$. The performances are evaluated on T_i. The set of parameters with the lowest average error across all k trials is chosen. Finally, the learning of the T-SVM is performed setting $S = T_1 \cup T_2 \cup \dots \cup T_k$ and $S^* = V$, and the accuracy is evaluated on the validation set V. It is worth noting that, in order to obtain reliable results, this strategy requires a reasonable number of labeled data; nevertheless, such a requirement is seldom satisfied in real applications. From a computational point of view, this strategy is quite expensive because the learning of the T-SVM has to be carried out k times; however, good performances can be obtained even if $k = 2$.

(ii) When the small number of labeled patterns does not permit one to define a reasonable validation set, it is possible to employ a simpler strategy. Two disjoints labeled sets, T_1 and T_2, can be defined: T_1 coincides with the training set S, whereas T_2, considered without its labels, corresponds to the unlabeled set S^*. The set of parameters that permits one to obtain the lowest average of error on T_2 is selected. The computational burden is lower with respect to that of the strategy at point (i), but at the price of a lower reliability of the results (they strongly depend on the definition of T_1 and T_2).

(iii) If the number of labeled samples is very small, the only two possible choices are the leave-one-out and resubstitution methods. However, leave-one-out can become particularly critical in the presence of strongly minoritary classes, especially when information classes are represented by very few patterns (in the limit case, in which only one pattern is available for a class, it cannot be applied). In such extreme cases, the parameters should be selected on the basis of the training error (resubstitution error). From a theoretical viewpoint, this can lead to poor generalization capability in inductive learning. However, it is worth noting that even if the distribution of the originally labeled data set and the distribution of the semilabeled data set are slightly different, it is reasonable to expect that they represent a similar problem. Hence, even if the transductive approach cannot optimize the model on the unlabeled patterns (the model selection is carried out on training samples), it is able to adapt the model parameters to all the available data (this thanks to a proper choice of both the unlabeled patterns and the weighting criterion).

T-SVM: Experimental Results

In order to assess the effectiveness of the T-SVM technique, we carried out several experiments on the data set used in the previous section.[4] For our experiments, we employed the sequential minimal optimization (SMO) algorithm (Platt, 1999) in the learning phase of both the I-SVMs and the proposed T-SVMs (making proper modifications), exploiting the improvements proposed by Keerthi, Shevade, Bhattacharyya, and Murthy (1999). For all the experiments, we used Gaussian RBF kernels as they were proved effective in ill-posed classification problems. In this way, only one parameter (i.e., the Gaussian width) had to be tuned. An OAA architecture made up of nine different binary classifiers was adopted both for I-SVMs and T-SVMs.

From the analysis of the experimental results reported previously, it is possible to observe that the classification accuracies decrease significantly when few training samples are taken into account (i.e., 5%-25% of the original training set). This confirms the need for improving the performances when few prior information is available. In this particular framework, we carried out experiments with the transductive approach. It should be underlined that this problem is particularly complex and ill-posed because the number of training patterns is only slightly higher (or even comparable) than the size of the feature space.

Concerning model selection, we carried out several experiments. We took into account as training set (i.e., T_1) the three different sets containing 5%, 10%, and 25% of the original

Table 4. Kappa coefficient and overall accuracy (OA[%]) obtained by inductive SVMs and the proposed T-SVMs on three different subsets containing 5%, 10%, and 25% of the original training set ($C^{*(0)}$, P=0.01·m).

Percentage of Training Samples	Number of Samples	Overall Accuracy		Kappa Coefficient	
		I-SVMs	Proposed T-SVMs	I-SVMs	Proposed T-SVMs
5%	237	73.41	76.20	0.68	0.71
10%	475	76.46	80.21	0.73	0.77
25%	1189	82.17	84.83	0.79	0.82

training samples, respectively, whereas we kept the same test set (i.e., T_2) described in Table 2. In each trial, we employed T_1 as the training set S, and T_2 (considered without its labels) as the unlabeled set S^*, respectively. The set of parameters that permits one to obtain the lowest average of error on T_2 was selected. The accuracies obtained by I-SVMs proved to be particularly stable with respect to the random selection of the labeled patterns, given a fixed percentage of samples to be chosen. Therefore, to test the proposed technique, we decided to use always the same subsets of labeled patterns. We carried out experiments for different values of $C^{*(0)}$, varying (at the same time) the number of P patterns labeled from both sides of the margin. The performances, both in terms of overall accuracy and Kappa coefficient, improved the ones obtained by the I-SVMs when $C^{*(0)}$ started assuming very low values (i.e., in the range between 0.05-0.5). This is a further proof that the investigated problem was very complex and it was necessary to assign a starting low cost to errors occurred on the transductive samples. Moreover, for the most part of the nine binary subproblems, it happened that a high number of unlabeled patterns fell into the margin bound. For this reason, we obtained the best results when we labeled only a small portion of the transductive patterns at each iteration. The optimal values proved to be $C^{*(0)}$=0.1 and P=0.01m. Table 4 reports the best results obtained.

As one can see, we obtained improvements around 0.04 for Kappa coefficient and 3%-4% for overall accuracy (OA[%]). These results confirm that semisupervised T-SVMs seem a promising approach to hyperspectral image classification as they can increase the classification accuracy with respect to the standard I-SVMs in very critical hyperspectral problems.

Composite Kernels for Integrating Contextual Information

The good classification performance demonstrated by kernel methods using the spectral signature as input features can be further increased by including contextual (or even textural) information in the classifier.

Formulation

For this purpose, a pixel entity $\mathbf{x}_i$ is redefined simultaneously both in the spectral domain using its spectral content, $\mathbf{x}_i^\omega \in \mathbb{R}^{N_\omega}$, where N_ω represents the number of spectral bands, and in the spatial domain by applying some feature extraction to its surrounding area, $\mathbf{x}_i^\omega \in \mathbb{R}^{N_s}$, which yields N_s spatial (contextual) features, for example, the local mean or standard deviation per spectral band. These separated entities lead to two different kernel matrices, which can be easily computed using any suitable kernel function that fulfils Mercer's conditions. At this point, one can sum spectral and contextual dedicated kernel matrices ($\mathbf{K}_w$ and $\mathbf{K}_s$, respectively), or even introduce the cross-information between textural and spectral features ($\mathbf{K}_{\omega s}$ and $\mathbf{K}_{s\omega}$) in the formulation. To do that, we consider the properties of Mercer's kernels. Let X be any input space, $\mathbf{x}_i \in X \subseteq \mathbb{R}^N$, and let κ_1 and κ_2 be valid Mercer's kernels over $X \times X$, with $\mathbf{A}$ being a symmetric positive semidefinite $N \times N$ matrix, and $\beta > 0$. Then, the following functions are valid kernels:

$$\kappa(\mathbf{x}_i, \mathbf{x}_j) = \kappa_1(\mathbf{x}_i, \mathbf{x}_j) + \kappa_2(\mathbf{x}_i, \mathbf{x}_j),\tag{8}$$

$$\kappa(\mathbf{x}_i, \mathbf{x}_j) = \beta\, \kappa_1(\mathbf{x}_i, \mathbf{x}_j),\tag{9}$$

and

$$\kappa(\mathbf{x}_i, \mathbf{x}_j) = \mathbf{x}_i' \mathbf{A} \mathbf{x}_j.\tag{10}$$

It is worth noting that, with ℓ being the training set size, the size of the training kernel matrix is $\ell \times \ell$ and each position (i, j) of matrix $\mathbf{K}$ contains the similarity among all possible pairs of training samples ($\mathbf{x}_i$ and $\mathbf{x}_j$) measured with a suitable kernel function κ fulfilling Mercer's conditions. This simple methodology yields a full family of composite methods for hyperspectral image classification (Camps-Valls, Gómez-Chova, Muñoz-Marí, Vila-Francés, & Calpe-Maravilla, 2006), which can be summarized as follows.

- **The stacked-features approach.** The most commonly adopted approach in hyperspectral image classification is to exploit the spectral content of a pixel, $\mathbf{x}_i \equiv \mathbf{x}_i^{\omega}$. However, performance can be improved by including both spectral and spatial information in the classifier. This is usually done by means of the stacked approach, in which feature vectors are built from the concatenation of spectral and spatial features. Let us define the mapping ϕ as a transformation of the concatenation $\mathbf{x}_i \equiv \{\mathbf{x}_i^s, \mathbf{x}_i^\omega\}$; then the corresponding stacked kernel matrix is:

$$\mathbf{K}_{\{s,\omega\}} \equiv \kappa(\mathbf{x}_i, \mathbf{x}_j) = \langle \phi(\mathbf{x}_i), \phi(\mathbf{x}_j) \rangle,\tag{11}$$

which does not include explicit cross-relations between $\mathbf{x}_i^s$ and $\mathbf{x}_j^\omega$.

- **The direct-summation kernel.** A simple composite kernel combining spectral and spatial information naturally comes from the concatenation of nonlinear transformations of $\mathbf{x}_i^s$ and $\mathbf{x}_j^\omega$. Let us assume two nonlinear transformations $\varphi_1(\cdot)$ and $\varphi_2(\cdot)$ into Hilbert spaces F_1 and F_2, respectively. Then, the following transformation can be constructed:

$$\phi(\mathbf{x}_i) = \{\varphi_1(\mathbf{x}_i^s), \varphi_2(\mathbf{x}_i^\omega)\},\tag{12}$$

and the corresponding dot product can be easily computed as follows:

$$\kappa(\mathbf{x}_i, \mathbf{x}_j) = \langle \phi(\mathbf{x}_i), \phi(\mathbf{x}_j) \rangle$$

$$= \langle \{\varphi_1(\mathbf{x}_i^s), \varphi_2(\mathbf{x}_i^\omega)\}, \{\varphi_1(\mathbf{x}_j^s), \varphi_2(\mathbf{x}_j^\omega)\} \rangle = \kappa_s(\mathbf{x}_i^s, \mathbf{x}_j^s) + \kappa_\omega(\mathbf{x}_i^\omega, \mathbf{x}_j^\omega). \qquad (13)$$

Note that the solution is expressed as the sum of positive definite matrices accounting for the spatial and spectral counterparts, independently. Also note that $dim(\mathbf{x}_i^\omega) = N_\omega$, $dim(\mathbf{x}_i^s) = N_s$, and $dim(\mathbf{K}) = dim(\mathbf{K}_s) = dim(\mathbf{K}_\omega) = \ell \times \ell$.

- **The weighted-summation kernel.** By exploiting the second property of Mercer's kernels, a composite kernel that balances the spatial and spectral content can also be created. Let us define (a weighted) concatenation of nonlinear transformations of $\mathbf{x}_i^s$ and $\mathbf{x}_i^\omega$, which finally yield the following composite kernel:

$$\kappa(\mathbf{x}_i, \mathbf{x}_j) = \kappa(\mathbf{x}_i^s, \mathbf{x}_j^s) + (1 - \mu) \cdot \kappa_\omega(\mathbf{x}_i^\omega, \mathbf{x}_j^\omega), \qquad (14)$$

where μ is a positive real-valued free parameter ($0 < \mu < 1$) that is tuned in the training process or selected by the user, and constitutes a trade-off between the spatial and spectral information to classify a given pixel. This composite kernel allows us to introduce *a priori* knowledge in the classifier by designing specific μ profiles per class, and also allows us to extract some information from the best tuned μ parameter.

- **The cross-information kernel.** The preceding classifiers can be modified to account for the cross-relationship between the spatial and spectral information. Assume a nonlinear mapping $\varphi(\cdot)$ to a Hilbert space F and three linear transformations $\mathbf{A}_k$ from F to F_k, for $k=1,2,3$. Let us construct the following composite vector:

$$\phi(\mathbf{x}_i) = \{\mathbf{A}_1 \varphi(\mathbf{x}_i^s), \mathbf{A}_2 \varphi(\mathbf{x}_i^\omega), \mathbf{A}_3(\varphi(\mathbf{x}_i^s) + \varphi(\mathbf{x}_i^\omega))\}, \qquad (15)$$

and compute the dot product:

$$K(\mathbf{x}_i, \mathbf{x}_j) = \langle \phi(\mathbf{x}_i), \phi(\mathbf{x}_j) \rangle = \phi(\mathbf{x}_i^s)' \mathbf{R}_1 \phi(\mathbf{x}_j^s) + \phi(\mathbf{x}_i^\omega)' \mathbf{R}_2 \phi(\mathbf{x}_j^\omega)$$

$$+ \phi(\mathbf{x}_i^s)' \mathbf{R}_3 \phi(\mathbf{x}_j^\omega) + \phi(\mathbf{x}_i^\omega)' \mathbf{R}_3 \phi(\mathbf{x}_j^s), \qquad (16)$$

where $\mathbf{R}_1 = \mathbf{A}'_1 \mathbf{A}_1 + \mathbf{A}'_3 \mathbf{A}_3$, $\mathbf{R}_2 = \mathbf{A}'_2 \mathbf{A}_2 + \mathbf{A}'_3 \mathbf{A}_3$, and $\mathbf{R}_3 = \mathbf{A}'_3 \mathbf{A}_3$ are three independent positive definite matrices. Similar to the direct-summation kernel, it can be demonstrated that equation (15) can be expressed as the sum of positive definite matrices, accounting for the textural, spectral, and cross-terms between textural and spectral counterparts:

$$K(\mathbf{x}_i, \mathbf{x}_j) = K_s(\mathbf{x}_i^s, \mathbf{x}_j^s) + K_\omega(\mathbf{x}_i^\omega, \mathbf{x}_j^\omega) + K_{s\omega}(\mathbf{x}_i^s, \mathbf{x}_j^\omega) + K_{\omega s}(\mathbf{x}_i^\omega, \mathbf{x}_j^s) \ . \qquad (17)$$

The only restriction for this formulation to be valid is that $\mathbf{x}_i^s$ and $\mathbf{x}_j^\omega$ need to have the same dimension ($N_\omega = N_s$).

Including Spatial Information through Composite Kernels

In this battery of experiments, we used the polynomial kernel ($d=\{1,..,10\}$) for the spectral features according to previous results (Camps-Valls & Bruzzone, 2005; Gualtieri et al., 1999), and used the RBF kernel ($\sigma =\{10^1,..,10^3\}$) for the spatial features according to the locality assumption in the spatial domain. In the case of the weighted summation kernel, μ was varied in steps of 0.1 in the range [0,1]. For simplicity and for illustrative purposes, μ was the same for all labeled classes in our experiments. For the stacked ($\mathbf{K}_{\{s,\,\omega\}}$) and cross-information ($\mathbf{K}_{s\omega}$, $\mathbf{K}_{\omega s}$) approaches, we used the polynomial kernel. The penalization factor in the SVM was tuned in the range $C =\{10^{-1},..,10^7\}$. Note that solving the minimization problem in all kinds of composite kernels requires the same number of constraints as in the conventional SVM algorithm, and thus no additional computational efforts are induced in the presented approaches. A one-against-one multiclassification scheme was adopted in both cases. For this purpose, we used the whole scene.

The most simple (but powerful) spatial features $\mathbf{x}_i^s$ that can be extracted from a given region are based on moment criteria. Here, we take into account the first two moments to build the spatial kernels. Two situations were considered: (a) using the mean of the neighbourhood pixels in a window per spectral channel ($dim(\mathbf{x}_i^s) = N^\omega = 200$), or (b) using the mean and standard deviation of the neighbourhood pixels in a window per spectral channel ($dim(\mathbf{x}_i^s) = 400$). The inclusion of higher order moments or cumulants did not improve the results in our case study. The window size was varied between 3×3 and 9×9 pixels in the training set.

Table 5 shows the validation results (averaged over 10 random realizations) from six kernel classifiers: spectral ($\mathbf{K}_\omega$), contextual ($\mathbf{K}_s$), the stacked approach ($\mathbf{K}_{\{s,\,\omega\}}$), and the three presented composite kernels. In addition, two standard methods are included for baseline comparison: bLOOC + DAFE + ECHO, which uses contextual and spectral information to classify homogeneous objects, and the Euclidean classifier (Tadjudin & Landgrebe, 1998), which only uses the spectral information. All models are compared numerically (overall accuracy, OA[%]) and statistically (Kappa test and Wilcoxon rank sum test).

Several conclusions can be obtained from Table 5. First, all kernel-based methods produce better (and statistically significant) classification results than previous methods (simple Euclidean and leave one out covariance estimator-based [LOOC-based] method), as previously illustrated in Gualtieri et al. (1999). It is also worth noting that the contextual kernel classifier $\mathbf{K}_s$ alone produces good results in both images, mainly due to the presence of large homogeneous classes and the high spatial resolution of the sensor. Note that the extracted spatial features $\mathbf{x}_i^s$ contain spectral information to some extent as we computed them per spectral channel, thus they can be regarded as contextual or local spectral features. However, the accuracy is inferior to the best spectral kernel classifiers (both $\mathbf{K}_\omega$ implemented here and in Gualtieri et al., 1999), which demonstrates the relevance of the spectral information for hyperspectral image classification. Furthermore, it is worth mentioning that all composite

Table 5. Overall accuracy, OA[%], and Kappa statistic on the validation set for different spatial and spectral classifiers. The best scores for each class are highlighted in bold-face font. The OA[%] that are statistically different (at 95% confidence level, as tested through paired Wilcoxon rank sum test) from the best model are underlined.

	OA[%]	Kappa
Spectral Classifiers †		
Euclidean (Tadjudin & Landgrebe, 1998)	48.23	—
bLOOC+DAFE+ECHO (Tadjudin & Landgrebe, 1998)	82.91	—
K_ω (Gualtieri et al., 1999)	87.30	—
K_ω developed in this chapter	88.55	0.87
Spatial-Spectral Classifiers		
Mean		
K_s	84.55	0.82
$K_{\{s,\omega\}}$	94.21	0.93
$K_s + K_\omega$	92.61	0.91
$\mu K_s + (1-\mu) K_\omega$	**95.97**	**0.94**
$K_s + K_\omega + K_{s\omega} + K_{\omega s}$	94.80	0.94
Mean and Standard Deviation‡		
K_s	88.00	0.86
$K_{\{s,\omega\}}$	94.21	0.93
$K_s + K_\omega$	95.45	0.95
$\mu K_s + (1-\mu) K_\omega$	**96.53**	**0.96**

† *Differences between the obtained accuracies reported in Gualtieri et al. (1999) and the presented here could be due to the random sample selection; however, they are not statistically significant.*

‡ *Note that by using mean and standard deviation features, $N_\omega \neq N_s$, and thus no cross-kernels, $K_{s\omega}$ or $K_{\omega s}$, can be constructed.*

kernel classifiers improved the results obtained by the usual spectral kernel, which confirms the validity of the presented framework. Additionally, as can be observed, there is superior performance of cross-information and weighted summation kernels with respect to the usual stacked approach. It is also worth noting that, as the spatial-features extraction method is refined (extracting the first two momenta), the classification accuracy increases, which, in turn, demonstrates the robustness of kernel classifiers to high-input space dimensions. Finally, two relevant issues should be highlighted from the obtained results: (a) optimal μ and window size seem to act as efficient alternative trade-off parameters to account for the spatial information (in our particular application, μ =0.2 and 7×7 for the subset scene; μ =0.4 and 5×5 for the whole scene), and (b) results have been significantly improved without considering any feature-selection step previous to model development.

Discussion and Conclusion

In this chapter, we have addressed the framework of kernel-based methods in the context of hyperspectral image classification. Many experiments carried out with standard kernel methods have been presented, and two kernel-based formulations recently introduced in the literature to account for both the semisupervised case and the efficient integration of spatial and spectral information have been considered.

Table 6 shows some qualitative aspects of the kernel-based methods analyzed in this chapter in terms of computational burden, sparsity, capability to provide probabilistic outputs, accuracy, and robustness to noise, to the input space dimension, and to few labeled samples. The table does not intend to be an exhaustive analysis of methods, but only to provide some guidelines. The following conclusions can be drawn for each method.

1. SVMs revealed to be excellent in terms of computational cost, accuracy, and robustness to common levels of noise (i.e., Gaussian, uniform, or impulsive), and ensures sparsity. The only drawback is that it cannot provide probabilistic outputs directly.

2. Reg-AB showed very good results (almost comparable to those offered by SVMs), improving the robustness of Reg-RBFNN, and working efficiently with a low number of labeled samples. In addition, model simplicity was ensured in the form of a few hypotheses.

3. KFD exhibited good accuracies but, in normal situations, they were on average inferior to those obtained with SVMs and Reg-AB. In addition, an important drawback of KFD is the computational burden induced in its training, which is related to the lack of sparsity of the solution. This is a particularly relevant impairment for hyperspectral remote sensing applications. Its main advantage is the ability to directly estimate the conditional posterior probabilities of classes.

4. The Reg-RBFNN offered an acceptable trade-off between accuracy and computational cost. Nevertheless, accuracies in all tests were lower than those provided by the other nonlinear models. Simplicity of the model, given by a low number of hidden neurons, was achieved.

Table 6. Qualitative comparison of the analyzed kernel-based methods. Different marks are provided: H (high), M (medium), or L (low).

CLASSIFIER	Computational Cost	Sparsity	Probabilistic Outputs	Overall Accuracy	Robustness to Noise	Robustness to High Dimension	Accuracy with Very Few Labeled Samples
KFD	H	L	H	H	H	M	M
SVMs	L	H	L	H	H	H	H
Reg-AB	M	H	H	H	H	M	H
Reg-RBFNN	L	H	L	H	M	M	M
T-SVM	H	H	L	H	H	H	H
Composite Kernels	L	H	L	H	H	H	H

5. Transductive SVM improved classification accuracy and stability with respect to the standard inductive kernel machines, especially when very few training samples are available. This came at the cost of an increased computational time.

6. The family of composite kernels offers an elegant kernel formulation to integrate contextual and spectral information, and opens a wide field for further developments to include the spatial or textural information naturally. At present, the classification results presented with this methodology are the state-of-the-art in the benchmark image of AVIRIS Indian Pines. The computational effort depends on the spatial-feature extraction step.

In conclusion, we can state that, in the standard situation and in our case studies, the use of SVMs is more beneficial, yielding better results than the other kernel-based methods, and ensuring sparsity (see a deeper discussion in Camps-Valls & Bruzzone, 2005) at a much lower computational cost. However, it is worth noting that in order to attain significant results, the standard algorithm of SVMs must be tailored to exploit the special characteristics of hyperspectral images.

References

Bischof, H., & Leona, A. (1998). Finding optimal neural networks for land use classification. *IEEE Transactions on Geoscience and Remote Sensing, 36*(1), 337-341.

Boser, B. E., Guyon, I. M., & Vapnik, V. N. (1992). A training algorithm for optimal margin classifiers. *Fifth Annual Workshop on Computational Learning Theory* (pp. 144-152).

Bruzzone, L., Chi, M., & Marconcini, M. (2005). Transductive SVMs for semisupervised classification of hyperspectral data. In *Proceedings of IGARSS 2005* (pp. 1-4).

Bruzzone, L., Chi, M., & Marconcini, M. (in press). A novel transductive SVMs for the semisupervised classification of remote-sensing images. *IEEE Transactions on Geoscience and Remote Sensing.*

Bruzzone, L., & Cossu, R. (2002). A multiple-cascade-classifier system for a robust and partially unsupervised updating of land-cover maps. *IEEE Transactions on Geoscience and Remote Sensing, 40*(9), 1984-1996.

Bruzzone, L., & Melgani, F. (2003). Classification of hyperspectral images with support vector machines: Multiclass strategies. *SPIE International Symposium Remote sensing IX* (pp. 408-419).

Camps-Valls, G., & Bruzzone, L. (2005). Kernel-based methods for hyperspectral image classification. *IEEE Transactions on Geoscience and Remote Sensing, 43*(6), 1351-1362.

Camps-Valls, G., Gómez-Chova, L., Calpe, J., Soria, E., Martín, J. D., Alonso, L., et al. (2004). Robust support vector method for hyperspectral data classification and knowledge discovery. *IEEE Transactions on Geoscience and Remote Sensing, 42*(7), 1530-1542.

Camps-Valls, G., Gómez-Chova, L., Calpe, J., Soria, E., Martín, J. D., & Moreno, J. (2003). *Kernel methods for HyMap imagery knowledge discovery.* SPIE International Symposium Remote Sensing, Barcelona, Spain.

Camps-Valls, G., Gómez-Chova, L., Muñoz-Marí, J., Vila-Francés, J., & Calpe-Maravilla, J. (2006). Composite kernels for hyperspectral image classification. *IEEE Geoscience and Remote Sensing Letters, 3*(1), 93-97.

Camps-Valls, G., Serrano-López, A., Gómez-Chova, L., Martín, J. D., Calpe, J., & Moreno, J. (2004). Regularized RBF networks for hyperspectral data classification. In *Lecture notes in computer science: International Conference on Image Recognition, ICIAR 2004.* Porto, Portugal: Springer-Verlag.

Chen, Y., Wang, G., & Dong, S. (2003). Learning with progressive transductive support vector machines. *Pattern Recognition Letters, 24*(12), 1845-1855.

Chi, M., & Bruzzone, L. (2005). A novel transductive SVM for semisupervised classification of remote sensing images. *SPIE International Symposium Remote Sensing.*

Cortes, C., & Vapnik, V. N. (1995). Support vector networks. *Machine Learning, 20,* 1-25.

Cristianini, N., & Shawe-Taylor, J. (2000). *An introduction to support vector machines.* Cambridge, UK: Cambridge University Press.

Dundar, M., & Langrebe, A. (2004). A cost-effective semisupervised classifier approach with kernels. *IEEE Transactions on Geoscience and Remote Sensing, 42*(1), 264-270.

Foody, G. M., & Mathur, J. (2004). A relative evaluation of multiclass image classification by support vector machines. *IEEE Transactions on Geoscience and Remote Sensing,* 1-9.

Giacinto, G., Roli, F., & Bruzzone, L. (2000). Combination of neural and statistical algorithms for supervised classification of remote-sensing images. *Pattern Recognition Letters, 21*(5), 399-405.

Gualtieri, J. A., Chettri, S. R., Cromp, R. F., & Johnson, L. F. (1999). Support vector machine classifiers as applied to AVIRIS data. In *Proceedings of the 1999 Airborne Geoscience Workshop.*

Gualtieri, J. A., & Cromp, R. F. (1998). Support vector machines for hyperspectral remote sensing classification. *The 27th AIPR Workshop, Proceedings of the SPIE, 3584* (pp. 221-232).

Huang, C., Davis, L. S., & Townshend, J. R. G. (2002). An assessment of support vector machines for land cover classification. *International Journal of Remote Sensing, 23*(4), 725-749.

Hughes, G. F. (1968). On the mean accuracy of statistical pattern recognizers. *IEEE Transactions on Information Theory, 14*(1), 55-63.

Joachims, T. (1999). Transductive inference for text classification using support vector machines. In *Proceedings of the International Conference on Machine Learning (ICML).*

Keerthi, S., Shevade, S., Bhattacharyya, C., & Murthy, K. (1999). *Improvements to Platt's SMO algorithm for SVM classifier design* (Tech. Rep.). Bangalore, India: Department of CSA, IISc.

Kwon, H., & Nasrabadi, N. (2004a). Hyperspectral anomaly detection using kernel RX-algorithm. *International Conference on Image Processing, ICIP'04* (pp. 3331-3334).

Kwon, H., & Nasrabadi, N. (2004b). Hyperspectral target detection using kernel matched subspace detector. *International Conference on Image Processing, ICIP'04* (pp. 3327-3330).

Landgrebe, D. (1992). *AVIRIS NW Indiana's Indian Pines 1992 data set.* Retrieved from http://dynamo.ecn.purdue.edu/~biehl/MultiSpec/documentation.html

Melgani, F., & Bruzzone, L. (2004). Classification of hyperspectral remote-sensing images with support vector machines. *IEEE Transactions on Geoscience and Remote Sensing, 42*(8), 1778-1790.

Platt, J. (1999). Fast training of support vector machines using sequential minimal optimization. In B. Schölkopf, C. J. C. Burges, & A. J. Smola (Eds.), *Advances in kernel methods: Support vector learning* (pp. 185-208). Cambridge, MA: MIT Press.

Richards, J. A., & Jia, X. (1999). *Remote sensing digital image analysis: An introduction* (3rd ed.). Berlin, Germany: Springer-Verlag.

Schölkopf, B., & Smola, A. (2002). *Learning with kernels: Support vector machines, regularization, optimization and beyond.* MIT Press Series.

Shahshahani, B. M., & Landgrebe, D. A. (1994). The effect of unlabelled samples in reducing the small sample size problem and mitigating the Hughes phenomenon. *IEEE Transactions on Geoscience and Remote Sensing, 32*(5), 1087-1095.

Shaw, G., & Manolakis, D. (2002). Signal processing for hyperspectral image exploitation. *IEEE Signal Processing Magazine, 50*, 12-16.

Song, X., Cherian, G., & Fan, G. (2005). A ν-insensitive SVM approach for compliance monitoring of the conservation reserve program. *IEEE Geoscience and Remote Sensing Letters, 2*(2), 99-103.

Srivastava, A. N., & Stroeve, J. (2003). Onboard detection of snow, ice, clouds and other geophysical processes using kernel methods. In *Proceedings of the ICML 2003 Workshop on Machine Learning Technologies for Autonomous Space Sciences.*

Swain, P. (1978). *Fundamentals of pattern recognition in remote sensing.* In P. Swain & S. M. Davis (Eds.) Remote sensing: The quantitative approach. (p. 136-188). New York: McGraw-Hill.

Tadjudin, S., & Landgrebe, D. (1998). *Classification of high dimensional data with limited training samples.* Unpublished doctoral dissertation, Purdue University, School of Electrical Engineering and Computer Science.

Vapnik, V. N. (1998). *Statistical learning theory.* New York: John Wiley & Sons.

Vapnik, V. N. (1999). An overview of statistical learning theory. *IEEE Transactions on Neural Networks, 10*(5), 988-998.

Yang, H., Meer, F. van der, Bakker, W., & Tan, Z. J. (1999). A back–propagation neural network for mineralogical mapping from AVIRIS data. *International Journal of Remote Sensing, 20*(1), 97-110.

Endnotes

[1] Other types of hyperspectral sensors exploit the emissive properties of objects by collecting data in the mid-wave and long-wave infrared (MWIR and LWIR) regions of the spectrum.

2   Indian Pines data set is available at: ftp://ftp.ecn.purdue.edu/biehl/PC_MultiSpec/
       ThyFiles.zip (Groundtruth) and ftp://ftp.ecn.purdue.edu/biehl/MultiSpec/92AV3C.lan
       (Hyperspectral data). More information can be found at the Prof. Landgrebe's Web
       site: http://dynamo.ecn.purdue.edu/~landgreb/publications.html

3   libSVM open source software is available from Chih-Jen Lin Web site together with
       paper, tools, and an interactive demo: http://www.csie.ntu.edu.tw/~cjlin/libsvm/

About the Authors

Gustavo Camps-Valls was born in València, Spain, in 1972. He received a BS in physics (1996), a BS in electronics engineering (1998), and a PhD in physics (2002) from the Universitat de València, Spain. He is currently an assistant professor with the Department of Electronics Engineering at the Universitat de València, teaching electronics, advanced time-series processing, and digital signal processing. His research interests are neural networks and kernel methods for hyperspectral data analysis, health sciences, and safety-related areas. He is the (co-)author of 30 journal papers, several book chapters, and more than 50 international conference papers. He is a referee of several international journals and has served on the scientific committees of several international conferences.

Manel Martínez-Ramón received a telecom engineering degree from Polytechnic University of Catalunya, Barcelona, Spain (1994), and a PhD in telecommunication from Universidad Carlos III de Madrid (1999). He is currently with the Department of Signal Theory and Communications, Universidad Carlos III de Madrid, Spain. Since 1996, he has taught about 20 different graduate and undergraduate subjects in the field of signal theory and communications. He has co-authored 15 journal papers and and the book *Support Vector Machines for Antenna Array Processing and Electromagnetics* (Morgan & Claypool Publishers, 2006). His current research is devoted to the applications of SVM to antenna array processing and to the analysis of functional magnetic resonance imaging (fMRI) of the human brain.

José Luis Rojo-Álvarez received a telecommunication engineering degree from the University of Vigo, Spain (1996), and a PhD in telecommunication from the Polytechnical University of

Madrid, Spain (2000). He is an assistant professor with the Department of Signal Theory and Communications, Universidad Rey Juan Carlos, Spain. His main research interests include statistical learning theory, digital signal processing, and complex system modeling, with applications both to cardiac signals and image processing, and to digital communications. He has published about 30 papers and more than 50 international conference communications on support vector machines (SVMs) and neural networks, robust analysis of time series and images, cardiac arrhythmia mechanisms, and Doppler echocardiographic images for hemodynamic function evaluation.

* * *

Felipe Alonso-Atienza was born in Bilbao, Spain, in May 1979. He received an MS in telecommunication engineering from the Universidad Carlos III de Madrid (2003). He is currently pursuing a PhD at Universidad Carlos III de Madrid, Spain, where he is doing research on digital signal processing, statistical learning theory, biological system modeling, and feature selection techniques and their application to biomedical problems, with particular attention to cardiac signals.

Gökhan H. Bakır received a diploma in computer engineering from the University of Siegen in 2000. He has worked since July 2002 under the supervision of Professor Schölkopf at the Max Planck Institute for Biological Cybernetics, Germany. He obtained a doctorate degree in computer engineering from the Technical University Berlin in 2006 (under Professor Schölkopf). His interests are in kernel methods and applications to robotics.

Lorenzo Bruzzone received an MS in electronic engineering (*summa cum laude*) and a PhD in telecommunications from the University of Genoa, Italy (1993 and 1998, respectively). He is currently head of the Remote Sensing Laboratory in the Department of Information and Communication Technology at the University of Trento, Italy. From 1998 to 2000, he was a postdoctoral researcher at the University of Genoa. From 2000 to 2001, he was an assistant professor at the University of Trento, and from 2001 to 2005, he was an associate professor at the same university. Since March 2005, he has been a full professor of telecommunications at the University of Trento, where he currently teaches remote sensing, pattern recognition, and electrical communications. His current research interests are in the area of remote-sensing image processing and recognition (analysis of multitemporal data, feature selection, classification, regression, data fusion, and neural networks). He conducts and supervises research on these topics within the frameworks of several national and international projects. Since 1999, he has been appointed evaluator of project proposals for the European Commission. Dr. Bruzzone is the author (or coauthor) of more than 150 scientific publications, including journals, book chapters, and conference proceedings. He is a referee for many international journals and has served on the scientific committees of several international conferences. Dr. Bruzzone is a member of the scientific committee of the India-Italy Center for Advanced Research. He ranked first place in the Student Prize Paper Competition of the 1998 IEEE International Geoscience and Remote Sensing Symposium (Seattle, July 1998). He was a recipient of the Recognition of *IEEE Transactions on Geoscience and Remote Sensing* Best Reviewers in 1999 and was a guest editor of a special issue of the journal on the subject of the analysis of multitemporal remote-sensing images (November 2003). Dr. Bruzzone was the general chair and co-chair of the First and Second IEEE International Workshop on the

Analysis of Multi-Temporal Remote-Sensing Images, respectively. Since 2003, he has been the chair of the SPIE Conference on Image and Signal Processing for Remote Sensing. He is an associate editor of *IEEE Transactions on Geoscience and Remote Sensing*. He is a senior member of IEEE and a member of the International Association for Pattern Recognition (IAPR) and the Italian Association for Remote Sensing (AIT).

Christos Christodoulou received his PhD in electrical engineering from North Carolina State University, Raleigh (1985). He served as a faculty member in the University of Central Florida, Orlando, from 1985 to 1998 and joined the University of New Mexico (USA) in 1999. He is a fellow of the IEEE and associate editor for the *IEEE Transactions on Antennas and Propagation* (AP) and the *IEEE AP Magazine*. He has published over 250 papers in journals, conference proceedings, and books. His research interests are in the areas of neural network and machine learning applications in electromagnetics, smart antennas, and MEMS.

Daniel Cremers received a master's degree in theoretical physics (Heidelberg, 1997) and a PhD in computer science (Mannheim, 2002). From 2002 until 2004, he was postdoctoral researcher in computer science at the UCLA, and from 2004 until 2005, with Siemens Corporate Research, Princeton. Since October 2005, he has been heading the Computer Vision Group at the University of Bonn, Germany. His research received numerous awards, among others, the 2004 Olympus Award, the UCLA Chancellor's Award for Postdoctoral Research, and the award of Best Paper of the Year 2003 (Pattern Recognition Society).

Nello Cristianini obtained a degree in physics from the University of Trieste (1996) and an MS in computational intelligence from Royal Holloway, University of London (1997). He obtained a PhD in engineering mathematics at the University of Bristol in 2000, then returned to Royal Holloway for postdoctoral work in computer science. In 2001, he was appointed a visiting lecturer at the University of California (U.C.) at Berkeley and a senior scientist with BIOwulf Technologies. In 2002, he took up the post of director of statistics and information services with Concurrent Pharmaceuticals in Cambridge, Massachusetts, and from there became an assistant and then associate professor in the statistics department at the University of California, Davis. In March 2006, he was appointed to the post of professor with the Department of Engineering Mathematics at Bristol. He has interests in all statistical and computational aspects of machine learning and pattern analysis, and in their application to problems arising in computational biology and linguistics. Since 2001 has been action editor of the *Journal of Machine Learning Research* (JMLR), and since 2005, associate editor of the *Journal of Artificial Intelligence Research* (JAIR). He co-authored the books *Introduction to Support Vector Machines* and *Kernel Methods for Pattern Analysis* with John Shawe-Taylor (both published by Cambridge University Press).

Tijl De Bie obtained a degree in electrical engineering at the Katholieke Universiteit (K. U.) Leuven, Belgium in June 2000 (*summa cum laude*). In 2005, he completed a PhD with the Department of Electrical Engineering (ESAT) of the same university under the supervision of Professor Bart De Moor. During his PhD, he visited different research groups in Imperial College London, U.C. Berkeley, and U.C. Davis. After his PhD research, he became a post doc in the ISIS research group at the University of Southampton and subsequently in the OKP research group on quantitative psychology at K. U. Leuven.

Bart L. R. De Moor obtained a PhD in electrical engineering at the Katholieke Universiteit Leuven, Belgium (1988), where he is now a full professor. He was a visiting research associate at Stanford University (1988-1990). His research interests are in numerical linear algebra and optimization, system theory, control and identification, quantum information theory, data mining, information retrieval, and bioinformatics, about which he (co-)authored more than 400 papers and three books. His work has won him several scientific awards. Since 2004, he has been a fellow of the IEEE. From 1991 to 1999, he was chief advisor of science and technology of several ministers of the Belgian federal and the Flanders regional governments.

Frank De Smet was born in Bonheiden, Belgium, in August 1969. He received an MS in electrical and mechanical engineering (1992) and a PhD (1998) from the Katholieke Universiteit Leuven, Belgium. He received a PhD in electrical engineering from the same university in 2004 with a dissertation titled *Microarrays: Algorithms for Knowledge Discovery in Oncology and Molecular Biology*. Currently, he is a medical advisor responsible for data analysis and a member of the medical direction of the National Alliance of Christian Mutualities, Brussels, Belgium.

M. Julia Fernández-Getino García received a master's degree and a PhD in telecommunication engineering, both from the Polytechnic University of Madrid, Spain (1996 and 2001, respectively). She is currently working as an associate professor at the Department of Signal Theory and Communications, Universidad Carlos III de Madrid, Spain. From 1996 to 2001, she held a research position with the Department of Signals, Systems and Radiocommunications, Polytechnic University of Madrid. She was on leave during 1998 at Bell Laboratories, Murray Hill, NJ; visited Lund University, Sweden, during two periods in 1999 and 2000; and visited Politecnico di Torino, Italy, in 2003 and 2004. Her research interests include multicarrier communications, signal processing, and digital communications. She has published about 30 international journal and conference papers in these areas.

Carlos Figuera was born in Madrid, Spain. He received his degree in telecommunication engineering at Universidad Politécnica of Madrid (2002). He has been with the Department of Theory of Signal and Communications at Universidad Carlos III de Madrid for 2 years, where he has been studying for a PhD. He is currently a research assistant in the Department of Theory of Signal and Communications, Universidad Rey Juan Carlos, Fuenlabrada, Spain. His research interests include signal processing for wireless communications and diversity theory for wireless ad hoc networks.

Blaž Fortuna has been a PhD student at Jožef Stefan Institute (JSI), Slovenia, since 2005 in the area of kernel methods and statistical learning. In the past, he achieved several awards at international computer science competitions. In recent years, he had several publications at international conferences and developed several software modules for scalable machine learning, ontology learning, and active learning, which are part of JSI's Text Garden software environment.

Aravind Ganapathiraju was born in Hyderabad, India, in 1973. He received his BS (1995) in electronics from Regional Engineering College, Trichy, India, and his MS (1997) and PhD

(2002) from Mississippi State University, USA, in computer engineering while specializing in signal processing and speech recognition. His work on applying support vector machines for speech recognition was one the first formal efforts at using this machine learning technique for speech recognition. He is currently the vice president of core technology at Conversay (http://www.conversay.com) and is responsible for research and development. His research interests include the optimization of speech-recognition algorithms for embedded applications, error correction in voice user interfaces, and noise robustness in speech front ends.

Ana García-Armada received a telecommunication engineer degree from the Polytechnic University of Madrid (Spain) in July 1994 and a PhD in electrical engineering from the same university in February 1998. She is currently working as an associate professor at Universidad Carlos III de Madrid, Spain, where she has occupied several management positions. She has participated in several national and international research projects, most of them related to orthogonal frequency division multiplexing (OFDM). She is the co-author of three books on wireless communications. She has published 12 papers in international journals and more than 40 papers in international conference proceedings. She has contributed to international organizations such as ITU and ETSI. She has performed research stays in ESA-ESTEC, Kansas University, Stanford University, and Bell Labs. Her research interests are the simulation of communication systems, and multicarrier and MIMO techniques.

Víctor P. Gil-Jiménez received a bachelor's degree in telecommunications with Honors from the University of Alcalá (1998), and a master's in telecommunications and PhD, both from the Universidad Carlos III de Madrid, Spain (2001 and 2005, respectively). He is an assistant professor at the Department of Signal Theory and Communications of the same university. He worked at the Spanish Antarctica Base in 1999 as communications staff. His research interests include multicarrier communications and signal processing for wireless systems.

Luis Gómez-Chova received his BS with first-class Honors in electronics from the Universitat de València, Spain (2000). He was awarded by the Spanish Ministry of Education with the National Award for Electronics Engineering. Since 2000, he has been with the Department of Electronic Engineering, enjoying a research scholarship from the Spanish Ministry of Education, and currently is a lecturer.

Gabriel Gómez-Pérez received a BS in physics (2002) and a BS in electrical engineering (2004), both from the Universitat de València, Spain. Currently, he is working at the Grupo de Procesado Digital de Señales (GPDS) and at the Visual Statistics Group (VISTA) of the Universitat de València. He is interested in machine learning algorithms (support vector machines and reinforcement learning) and image processing.

Juan Gutiérrez received a degree in physics (electricity, electronics, and computer science) in 1995 from the Universitat de València. He is with the Department of Computer Science, Universitat de València, Spain, where he is an assistant professor. Currently, he is with the VISTA at the Universitat de València (http://www.uv.es/vista/vistavalencia). His current research interests include regularization theory, models of low-level human vision, and the representation and analysis of images.

Jon Hamaker was born in Birmingham, Alabama, USA, in 1974. He received a BS degree in electrical engineering in 1997 and an MS degree in computer engineering in 2000, both from Mississippi State University. He joined Microsoft Corporation in 2004 after pursuing graduate work in the application of kernel machines to speech recognition. He is currently a development lead at Microsoft, where he leads a team focused on the development of core speech-recognition technology for all Microsoft platforms. His primary research interest is in the application of machine learning to speech recognition in constrained environments. Further interests include noise-robust acoustic modeling and discriminative modeling.

Gregory L. Heileman received a BA from Wake Forest University (1982), an MS in biomedical engineering and mathematics from the University of North Carolina - Chapel Hill (1986), and a PhD in computer engineering from the University of Central Florida (1989). In 1990, he joined the Department of Electrical and Computer Engineering at the University of New Mexico, Albuquerque (USA), where he is currently professor and associate chair. In 1998, he held a research fellowship at the Universidad Carlos III de Madrid, and in 2005 he held a similar position at the Universidad Politécnica de Madrid. His research interests are in digital-rights management, information security, the theory of computing and information, machine learning, and data structures and algorithmic analysis. He is the author of *Data Structures, Algorithms and Object-Oriented Programming* (McGraw-Hill, 1996).

Timo Kohlberger received a master's degree in computer engineering (University of Mannheim, 2001) and his PhD in the CVGPR Group of Dr. Christoph Schnörr (University of Mannheim, 2006). Since November 2005, he has been with Siemens Corporate Research, Princeton (USA). His current areas of research are 4-D shape priors in variational image segmentation as well as the parallelization of nonlinear PDE-based image filtering techniques. During his studies, he was supported by the German National Academic Foundation.

Vladimir Koltchinskii is a professor in mathematics at the Georgia Institute of Technology (USA). He received a PhD in mathematics from Kiev University, Ukraine, in 1982. His background is in probability and statistics, and he has been working on a variety of pure and applied problems. He is an associate editor of the *Annals of Statistics* and a fellow of the Institute of Mathematical Statistics. Koltchinskii has published 100 research articles, many of them in the leading journals in statistics and probability. His research has been supported by NSF, NSA, and NIH grants. For the last several years, his work has been focused primarily on the development of mathematical foundations of statistical learning theory, in particular, on generalization error bounds and model-selection techniques in pattern classification. On a more applied side, Koltchinskii has been involved in research projects related to statistical learning methods in robust control and brain imaging.

Jesús Malo received an MS in physics in 1995 and a PhD in physics in 1999, both from the Universitat de València. He was the recipient of the Vistakon European Research Award in 1994. In 2000 and 2001, he worked as a Fulbright postdoc at the Vision Group of the NASA Ames Research Center, and at the Lab of Computational Vision of the Center for Neural Science, New York University. Currently, he is with the Visual Statistics Group at the Universitat de València, Spain (http://www.uv.es/vista/vistavalencia). He is a member of the Asociación de Mujeres Investigadoras y Tecnólogas (AMIT). He is interested in models of low-level human vision, their relations with information theory, and their applications to image processing and vision science experimentation. His interests also include (but are not limited to) Fourier, Matlab, modern art, independent movies, chamber music, Lou Reed, Belle and Sebastian, The Pixies, comics, Faemino y Cansado, la Bola de Cristal, and beauty in general.

Mattia Marconcini was born in Verona, Italy, in 1980. He received BS and MS degrees in telecommunication engineering (*summa cum laude*) from the University of Trento, Italy (2002 and 2004, respectively). He is currently pursuing a PhD in information and communication technologies at the University of Trento. He is presently with the Pattern Recognition and Remote Sensing Group, Department of Information and Communication Technologies, University of Trento. His current research activities are in the area of machine learning and remote sensing. In particular, his interests are related to semisupervised, partially supervised, and context-sensitive classification problems. He conducts research on these topics within the frameworks of several national and international projects.

Tomasz Markiewicz was born in Poland in 1976. He received MS and PhD degrees in electrical engineering from the Warsaw University of Technology, Poland (2001 and 2006, respectively). His scientific interest is in neural networks and biomedical signal and image processing.

Carlos E. Martínez-Cruz was born in Santa Tecla, El Salvador, in May 1972. He received an MS degree in electrical engineering from Universidad de El Salvador (1996) where he worked as an assistant professor until 2004. He is currently pursuing a PhD at Universidad Carlos III de Madrid, Spain. His research interests are in digital signal processing and machine learning.

Francesca Odone received a degree in information science in 1997 and a PhD in computer science in 2002, both from the University of Genova, Italy. She visited Heriot-Watt University, Edinburgh, in 1997 as a research associate and in 1999 as a visiting student. She has been *ricercatore* at INFM (National Institute of Solid State Physics) and research associate with the Department of Mathematics of the University of Ferrara. Today she is *ricercatore* with the Department of Computing and Information Science, Università degli Studie di Genova. She published papers on computer vision applied to automation, motion analysis, image matching, image classification, and view-based object recognition. Her present research focuses on statistical learning and its application to image understanding and bioinformatics.

Fabian Ojeda was born in Anserma (Caldas), Colombia. In 2003, he completed a BS in electronic engineering from the National University of Colombia, Manizales. He received an MS in artificial intelligence from the Katholieke Universiteit Leuven, Belgium (2005). Currently he is pursuing a PhD in electrical engineering (ESAT-SCD Division) at the Katholieke Universiteit Leuven, Belgium.

Stanislaw Osowski was born in Poland in 1948. He received MS, PhD, and DSc degrees from the Warsaw University of Technology, Poland (1972, 1975, and 1981, respectively), all in electrical engineering. Currently, he is a professor of electrical engineering at the Institute of the Theory of Electrical Engineering, Measurement and Information Systems, Warsaw

University of Technology. His research and teaching interest are in the areas of neural networks, optimization techniques, and their application in biomedical signal and image processing. He is an author or co-author of more than 200 scientific papers and 10 books.

Joseph Picone is currently a professor in the Department of Electrical and Computer Engineering at Mississippi State University (USA), where he also directs the Intelligent Electronic Systems program at the Center for Advanced Vehicular Systems. His principal research interests are the development of new statistical modeling techniques for speech recognition. He has previously been employed by Texas Instruments and AT&T Bell Laboratories. Dr. Picone received his PhD in electrical engineering from Illinois Institute of Technology in 1983. He is a senior member of the IEEE

Nathalie L. M. M. Pochet was born in 1977 in Belgium. She received MS degrees in industrial engineering in electronics (2000), artificial intelligence (2001), and bioinformatics (2002). She is expected to obtain a PhD in electrical engineering in 2006 at ESAT-SCD, K. U. Leuven, Belgium, with a dissertation titled *Microarray Data Analysis Using Support Vector Machines and Kernel Methods*. Recently, she received an award with a fellowship to perform postdoctoral research as a Henri Benedictus and BAEF fellow (of the King Baudouin Foundation and the Belgian American Educational Foundation) at the Bauer Center for Genomics Research at Harvard University, USA.

Stefan Posse is director of MR research at the MIND Institute and a tenured associate professor of psychiatry and electrical and computer engineering at the University of New Mexico (USA). He obtained his PhD in physics at the University of Berne, Switzerland. After postdoctoral training at the NIH, he moved to Germany to establish an MR research group at the Research Center Juelich and obtained his habilitation at the University of Duesseldorf. He subsequently held tenure at Wayne State University School of Medicine in Michigan before moving to New Mexico. His NIH-funded research includes the development and application of real-time functional MRI and high-speed MR spectroscopic imaging in the human brain.

Craig Saunders obtained a PhD in machine learning at Royal Holloway, University of London (2000). Shortly after completion of his PhD, he was appointed to a lectureship at Royal Holloway. In 2004, he moved to the ISIS research group at the University of Southampton, UK. He is interested in all aspects of machine learning, but recently has focused on kernel methods. He has published several papers within the field, and has organized many international workshops on kernel methods and support vector machines. His current interests are in constructing kernels for discrete objects such as strings and graphs, and also developing algorithms that allow for prediction in structured output spaces.

Bernhard Schölkopf received an MS in mathematics and the Lionel Cooper Memorial Prize from the University of London (1992), followed in 1994 by a diploma in physics from the Eberhard-Karls-Universität, Tübingen. Three years later, he obtained a doctorate in computer science from the Technical University Berlin. His thesis on support vector learning won the annual dissertation prize of the German Association for Computer Science (GI). In 1998, he won the prize for the best scientific project at the German National Research Center for Computer Science (GMD). He has researched at AT&T Bell Labs, at GMD FIRST in Berlin, at the Australian National University in Canberra, and at Microsoft Research Cambridge (UK). He has taught at Humboldt University and the Technical University Berlin, and also at the Eberhard-Karls-Universität of Tübingen. In July 2001, he was elected scientific member of the Max Planck Society and director at the MPI for Biological Cybernetics, Germany. In October 2002, he was appointed honorary professor of machine learning at the Technical University Berlin.

John Shawe-Taylor obtained a PhD in mathematics at Royal Holloway, University of London (1986). He subsequently completed an MS in the foundations of advanced information technology at Imperial College. He was promoted to professor of computing science in 1996. He has published over 150 research papers. In 2003, he moved to the University of Southampton (UK), where he heads the ISIS research group. He has pioneered the development of the well-founded approaches to machine learning inspired by statistical learning theory (including support vector machines, boosting, and kernel principal components analysis), and has shown the viability of applying these techniques to document analysis and computer vision. He has coordinated a number of European-wide projects investigating the theory and practice of machine learning, including the Neural and Computational Learning (NeuroCOLT) projects and the Kernel Methods for Images and Text (KerMIT) project. He is currently the coordinator of the Network of Excellence in Pattern Analysis, Statistical Modeling and Computational Learning (PASCAL) involving 57 partners. He is coauthor of *Introduction to Support Vector Machines*, the first comprehensive account of this new generation of machine learning algorithms. A second book titled *Kernel Methods for Pattern Analysis* was published in 2004.

Johan A. K. Suykens is an associate professor with K. U. Leuven, Belgium. His research interests are mainly in the areas of the theory and application of neural networks and nonlinear systems. He is an associate editor for the *IEEE Transactions on Neural Networks* and the *IEEE Transactions on Circuits and Systems*. He received the IEEE Signal Processing Society 1999 Best Paper Senior Award and the International Neural Networks Society (INNS) 2000 Young Investigator Award. He has served as director and organizer of the NATO Advanced Study Institute on Learning Theory and Practice (Leuven, 2002) and as a program co-chair for the International Joint Conference on Neural Networks (IJCNN) 2004. More information is available at http://www.esat.kuleuven.ac.be/sista/members/suykens.html.

Alessandro Verri received both a master's degree and a PhD in physics from Universitià degli Studie di Genova, Italy (1984 and 1989, respectively). Since 1989, he has been with Universitià degli Studie di Genova where he is a professor with the Department of Computer and Information Science. Currently, he is interested in the mathematical and computational aspects of learning theory and computer vision. He has been a visiting scientist and professor at MIT, INRIA (Rennes), ICSI (Berkeley), and Heriot-Watt University (Edinburgh). He has published papers on stereopsis, motion analysis in natural and machine vision systems, shape representation and recognition, 3-D object recognition, and learning theory. He is the co-author of a textbook on computer vision with Dr. E. Trucco (Prentice Hall).

Jean-Philippe Vert is senior researcher and director of the Center for Computational Biology at the Ecole des Mines de Paris. He holds degrees from Ecole Polytechnique and Ecole des Mines, and an MS and PhD in mathematics from Paris 6 University. He joined Ecole des

Mines as a principal investigator after 2 years as associate researcher in Kyoto University's Bioinformatics Center. His interest is probabilistic and machine learning approaches to the analysis and modeling of biomedical data.

Vincent Wan received a BA in physics from the University of Oxford in 1997. In 1998 and 1999, he worked on hybrid speech recognition at the University of Sheffield, UK, then spent 2000 working at the Motorola Human Interface Labs at Palo Alto, California, on speech and handwriting recognition. In 2003, he received his PhD on speaker verification and support vector machines from the University of Sheffield, where he is presently holding a postdoctoral position at the Department of Computer Science. His interests include machine learning, biometrics, and speech processing.

Jason Weston completed his PhD at Royal Holloway in 1999 (under Vladimir Vapnik) studying kernel learning algorithms and support vector machines. He now works in NEC Research Labs, Princeton (USA). His areas of interest are scaling up kernel learning algorithms, structured learning, semisupervised learning, and applications to bioinformatics. He is author of more than 50 papers in the field of machine learning and bioinformatics.

Index